Myopia and Nearwork

MYOPIA AND NEARWORK

Mark Rosenfield MCOptom, PhD, FAAO
State College of Optometry,
State University of New York, New York, USA

Bernard Gilmartin FCOptom, PhD, FAAO
Department of Vision Sciences, Aston University,
Birmingham, UK

With a Foreword by Ernst Goldschmidt

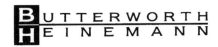

OXFORD BOSTON JOHANNESBURG MELBOURNE NEW DELHI SINGAPORE

Butterworth-Heinemann
Linacre House, Jordan Hill, Oxford OX2 8DP
225 Wildwood Avenue, Woburn, MA 01801–2041
A division of Reed Educational and Professional Publishing Ltd

Ⓡ A member of the Reed Elsevier plc group

First published 1998

British Library Cataloguing in Publication Data
Rosenfield, Mark
  Myopia and nearwork
  1. Myopia – Etiology
  I. Title   II. Gilmartin, Bernard
  617.7'55

ISBN 0 7506 3784 6

Library of Congress Cataloguing in Publication Data
Myopia and nearwork/(edited by) Mark Rosenfield, Bernard Gilmartin.
  p. cm.
  Includes bibliographical references and index.
  ISBN 0 7506 3784 6
  1. Myopia – Etiology.   2. Eye – Accomodation and refraction.
  I. Rosenfield, Mark.   II. Gilmartin, Bernard.
  (DNLM: 1. Myopia – etiology.   WW 320 M9964)
  RE938.M95
  617.7'55–dc21

                                                                98–10422
                                                                CIP

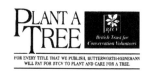

FOR EVERY TITLE THAT WE PUBLISH, BUTTERWORTH-HEINEMANN
WILL PAY FOR BTCV TO PLANT AND CARE FOR A TREE.

Typeset by Interactive Sciences Ltd, Gloucester
Printed and bound in Great Britain by The Bath Press

Contents

There are few subjects in ophthalmology capable of triggering the impassioned responses, often visceral rather than cerebral, that the subject of nearwork and myopia genesis evokes.

(Curtin, B.J. *The Myopias. Basic Science and Clinical Management.* Harper & Row, 1985, p. 120)

Contributors

Martin H. Birnbaum
State College of Optometry, State University of New York, USA

Marion H. Edwards
Department of Optometry and Radiography, The Hong Kong Polytechnic University, Hong Kong

William F. Harris
Department of Optometry, Rand Afrikaans University, Johannesburg, South Africa

Bernard Gilmartin
Department of Vision Sciences, Aston University, Birmingham, UK

David A. Goss
School of Optometry, Indiana University, Bloomington, Indiana, USA

Theodore Grosvenor
Professor Emeritus, School of Optometry, Indiana University, Bloomington, Indiana, USA; Visiting Scholar, Department of Optometry and Vision Science, University of Auckland, Auckland, New Zealand

Donald O. Mutti
School of Optometry, University of California, Berkeley, California, USA

Mark Rosenfield
State College of Optometry, State University of New York, USA

Earl L. Smith III
College of Optometry, University of Houston, Texas, USA

Christine F. Wildsoet
New England College of Optometry, Boston, Massachusetts, USA

Karla Zadnik
College of Optometry, Ohio State University, Columbus, Ohio, USA

Preface

The prevalence of myopia has increased in recent decades such that at least 25% of individuals in modern industrialized societies are myopic, and in some Asian societies, for example Taiwan, the prevalence approaches 75% of the population depending on the age group and occupational category. This increase, together with the substantial economic, social and psychological costs associated with myopia, has fuelled academic and clinical debate as to why the emmetropic state, achieved at some point in the continuum of refractive development, is not retained in many individuals.

Whilst the higher degree of concordance in myopia onset and development for uniovular twins is a compelling argument for the predominance of genetics in the aetiology of myopia, a significant and increasing proportion of myopia occurs after the cessation of bodily growth. Furthermore, the incidence of late- or young-adult onset myopia is often reported as being directly linked to an occupational requirement for significant amounts of near vision, which has led to the conjecture that the condition is attributable principally to the influence of the visual environment.

In addition, myopia induced in animals, invariably neonates, by various forms of visual deprivation has identified local and central control processes for eye growth which appear to occur independently of genetic programming, although it has yet to be established whether the link between normal eye growth in humans and induced myopia in animals is analogous.

It is these two aspects of research into human and animal myopia which instigated our desire to re-examine the evidence as to whether a specific feature of the visual environment, i.e., nearvision which is sustained and carries a high level of cognitive demand, is a genuine aetiological factor in the onset and development of myopia.

The evidence is gathered from a group of individuals who have specialized in diverse aspects of myopia research encompassing epidemiology, socio-economics, ocular biometry, animal myopia, oculomotor function and clinical management. In this regard, the book is a unique compilation of data and opinion on the issue of myopia and nearwork. The final chapter provides an overview and assimilation of the evidence, and speculates on a possible model for nearwork-induced myopia based on retinal defocus and accommodative adaptation.

We envisage that this book will appeal to all who, like ourselves, are perplexed by the issue of myopia and nearwork. At the very least we would hope to furnish the harassed ophthalmic and optometric practitioner with something substantial to counter the questions on myopia asked by the newly myopic patient; at most it would be gratifying if our efforts to juxtapose and collate the work of our contributors were to generate some special insight into the topic. A special reward would be for the book to act as a catalyst for an aspiring graduate student to undertake research into myopia and nearwork despite the intricacy of an issue first identified by Kepler almost four centuries ago.

We have greatly enjoyed working with our contributors and appreciate their willingness to enter into the spirit of the project. The inexorable increase in near vision in the workplace, mediated by advances in electronic displays, will ensure that efforts to clarify the connection between nearwork and myopia will continue into the twenty-first century.

Mark Rosenfield
Bernard Gilmartin

Foreword

The aetiology of myopia has excited an immense amount of speculation and controversy ever since ophthalmology became a science, and the theories which have been put forward to explain its development are as ingenious, fanciful and contradictory as have accumulated around any subject in medicine. Unfortunately, their enthusiastic implementation in practice has too often involved far-reaching social and economic consequences, the rational basis for which has usually been insubstantial.

The theory that nearwork is a determining factor in the aetiology of myopia depends mainly on statistical evidence. From all parts of the world figures have been published showing that myopia is rare before school age, gradually increases during school life and reaches its highest prevalence in the years of most intense study at the universities. Among university students in Hong Kong and Taiwan over 90% are myopic and the average degree of myopia is 4–5 dioptres. A similar extreme prevalence was seen in the educational elite of Europe in the late nineteenth-century, and there seems to be a tendency that particularly high incidences of myopia are associated with stressful educational systems in which there are high demands on the child and young adult to learn. It is a widely held opinion that you harm your eyes by continuous reading but all attempts which have been made to reduce accommodative fatigue by introducing pauses during reading and teaching, by eye exercises etc. have not been successful with regard to reducing the number of children developing myopia. The amount of accommodation during close work can also be reduced by optical or pharmaceutical initiatives, but again data are inconclusive.

No general arrangements around school children have reduced the amount of myopia, but certainly better tables in schools, better lighting, more breaks, more sport etc. may have benefited the general health of children mentally, as well as physically.

The present book reflects all available evidence for an association between myopic development and the performance of nearwork. In addition it gives the reader an impressive view of myopia research from centres around the world. In modern myopia research the role of optometry is substantial.

Looking at available epidemiologic data on myopia, the development seems more strongly associated with the process of learning and memorising than with nearwork as such. As a consequence, computer games appear to have little or no influence on refraction in contrast with intensive intellectual activities. More research in this area is needed, but relevant protocols are difficult to establish.

The 10 chapters cover the topic, reviewing myopia research of the 1990s. Together with the huge amount of relevant references and the fine editing which has avoided overlap, this book makes an outstanding contribution to the myopia literature.

Ernst Goldschmidt
Danish Institute for Myopia Research

Myopia: definitions, classifications and economic implications

Marion H. Edwards

1.1 Definitions

Myopia is that form of refractive error wherein parallel rays of light come to a focus in front of the sentient layer of the retina when the eye is at rest (Duke-Elder and Abrams, 1970). The state of accommodation of the eye affects the refractive state of the eye and definitions of myopia have varied slightly in the way in which this is described. Helmholtz (who completed the first edition of his Treatise in 1866) defined myopia in terms of the position of the far point plane (objects situated in this plane are focused on the retina), this being in front of the eye in myopia, and pointed out that light entering the eye had to be divergent in order to be focused on the retina of the myopic eye.

The essential elements of myopia are shown in Figures 1.1 to 1.3. They are: that parallel light entering the relaxed eye is brought to a focus (at F'_e) anterior to the retina (at M') as shown in Figure 1.1; that the far point plane of the eye (M_R),which is conjugate with the retina, lies in front of the eye (as in Figure 1.2), and that myopia can be corrected optically by making light entering the eye divergent such that the second focal point of the correcting lens (F') coincides with the far point of the eye (as shown in Figure 1.3).

Modern lexicographers have offered similar definitions of myopia:

> The refractive condition of the eye represented by the location of the conjugate focus of the retina at some finite point in front of the eye, when accommodation is said to be relaxed, or the extent of that condition represented in the number of diopters of concave lens power required to compensate to the optical equivalent of emmetropia. The condition may also be represented as one in which parallel rays of light entering the eye, with accommodation relaxed, focus in front of the retina. (Cline *et al.*, 1989)

> Refractive condition of the eye in which the images of distant objects are focused in front of the retina when the accommodation is relaxed. Thus distance vision is blurred. In myopia the point conjugate with the retina, that is the far point of the eye, is located at some finite point in front of the eye. (Millodot, 1993)

1.2 Difficulties in the quantification of myopia

1.2.1 Statistical analysis of refractive data

Myopia often exists in the company of astigmatism, and the tripartite nature of refraction (which has a spherical component plus a cylindrical component comprising power and axis) complicates statistical analyses of refractive error and its development. Vision scientists investigating myopia have the choice of considering the spherical error in one meridian, of averaging the power in the two principal meridians, or of trying to also represent astigmatism in some way. Most studies of myopia report the average refractive error in the two principal meridians of the eye, this being called the spherical equivalent refractive error (SE), a misnomer as it in no way provides a spherical lens which is equivalent to a sphero-cylinder. Unfortunately much information is lost in this process, in particular information regarding the amount and

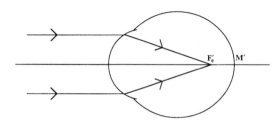

Figure 1.1 In myopia parallel light entering the eye is brought to a focus anterior to the retina

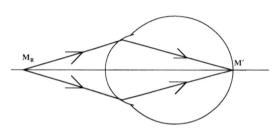

Figure 1.2 In the relaxed myopic eye light from the far point plane is brought to a focus on the retina

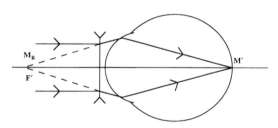

Figure 1.3 A correcting lens is selected such that its second focal point coincides with the far point. Parallel light is then brought to a focus on the retina

axis of astigmatism. For example, the following very different refractive errors all produce the same SE of −4.00 D. In the first case, although the SE indicates myopia, the refractive problem is essentially astigmatism:

−1.00 DS / −6.00 DC × 180
−3.00 DS / −2.00 DC × 90
−4.00 DS

A number of researchers have addressed the problem of the mathematical manipulation and statistical analysis of refractive error data. Saunders (1980) suggested a method for determining the mean of refractive errors by applying theorems relating to the curvature of a surface. Harris has emphasized that the best way to represent refractive error, a three-dimensional concept, is in three-dimensional space (Harris, 1991, 1997). Using a three-dimensional graph, refraction becomes a single point in space and changes in refraction are represented by the locus of the point.

Harris (1988) described the use of matrix algebra to express in sphero-cylinder format the mean, variance and standard deviation of refractive error. Matrix algebra methods have also been applied to ophthalmic lens decentration problems (Long, 1976) and to obliquely crossed sphero-cylinder lens combinations (Keating, 1981a, 1981b). While matrix algebra is not particularly complex, it is not widely taught in schools and despite its obvious advantages has not been adopted in studies of myopia (an exception being the Orinda Longitudinal Study of Myopia, *see* Zadnik *et al.*, 1993). For a more detailed account of the use of matrices to calculate average power, *see* Appendix.

1.2.2   Defining when myopia first exists

Refractive error is a continuous scale from hyperopia through emmetropia to myopia, and the point at which myopia can be first considered to exist is somewhat arbitrary. For example, recent studies have variously used an SE of −0.50 D (Garner *et al.*, 1990; Yap *et al.*, 1994; Edwards and Brown, 1996), greater than −0.50 D (Rosenfield and Gilmartin, 1987; Lam *et al.*, 1994), and −0.75 D or more in both primary meridians (Zadnik *et al.*, 1993) to define the onset of myopia. Occasionally the definition of myopia used is not stated at all.

The definition of myopia becomes particularly important where prevalence or incidence is being studied, and if the population being investigated is one in which myopia is just developing (say 8- to 14-year-old children), then the way in which myopia is defined may make a considerable difference to the results.

1.2.3   Effects of cycloplegic drugs on refractive outcomes

The use of a cycloplegic drug also affects refractive outcomes. The effects are greater when hyperopia, rather than myopia, is being studied, and are also greater the younger the subject (Young *et al.*, 1971; Hiatt *et al.*, 1973; Shultz *et al.*, 1975; Chan and Edwards, 1994). Because of the risks associated with its use and the availability of safer alternatives, atropine, which was widely used in the past, is seldom used in modern studies. If comparisons are to be made between studies, the use, or otherwise, of a cycloplegic, and the particular drug used, must be taken into account. The enlarged pupils which are a byproduct of cycloplegia often introduce spherical aberration which may make retinoscopy more difficult, and so the use of a cycloplegic *per se* does not guarantee accuracy of refraction.

1.2.4 Establishing criteria for refractive change

Where myopia progression is being studied, it is necessary to establish and apply criteria to determine whether a measured change is likely to be real, or whether it could have occurred by chance because of the nature of refractive error and of the measurement process. This can be done by taking two sets of measures of refraction for the same subjects (test and retest), under exactly the same conditions, and determining the 95 per cent confidence limits for the difference between the test and retest measures. If the difference has a normal distribution, then in 95 per cent of repeated measures the discrepancy between test and retest values will be equal to, or less than the standard deviation of the difference multiplied by 1.96. A change in refraction greater than this value (which is expressed in dioptres) can be considered a real change.

The correlation coefficient, on its own, is not a useful statistic to compare test and retest results, being a measure of the relationship, rather than the agreement; between two measures. A perfect correlation, along with a regression line with a slope of unity for the paired data, indicates perfect agreement; however, these statistics cannot be used to develop clinical criteria for change in individual subjects.

When the difference between two measures is likely to vary with the magnitude of the measures, the method recommended by Bland and Altman (1986), whereby the difference between the test and retest result is plotted against the mean of the test and retest result, is particularly useful. It is quite likely that the difference between measurements of refractive error will be greater for large refractive errors than for smaller errors and use of

the Bland and Altman technique would alert the researchers to this. It may then be deemed desirable to use different criteria for change for different ranges of refractive error.

1.2.5 Method of measurement used

Refraction may be measured in a number of different ways and each method generally has advantages and disadvantages. For example, measurements obtained using an autorefractor with a target at virtual infinity may be affected by proximal accommodation (*see* instrument myopia in this chapter) if a cycloplegic agent is not used. On the other hand, autorefraction may be the technique of choice when examining 4-year-old children in whom full cycloplegia has been attained.

If a subjective refraction technique is used, then end-point criteria should be stated, e.g. minimum minus power for best visual acuity. Similarly, clear end-point criteria should be given for the measurement of vision and visual acuity. Whatever method is used to measure refraction, ideally information should be provided regarding the reliability (repeatability and/or reproducibility) of the data thereby obtained, and this can be done using the standard deviation of the difference multiplied by 1.96 as described above (see also ISO 5725–1: 1994). Repeatability is the agreement between repeated measures taken under identical conditions. Reproducibility is the agreement between repeated measures when some aspect such as the location where the measurements are taken, or the person taking the measurements, is different. The reproducibility of subjective measures of refraction are likely to be lower than the repeatability when the refractionist is different and appropriate objective measures of refraction may therefore be preferable to subjective measures in a study of myopia where more than one person is measuring refraction.

If it is wished to express repeatability in terms of the mean difference between test and retest measurements, then the absolute mean should be used, as algebraic differences will tend to cancel each other out. The algebraic mean, however, can be used to determine if there is a bias between the test and retest readings.

1.3 Classifications of myopia

Over the past century a plethora of classifications of myopia have been offered and have particularly tended to reflect contemporary ideas on the aetiology or the course of the condition.

1.3.1 Pathological, physiological and intermediate myopia

Perhaps the most clearly recognizable type of myopia is that which is variously called pathological (or pathologic), progressive or degenerative, the latter two names characterizing the course and the fundus appearance of the condition respectively. The term malignant has also been applied to this type of myopia, but adds nothing to our understanding of the condition, and is liable to unnecessarily alarm any myope who hears the word used. With regard to the use of 'malignant' as a classification, Curtin (1985) points out that the poor visual prognosis which exists in cases where a posterior staphyloma involves the macular area is 'hardly justification for a diagnosis that is so devoid of hope and conjures up thoughts of ocular tumors'.

Pathological myopia typically first presents at an early age (often during the pre-teen years), advances rapidly and is accompanied by characteristic chorio-retinal degeneration. Depending on the extent of the fundus changes (in particular the development of a posterior staphyloma) normal vision may, or may not, be attainable with spectacles or contact lenses. Axial length is always abnormally large (Curtin, 1985).

Pathological myopia is an important clinical entity because quality of life may be adversely affected as a result of retinal changes, and in particular, progressive myopes are at risk for retinal detachment. It is generally believed that the aetiology of this type of myopia is different from that of the other myopias, and in particular, environment factors such as nearwork have not been implicated in its onset or development.

Fortunately progressive myopia now seems to be less common, at all ages, than in the past (Goldschmidt, 1968; Adams *et al.*, 1989), perhaps because of a lower incidence of childhood febrile diseases such as measles, which have been associated with the onset of myopia in early childhood (Hirsch, 1957). The theory that a raised body temperature causes weakening of the sclera with the subsequent development of myopia has some experimental support. Maurice and Mushin (1966) raised the body temperature and intraocular pressure (IOP) of rabbits and myopia subsequently developed in young rabbits (but not in older animals), provided the body temperature was above 41 °C and the IOP was above 40 mmHg. Tokoro

(1970) and Mohan *et al.* (1977) have also induced myopia in rabbits by raising the body temperature and the IOP. These experimental conditions included a high IOP as well as a raised body temperature, and it is not clear whether a high IOP occurs in childhood febrile diseases.

The use of the term pathological to describe one type of myopia suggests that other types are not pathological in character, and the term physiologic (sic) has been used by Curtin (1985) to describe myopias in which the components of refraction all lie within the ranges found in emmetropia.* In clinical practice the components of refraction are not normally measured and so it is difficult to make a diagnosis of physiological myopia based on this definition. Duke-Elder (1949) called this type of myopia 'simple' myopia, terming other myopias 'degenerative'.

Curtin (1979) states that 'it is the type and degree [of retinal changes] that determine the diagnosis of pathologic myopia'; eyes with physiological myopia, by definition, do not have any of the fundus characteristics of pathological myopia. The clinical diagnosis of physiological myopia can therefore be made on the basis of fundus appearance. In practice, however, the dividing line between physiological and pathological myopia is not always sharp, as myopic crescents (which are among the fundus changes which typify pathological myopia) can be found in eyes which would otherwise be diagnosed as having physiological myopia. This overlap between pathological and physiological myopia was recognized by Otsuka (1967), who proposed that such cases be described as intermediate. Myopic eyes with an axial length within the range found in emmetropia, and without a temporal crescent (or, Curtin (1979) suggests, with a crescent not wider than one-tenth of the optic disc diameter) are classified as physiological.

For eyes with axial length within the emmetropic range but which have a temporal crescent wider than one tenth of the optic disc diameter, the classification is one of intermediate myopia. Temporal crescents are more common in Chinese eyes than in Caucasian eyes, and Hendicott and Lam (1991) found that 84 per cent of Chinese eyes with a refraction between 2 D and 4 D, and all eyes with

---

* Sorsby *et al.* (1957) found the ranges for the components in emmetropia to be: axial length 21–26 mm; corneal power 39–48 D and crystalline lens power 17–26 D. Axial length, however, was not measured independently, being calculated from optical measurement of corneal radius, anterior chamber depth and lens radii and thickness. Refractive indices were assumed.

a refractive error greater than 4 D, or an axial length greater than 25.5 mm had a myopic crescent. In contrast, Curtin and Karlin (1971) found that crescents occurred in 100 per cent of eyes of axial length greater than 28.5 mm. It is interesting to speculate as to whether the difference in distribution of temporal crescents in Chinese compared with Caucasian eyes and the high prevalence of myopia in Chinese eyes have the same cause.

Classification into pathological, intermediate or physiological provides information regarding the degree of myopia, its likely course, the fundus appearance and some idea of the visual prognosis.

1.3.2 Correlation versus component ametropia

Emmetropia can be associated with a range of axial lengths (Steiger, 1913; Sorsby *et al.*, 1957), the components of refraction being correlated to produce a zero refractive error. Sorsby *et al.* (1957) found that spherical errors within the range ±4 D are the result of imperfect correlation (thus, 'correlation' ametropia) and suggested that up to 98 per cent of refractive errors fall within this range. They found that high refractive error is due to one or more components, usually the axial length, being outside the range associated with emmetropia; Sorsby *et al.* termed this type of error 'component' ametropia.

Hirsch (1950) suggested that refractive error can be divided into three distributions. The alpha group follows a normal distribution, with a mean of +0.50 D, and represents normal biological variation. The beta group has a peak at −4.00 D and Hirsch suggested that this myopia is inherited, while myopias between 9.00 D and 15.00 D fall into the gamma group. The alpha and beta groups are similar to the correlation and component groups of Sorsby *et al.* (1957).

1.3.3 Classification by degree of myopia

A simple classification of myopia, though not a particularly informative one, is by degree. Hine (1949) classified myopia of less than 3 D as low, of 3 D to 6 D as moderate, and of more than 6 D as high. Hirschberg (cited by Weymouth and Hirsch, 1991) proposed a classification similar to Hine's except with the additional category of very high myopia for refractive errors greater than 15 D.

Classification by degree, while often used by clinicians, is quite arbitrary and if used in research then it is necessary to clearly define the divisions being used and to present results in such a way as to permit comparison with results from studies using different divisions. It is also necessary to state whether myopia is being quantified by the refractive error in the least minus meridian, the most minus meridian or the average of these two meridians.

1.3.4 Axial versus refractive myopia

The posterior focal length of an eye is a function of the corneal power, the anterior chamber depth and the crystalline lens power. The refractive state depends on the balance between the axial length and the focal length. If the focal length is less than the axial length then the situation described in the first paragraph of this chapter exists and the eye is myopic. If the focal length is greater than the axial length then the eye is hyperopic and if the focal length is the same as the axial length then the ideal situation exists (at least for distance vision) and the eye is said to be emmetropic.

A further classification of refractive error is according to whether the focal length or the axial length can be said to be abnormal. If the axial length is abnormal then the condition is axial, however, this classification becomes less clear cut in the light of the knowledge that a wide range of axial lengths can still result in emmetropia (Steiger, 1913; Sorsby *et al.*, 1957). There is therefore no 'normal' axial length. Axial length is the component which correlates most closely with refractive error. Stenstrom (Stenstrom, 1946, translated by Woolf, 1948) found a correlation coefficient of −0.76, which increased to −0.87 when corneal radius was controlled (Hirsch and Weymouth, 1947) and Lam *et al.* (1994) found a correlation of −0.62 for adult female and −0.66 for adult male Chinese. Sorsby *et al.* (1957) found that axial lengths within the range found in emmetropia are exceptional in refractive errors of more than ±4 D; thus higher refractive errors tend to be axial in nature. The type of myopia which develops in young adults (*see* Age of Onset classification below) is also axial in nature (Adams, 1987).

If the focal length is abnormal then the condition is refractive, and may be further sub-classified according to the component at fault. Lenticular myopia can be associated with the development of cataract and transient lenticular myopia may also occur in diabetes mellitus. Both of these types of lenticular myopia could also be classified as index myopia. Curvature myopia occurs in keratoconus in which the cornea becomes cone shaped and greatly steepened. Clinically it is seldom possible to sub-classify refractive myopia except in the extreme cases given above.

1.3.5 Congenital versus acquired myopia

Congenital myopia occurs in premature babies (Fletcher and Brandon, 1954; Graham and Gray, 1963) and decreases rapidly after birth (Linfield, 1993) except when retrolental fibroplasia is present (Fletcher and Brandon, 1954). Myopia also occurs in full-term babies and again there is a trend for reduction in myopia in the first year of life (Gwiazda *et al.*, 1993). Infant myopia seems to be the only type of myopia which tends to decrease in this way, raising questions about the nature and duration of emmetropization in humans.

Myopia that develops after very early infancy (it is rarely possible to determine if myopia is actually present at birth) has been termed acquired myopia, and most myopia can therefore be thus classified. Although both Cline *et al.* (1989) and Millodot (1993) define acquired myopia as myopia appearing after infancy, an acquired type of myopia, associated with neonatal lid closure, occurs in infants (Hoyt *et al.*, 1981) and is presumably analogous to the myopia produced experimentally by lid fusion in animals (Wiesel and Raviola, 1977).

Weymouth and Hirsch (1991) suggested that 'acquired' is an inappropriate term, as its use seems to 'support the theory that the use of the eyes is responsible for myopia' and that 'until the evidence for an active acquisition of myopia is examined, we should be wary of this term'. There is now increasing evidence that myopia can be the result of environmental factors and the use of this classification may increase.

1.3.6 Age at onset

Grosvenor (1987) has proposed a myopia classification based on age-related prevalence (in Western populations) and age of onset. In Grosvenor's schema, children born with myopia, and who remain myopic during infancy and childhood, have congenital myopia. This is in line with other definitions of congenital myopia. Myopia with onset during the period from about age 6 years through the teenage years is classified as youth-onset, and

Grosvenor suggests that a large percentage of such cases have relatively small amounts of myopia and are likely to become emmetropic in future years. Myopia with onset between the age of 20 and 40 years is classified as early adult-onset, and again Grosvenor apparently anticipates that many of these will become emmetropic in later years, though why this should happen is not explained. Myopia with onset after 40 years is classified as late adult-onset.

There is an accumulating body of evidence that the accommodation–vergence system in persons who develop myopia between the ages of about 18 and 25 years is different from that found in emmetropes and in persons who develop myopia in the pre-teens or early teens (Bullimore and Gilmartin, 1987; McBrien and Millodot, 1988; Gilmartin and Bullimore, 1991; Woung *et al.*, 1993). These are important findings as they suggest that the causes of these types of myopia are different; however, these researchers classified the former as late-onset myopia (LOM) and the latter as early-onset myopia (EOM). The terms juvenile-onset and adolescent-onset have also been used to describe myopia that starts before the age of about 18 years. It would be beneficial for vision scientists to agree the age ranges and terminology; and it may be that the classification that should be used will become clearer as more work is done using these types of age divisions. If age-related prevalence is to be a basis for the classification then the prevalence in Chinese and Japanese eyes, which probably accounts for the majority of the world's cases of myopia, should be considered.

Goldschmidt (1968) recognized that the causes of early-onset and late-onset myopia are likely to be different. At that time he suggested that early-onset myopia is genetically determined, while late-onset myopia is the result of some environmental factor or factors. However, Goldschmidt (1997) now believes that environmental factors also play a role in early-onset myopia.

1.3.7 Heredity versus environmental causes

Studies of refraction in siblings raised together, and of refraction in several generations of families, suffer from the problem of separating genetic and environmental influences. It has been shown that the concordance of refractive error is greater in uniovular than in binovular twins (Sorsby *et al.*, 1962; Sorsby and Fraser, 1964; Chen *et al.*, 1985), thus demonstrating the existence of a genetic input into refractive error. Angle and Wissmann (1980) found that measures of nearwork explained only a small part of variance in myopia in a group of 12–17-year-old children, and concluded that myopia is the result of biological processes that are little influenced by eye use. They did point out, however, that the indicators of nearwork used might have missed a critical environmental factor or factors. The work of Sorsby and others led to a conviction that that 'heredity is the basic determinant of ocular refraction' (Curtin, 1979), the only unknown being the exact mode of inheritance (*see* Goss *et al.*, 1988, for a review of genetic factors in myopia).

There is now strong evidence from animal studies that myopia can result from manipulation of environmental factors (e.g. Young, 1961, 1963; Wiesel and Raviola, 1977; Wallman *et al.*, 1978; and *see also* Chapter 4). The idea that the way in which we live can affect the development of myopia is not new; Cohn's use–abuse theory (Cohn, 1886, and *see also* Chapter 5) was based on the assumption that accommodation at school, along with other factors, led to myopia (hence 'school myopia'). Lam *et al.* (1994) have shown that the prevalence of myopia is lower in older than in younger people in Hong Kong and as the genetic composition of these two groups is similar, this is evidence of a factor other than heredity in the development of myopia. Zylbermann *et al.* (1993) compared the prevalence of myopia in Jews in Jerusalem, a sample genetically rather homogeneous. They found that myopia was more prevalent, and occurred in higher amounts, in Orthodox boys compared with Orthodox girls. Orthodox boys spend up to 16 hours a day reading religious texts, whereas the education received by the girls in the Orthodox community is similar to that in Western countries.

Animal studies have resulted in sub-classification of environmentally induced myopia. Myopia produced by depriving a young animal of form vision is known as form-deprivation myopia, or more usually, deprivation myopia. Myopia induced when a young animal compensates for a negatively powered ophthalmic lens has been termed lens-compensation (or compensational) myopia.

Unilateral myopia is an interesting phenomenon, if only because it is so difficult to explain in the light of what we presently know of the causes of myopia. Based on the hereditary/environmental classification, the only explanation for unilateral myopia is that there is a genetic programming which affects the two eyes differently, or which affects the susceptibility of two eyes to some environmental factor (or factors) differently.

1.3.8 Pseudomyopia (false myopia, hypertonic myopia, functional myopia)

As mentioned at the beginning of this chapter, definitions of myopia almost invariably include a reference to the state of accommodation of the eye. If accommodation is in play then the refractive status will appear more myopic than it actually is. Spasm of accommodation, especially if long periods of fine work are undertaken at a short working distance, may result in a condition, most commonly termed pseudomyopia, in which an individual who is actually hyperopic or emmetropic, appears to be myopic. The use of a cycloplegic will reveal the true refractive status.

1.3.9 The 'empty field' myopias (dark focus myopia, night myopia, twilight myopia, empty field myopia, sky myopia)

Leibowitz and Owens (1975) term the myopias that occur in reduced light conditions 'anomalous myopias' and believe that they represent a maladaption of the visual system. These myopias, also called empty field myopias, are temporary states characterized by the absence of light (dark focus myopia), reduced luminance levels (night myopia at scotopic lighting levels and twilight myopia at mesopic levels) or by the absence of an accommodative stimulus (empty field myopia). In these situations the eye is focused, not at the far point, but at a more myopic position which is dependent on the tone of the ciliary muscle (Leibowitz and Owens, 1975). The difference between the normal distance focus in photopic conditions and the anomalous focus decreases as the ambient light level increases. Dark focus myopia has a value of about 1 D in young people, and decreases with increasing age and with increasing ambient light (for a review *see* Charman, 1996).

These states of tonic accommodation (Rosenfield *et al.*, 1993, 1994) are of some practical significance as they raise the question of the optimal refractive correction for drivers at night (Charman, 1996) and in fog, and of pilots. There are also differences related to tonic accommodation between myopes and non-myopes which may have some bearing on the development of myopia (*see* Chapter 5).

1.3.10   Instrument myopia

There is a long-recognized tendency for operators of optical instruments such as microscopes to over-accommodate (Richards, 1976; Wesner and Miller, 1986). While an instrument does not provide a true empty field, it may provide an inadequate stimulus to accurate accommodation and so mimic an empty field state.

Leibowitz and Owens (1975) compared the dark focus position with the accommodation for a target in a microscope and found that the latter value was higher in 24 out of 30 subjects. Proximal accommodation is that accommodation which results from awareness of the physical proximity of a target even though the target may optically be at infinity; it can be reduced with training. Instrument myopia can also be improved by training and the difference observed by Leibowitz and Owens may have been due to an element of proximal accommodation, when viewing through a microscope.

The measurement of refractive error using an autorefractor is also affected by instrument myopia and may lead to inaccurate results especially when the subject being measured has a large amplitude of accommodation.

1.4   Social and economic significance of myopia

Myopia, even in quite low amounts, must have been a great disadvantage to (especially male) members of primitive hunter–gatherer communities. Fortunately, in modern societies efficient vision aids mean that most myopes are little inconvenienced by the condition. Some occupations, mainly in the disciplined services and commercial aviation, are still restricted or closed to individuals with myopia. For such occupations there are two concerns. The first is that where myopia is very common in the community, the pool of applicants is reduced by the unaided vision requirements associated with the job. The second is that applicants who meet the vision requirements and are accepted for training may develop late-onset myopia (*see* Diamond, 1957 for an account of the development of late-onset myopia in pilots). This can be devastating for a young person starting a career, and costly for the organization.

In places such as Hong Kong, where myopia is prevalent, these problems have sometimes led to an easing of vision requirements and sometimes, paradoxically, to a tightening. The Royal Hong Kong Police Force previously insisted that all police officers should have good unaided vision. The prevalence of myopia, however, is higher now than some years ago (Lam *et al.*, 1994) and this promoted a gradual relaxation of vision requirements. Firstly inspectorate level officers were permitted to wear glasses, and now officers at all grades may wear spectacles, and unaided vision is not a consideration. For certain active duty roles perfect unaided vision is still preferred and officers with myopia may be disadvantaged.

In contrast, the Hong Kong airline Cathay Pacific requires young Chinese recruited for pilot training to have uncorrected vision of 6/9 in each eye. This is more stringent than international requirements – the International Civil Aviation Organization (ICAO) requirements for an Airline Transport Pilot Licence is corrected vision of 6/9 in each eye, unaided vision of not less than 6/60 in each eye and refractive error within the range +3 to −3 D. The airline management takes this more stringent approach to unaided vision because they believe that the progression of myopia is less predictable in Chinese than in Caucasians. Similarly the Hong Kong Government Flying Service requires new recruits for flying duties to have unaided vision of 6/6 in each eye. Older applicants who are already qualified pilots, on the other hand, are required only to meet the ICAO requirements.

The Hong Kong Fire Service requires newly recruited firefighters to have unaided vision of 6/9 in each eye. Spectacles cannot be worn with a face mask or breathing apparatus and myopia is the main medical reason for rejecting applicants.

Concerns regarding the economic and social costs of myopia led the US Air Force School of Aerospace Medicine to sponsor a major study of the prevalence of progression of myopia (Adams *et al.*, 1989). This study recommended, among other things, that the uncorrected vision requirements for military pilots should be reduced and that the feasibility of wearing spectacles or contact lenses while flying should be examined. It also recommended that research should be carried out into prophylactic measures to reduce the shift towards myopia in young adults, and that the difference in job performance when vision aids are worn should be evaluated.

Myopes tend to be high achievers at school compared to non-myopes (Hirsch, 1959; Grosvenor, 1970) and Young *et al.* (1970) found that this was also true in an Eskimo (Inuit) community in which there was a particularly high prevalence of myopia. It seems that in the process of becoming high achievers, students also develop myopia. Physiological myopia may be a slight advantage for some close work occupations, especially for pre-presbyopes and early presbyopes, however, this is offset by the need to wear spectacles for driving.

In most myopes corrected vision is normal, and the direct costs of the condition relate to the expense of regular eye examinations and related professional services, the cost of spectacles (and in many cases also of contact lenses and contact lens solutions), the cost of the treatment of squint associated with myopia, and, in recent years, the cost of refractive surgery. There are also indirect costs related to loss of productivity or leisure time while undergoing eye examination or selecting or collecting eyecare products.

Javitt and Chiang (1994) calculated that for the myopic population of the United States in the year 1990, the direct costs of professional services and eyecare products and the indirect costs related to loss of productivity were US$4.8 billion. They also calculated that the lifetime costs of excimer laser surgery for 5 per cent of the US myopic population were US$5.9 billion, compared with $4.6 billion for spectacles or contact lenses.

No attempt will be made here to quantify the costs associated with myopia, as they vary considerably from country to country and even within countries. Some of these, such as contact lens wear and refractive surgery, are themselves not without risk; others, such as a regular eye examination, might aid the diagnosis of other eye conditions and could thus be considered desirable. There are other risks associated with wearing spectacles, such as eye damage from broken spectacle lenses in the event of an accident. Generally speaking, the minus lenses worn by myopes are more likely to break, when made of glass, than the thicker lenses worn by hyperopes.

In the event of an accident rigid contact lenses may break and embed in the cornea. Such an accident would almost certainly cause eye damage in the absence of contact lenses, and in some cases contact lenses may lessen the damage by spreading the impact.

Should prophylaxis against myopia be developed then this would have cost implications depending on the nature of the treatment. It seems most likely that prophylaxis will take the form of spectacles to be worn or drugs to be instilled to prevent the development or the progression of myopia, and more frequent eye examinations will

probably be needed to monitor closely refractive changes. Presumably the prophylaxis will be needed only during childhood and early adulthood when myopia typically starts and progresses. Thereafter the costs involved would decrease considerably. Successful refractive surgery has the effect of removing or reducing the need for spectacle wear, but periodic follow-up is needed and the long-term effects of this type of surgery are still unknown.

The cost of myopia to a community is related to the prevalence of the condition and this varies considerably around the world. For example, the prevalence reported for secondary school children ranges from 4.3 per cent in Melanesian children at age 15–16 years (Garner *et al.*, 1990) to 80.6 per cent in junior high school girls aged 14 to 15 years in Taiwan (Lin *et al.*, 1988). It is difficult to obtain unbiased samples for prevalence estimates and modern reports should include consideration of what sample bias may have been introduced, for example, by the need to obtain informed consent. This requirement probably tends to increase the prevalence found as myopes, or people with myopes in the family, may be more likely to take part in an investigation of myopia. Examples of samples that are unlikely to represent the population at large are army conscripts, university students and people attending an eye hospital clinic. Where a single prevalence is given for a range of ages it is necessary to give a weighted average which accounts for the number of subjects in each age group.

On a case by case basis, the costs of progressive myopia are much greater than those of physiological and intermediate myopia in both human and economic terms. At the simplest level, the cost of high minus spectacle lenses, especially when produced in high refractive index material, is greater than lower power lenses. More frequent eye examinations are required, because of the risk of retinal detachment, a dreaded sequela of progressive myopia which results in hospitalization and retinal surgery. Time is lost from work, medical costs, either direct or indirect, are considerable and if the visual outcome is not good, then the cost of sub-normal vision is borne by the individual, his or her family and by society. These include medical expenses, reduced productivity and the cost of social benefits.

Myopic degeneration is the second highest cause of low vision in Hong Kong (Yap *et al.*, 1990). Recent data on world blindness (Thylefors *et al.*, 1995) do not shed much light on the extent of blindness due to pathological myopia. In data collected between 1984 and 1989, refractive errors were found to be the second highest cause of blindness in India; similarly data collected in 29 provinces of China in 1987 show refractive errors as the highest cause of blindness after cataract. It seems likely that pathological myopia is the main source of blindness due to refractive error. It is not possible from the data provided to determine the prevalence of blindness due to retinal detachment associated with pathological myopia and so the prevalence of blindness due to myopia may be underestimated.

Glaucoma is significantly more prevalent in myopic eyes, particularly in pathological myopia, and the incidence of cataract in myopia is twice that in the normal population (Curtin, 1979), further increasing the personal, social and economic costs of myopia.

Acknowledgements

I should like to thank the Royal Hong Kong Police Force, the Hong Kong Fire Services Department, the Hong Kong Government Flying Service and Cathay Pacific Airlines for their assistance and Professor William Harris, May Wu and Carly Lam for their advice.

References

Adams, A. J. (1987) Axial elongation, not corneal curvature, as a basis of adult onset myopia. *Am. J. Optom. Physiol. Opt.* **64**, 150–155.

Adams, A. J., Baldwin, W. R., Biederman, I. *et al.* (1989) *Myopia: Prevalence and Progression.* Working Group on Myopia Prevalence and Progression, Committee on Vision, Commission on Behavioral and Social Sciences and Education, National Research Council. National Academy Press.

Angle, J. and Wissmann, D. A. (1980) The epidemiology of myopia. *Am. J. Epidemiol.* **111**, 220–228.

Bland, J. M. and Altman, D. G. (1986) Statistical methods for assessing agreement between two methods of clinical measurement. *Lancet*, **i**, 307–310.

Bullimore, M. A. and Gilmartin, B. (1987) Aspects of tonic accommodation in emmetropia and late-onset myopia. *Am. J. Optom. Physiol. Opt.* **64**, 499–503.

Chan, O. Y. C. and Edwards, M. (1994) Comparison of cycloplegic and noncycloplegic retinoscopy in Chinese pre-school children. *Optom. Vis. Sci.* **71**, 312–318.

Charman, W. N. (1996) Night myopia and driving. *Ophthal. Physiol. Opt.* **16**, 474–485.

Chen, C. J., Cohen, B. H. and Diamond, E. L. (1985) Genetic and environmental effects on the development of myopia in Chinese twin children. *Ophthalmol. Pediat. Genet.* **6**, 113–119.

Cline, D., Hofstetter, H. W. and Griffin, J. R. (1989) *Dictionary of Visual Science*, 4th edn. Chilton Trade Book Publishing.

Cohn, N. (1886) *The Hygiene of the Eye in Schools* (English translation by W. P. Turnbull). Simpkin, Marshall & Co.

Curtin, B. J. (1979) Physiologic vs pathologic myopia: genetics vs environment. *Ophthalmology*, **86**, 681–691.

Curtin, B. J. (1985) *The Myopias: Basic Science and Clinical Management.* Harper & Row.

Curtin, B. J. and Karlin, D. B. (1971) Axial length measurements and fundus changes of the myopic eye. *Am. J. Ophthalmol.* **71**, 42–53.

Diamond, S. (1957) Acquired myopia in airline pilots. *J. Av. Med.* **28**, 559–568.

Duke-Elder, W. S. (1949) *Textbook of Ophthalmology.* C. V. Mosby.

Duke-Elder, S. and Abrams, D. (1970) *System of Ophthalmology*, vol. V: *Ophthalmic Optics and Refraction.* C. V. Mosby.

Edwards, M. H. and Brown, B. (1996) IOP in myopic children: the relationship between increases in IOP and the development of myopia. *Ophthal. Physiol. Opt.* **16**, 243–246.

Fletcher, M. C. and Brandon, S. (1954) Myopia of prematurity. *Am. J. Ophthalmol.* **40**, 474–481.

Garner, L. F., Chung, K. M., Grosvenor, T. P. and Mohidin, N. (1990) Ocular dimensions and refractive power in Malay and Melanesian children. *Ophthal. Physiol. Opt.* **10**, 234–238.

Gilmartin, B. and Bullimore, M. A. (1991) Adaptation of tonic accommodation to sustained visual tasks in emmetropia and late-onset myopia. *Optom. Vis. Sci.* **68**, 22–26.

Goldschmidt, E. (1968) On the aetiology of myopia. *Acta Ophthalmol.* Suppl. 98, 1–172.

Goldschmidt, E. (1997) Epidemiology of myopia. Scandinavian and Hong Kong experiences. In: *Myopia Updates* (T. Tokoro, ed.). Springer, pp. 3–12.

Goss, D. A., Hampton, M. J. and Wickham, M. G. (1988) Selected review on genetic factors in myopia. *J. Am. Optom. Assoc.* **59**, 875–884.

Graham, M. V. and Gray, O. P. (1963) Refraction of premature babies' eyes. *Br. Med. J.* **12**, 1452–1454.

Grosvenor, T. (1987) A review and a suggested classification system for myopia on the basis of age-related prevalence and age of onset. *Am. J. Optom. Physiol. Opt.* **64**, 545–554.

Grosvenor, T. (1970) Refractive state, intelligence test scores, and academic ability. *Am. J. Optom. Arch. Am. Acad. Optom.* **47**, 355–361.

Gwiazda, J., Thorn, F., Bauer, J. and Held, R. (1993) Emmetropization and the progression of manifest refraction in children followed from infancy to puberty. *Clin. Vis. Sci.* **8**, 337–344.

Harris, W. F. (1988) Algebra of sphero-cylinders and refractive error, and their means, variance and standard deviation. *Am. J. Optom. Physiol. Opt.* **65**, 794–802.

Harris, W. F. (1991) Representation of dioptric power in Euclidean 3-space. *Ophthal. Physiol. Opt.* **11**, 130–136.

Harris, W. F. (1997) Dioptric power: its nature and its representation in three- and four-dimensional space. *Optom. Vis. Sci.* **74**, 349–366.

Hendicott, P. and Lam C. (1991) Myopic crescent, refractive error and axial length in Chinese eyes. *Clin. Exp. Optom.* **74**, 168–174.

Hiatt, R. L., Braswell, R., Smith, L. and Patty, J. W. (1973) Refraction using mydriatic, cycloplegic and manifest techniques. *Am. J. Ophthalmol.* **76**, 739–744.

Hine, M. L. (1949) *May and Worth's Manual of Diseases of the Eye*, 3rd edn. Baillière, Tindall & Cox.

Hirsch, M. J. (1950) An analysis of inhomogeneity of myopia in adults. *Am. J. Optom. Arch. Am. Acad. Optom.* **27**, 562–571.

Hirsch, M. J. (1957) The relationship between measles and myopia. *Am. J. Optom. Arch. Am. Acad. Optom.* **34**, 289–296

Hirsch, M. J. (1959) The relationship between refractive state of the eye and intelligence test scores. *Am. J. Optom. Arch. Am. Acad. Optom.* **36**, 12–21.

Hirsch, M. J. and Weymouth, F. W. (1947) Notes on ametropia–a further analysis of Stenstrom's data. *Am. J. Optom. Arch. Am. Acad. Optom.* **24**, 601–608.

Hoyt, C. S., Stone, R. D., Fromer, C. and Billson, F. A. (1981) Monocular axial myopia associated with neonatal eyelid closure in human infants. *Am. J. Ophthalmol.* **91**, 197–200.

ISO 5725–1:1994(E) *Accuracy (trueness and precision) of measurement methods and results–Part 1: General principles and definitions*. International Organization for Standardization.

Javitt, J. C. and Chiang, Y-P. (1994) The socioeconomic aspects of laser refractive surgery. *Arch. Ophthalmol.* **112**, 1526–1530.

Keating, M. P. (1981a) A system matrix for astigmatic optical systems: I. Introduction and dioptric power relations. *Am. J. Optom. Physiol. Opt.* **58**, 810–819.

Keating, M. P. (1981b) A system matrix for astigmatic optical systems: II. Corrected systems including an astigmatic eye. *Am. J. Optom. Physiol. Opt.* **58**, 919–929.

Lam, C. S. Y., Goh, W. S. H., Tang, Y. K. *et al.* (1994) Changes in refractive trends and optical components of Hong Kong Chinese aged over 40 years. *Ophthal. Physiol. Opt.* **14**, 383–388.

Leibowitz, H. W. and Owens, D. A. (1975) Anomalous myopias and the intermediate dark focus of accommodation. *Science* **189**, 646–648.

Lin, L. L.-K., Chen, C-J., Hung, P-T. and Ko, L-S. (1988) Nation-wide survey of myopia among schoolchildren in Taiwan, 1986. *Acta Ophthalmol.* Suppl. 185, 29–33.

Linfield, P. B. (1993) Myopia and the trend towards emmetropia in new born premature babies. *Invest. Ophthalmol. Vis. Sci.*, **34** (Suppl.), 1353.

Long, W. F. (1976) A matrix formalisation for decentration problems. *J. Optom. Physiol. Opt.* **53**, 27–33.

Maurice, D. M. and Mushin, A. S. (1966) Production of myopia in rabbits by raised body-temperature and increased intraocular pressure. *Lancet*, **ii**, 1160–1162.

McBrien, N. A. and Millodot, M. (1988) Differences in adaptation of tonic accommodation with refractive state. *Invest. Ophthalmol. Vis. Sci.* **29**, 460–469.

Millodot, M. (1993) *Dictionary of Optometry*. 3rd edn. Butterworth-Heinemann.

Mohan, M., Rao, V. A. and Dada, V. K. (1977) Experimental myopia in the rabbit. *Eye Res.* **25**, 33–38.

Otsuka, J. (1967) Research on the etiology and treatment of myopia. *Acta Soc. Ophthalmol. Japn* **71** (Suppl), 7–212.

Richards, O. W. (1976) Instrument myopia–microscopy. *Am. J. Optom. Physiol. Opt.*, **53**, 658–663.

Rosenfield, M. and Gilmartin, B. (1987) Effect of a near-vision task on the response AC/A of a myopic population. *Ophthal. Physiol. Opt.* **7**, 225–233.

Rosenfield, M., Ciuffreda, K. J., Hung, G. K. and Gilmartin, B. (1993) Tonic accommodation: a review. 1. Basic aspects. *Ophthal. Physiol. Opt.* **13**, 266–284.

Rosenfield, M., Ciuffreda, K. J., Hung, G. K. and Gilmartin, B. (1994) Tonic accommodation: a review. 2. Accommodative adaptation and clinical aspects. *Ophthal. Physiol. Opt.* **14**, 265–277.

Saunders, H. (1980) A method for determining the mean value of refractive errors. *Br. J. Physiol. Opt.* **34**, 1–11.

Shultz, L. (1975) Variation in refractive change induced by cyclogyl upon children with differing degrees of ametropia. *Am. J. Optom. Physiol. Opt.* **52**, 482–484.

Sorsby, A. and Fraser, G. R. (1964) Statistical note on the components of ocular refraction in twins. *J. Med. Genet.* **1**, 47–49.

Sorsby, A., Benjamin, B., Davey, J. B., Sheridan, M. and Tanner, J. M. (1957) *Emmetropia and Its Aberrations*. Medical Research Council Special Reports Series. No 293. HMSO.

Sorsby, A., Benjamin, B. and Sheridan, M. (1962) *Refraction and Its Components in Twins*. Medical Research Council Special Reports Series No 303. HMSO.

Steiger, A. (1913) *Die Entstehung der Sphärischen Refraktionen des Menschlichen Auges*. Karger.

Stenström, S. ([1946] 1948) Investigation of the variation and the covariance of the optical elements of human eyes. (English translation by D. Woolf) *Am. J. Optom. Arch. Am. Acad. Optom.* **25**, 438–449.

Tokoro, T. (1970) Experimental myopia in rabbits. *Invest. Ophthalmol. Vis. Sci.* **9**, 926–934.

Thylefors, B., Négrel, A.-D., Pararajasegaram, R. and Dadzie, K. Y. (1995) Available data on blindness (update 1994) *Ophthal. Epidemiol.* **2**, 5–39.

Wallman, J., Turkel, J. and Trachtman, J. (1978) Extreme myopia produced by modest change in early visual experience. *Science* **201**, 1249–1251.

Wesner, M. F. and Miller, R. J. (1986) Instrument myopia conceptions, misconceptions, and influencing factors. *Doc. Ophthalmol.* **62**, 281–308.

Weymouth, F. W. and Hirsch, M. J. (1991) Theories, definitions, and classifications of refractive errors. In: *Refractive Anomalies: Research and Clinical Applications* (T. Grosvenor and M. C. Flom, eds) Butterworth–Heinemann, pp. 1-14.

Wiesel, T. N. and Raviola, E. (1977) Myopia and eye enlargement after neonatal lid fusion in monkeys. *Nature*, **266**, 66–68.

Woung, L. C., Ukai, K., Tsuchiya, K. and Ishikawa, S. (1993). Accommodation adaptation and age of onset of myopia. *Ophthal. Physiol. Opt.* **13**, 366–370.

Yap, M., Cho, J. and Woo, G. (1990) A survey of low vision patients in Hong Kong. *Clin. Exp. Optom.* **73**, 19–22.

Yap, M., Wu, M., Wang, S. H. *et al.* (1994) Environmental factors and refractive error in Chinese schoolchildren. *Clin. Exp. Optom.* **77**, 8–14.

Young, F. A. (1961) The effect of restricted visual space on the primate eye. *Am. J. Ophthalmol.*, **52**, 799–806.

Young, F. A. (1963) The effect of restricted visual space on the refractive error of the young monkey eye. *Invest. Ophthalmol. Vis. Sci.* **2**, 571–577.

Young, F. A., Leary, G. A., Baldwin, W. R. *et al.* (1970) Refractive errors, reading performance, and school achievement among Eskimo children. *Am. J. Optom. Arch. Am. Acad. Optom.* **47**, 384–390.

Young, F. A., Leary, G. A., Baldwin, W. R. *et al.* (1971) Comparison of cycloplegic and non-cycloplegic refractions of Eskimos. *Am. J. Optom. Arch. Am. Acad. Optom.* **48**, 814–824.

Zadnik, K., Mutti, D. O., Friedman, N. E. and Adams, A. J. (1993) Initial cross-sectional results from the Orinda Longitudinal Study of Myopia. *Optom. Vis. Sci.* **70**, 750–758.

Zylbermann, R., Landau, D. and Berson, D. (1993). The influence of study habits on myopia in Jewish teenagers. *J. Pediatr. Ophthalmol. Strab.* **30**, 319–322.

2

Prevalence of myopia

Karla Zadnik and Donald O. Mutti

Whilst excessive nearwork has classically been cited as a risk factor for myopia, it is a complex variable to examine and especially to quantify. Throughout the studies reviewed in this chapter, nearwork is either measured by the use of non-standardized surveys, or alternatively it is assessed indirectly by examining those activities that require nearwork, such as the number of years of education completed. Furthermore, the performance of nearwork cannot be considered in isolation. Varying levels of nearwork may be required according to one's culture, nationality, residence, occupational requirements, age, gender, educational level, socio-economic status and intellectual ability. Unfortunately for both the clinician and the researcher attempting to consider the importance of nearwork in the risk of becoming myopic, each of these factors is also associated with myopia. This has created a challenge that, for the most part, has not been met in trying to untangle what are the primary risk factors and what are the secondary, potentially confounding associations. The following review of the many studies which associate nearwork and other classic risk factors with myopia attempts to convey both the efforts that have already been made as well as some of the more promising avenues for future research in this area.

2.1 Nearwork and myopia are associated

Nearwork has been linked to myopia for more than a century (Ware, 1813; Cohn, 1886; Angle and

Wissmann, 1980; Richler and Bear, 1980; Rosner and Belkin, 1987). Although much has been made of the potential causative role for accommodation in the development of myopia (*see* Chapter 5) (Young *et al.*, 1969; Angle and Wissmann, 1980; Richler and Bear, 1980; McBrien and Barnes, 1984), studies of myopia and nearwork all report associations, i.e., not necessarily causation. There are associations of nearwork with both the prevalence and degree of myopia. Many factors appear to influence these associations, including geographic considerations, occupation, age, gender, education, and intelligence.

Examples of the association between myopia and nearwork include an increased prevalence of myopia among the first school-educated Eskimos, where the prevalence of myopia in grandchildren is greater than that in their grandparents (Young *et al.*, 1969). Also, a decreased prevalence of myopia was observed in Japan during the Second World War, when schooling (and, presumably, intensive nearwork) was halted (National Research Council, 1989). Several studies have also reported an association between myopia, intelligence, and nearwork, with myopes undertaking more nearwork and having higher IQs or superior levels of school achievement (Richler and Bear, 1980; Rosner and Belkin, 1987). Furthermore, many eye care practitioners have observed adult-onset myopia or adult progression of myopia in college student populations (National Research Council, 1989).

Although there is an extensive literature on myopia in general, which has been reviewed in a number of comprehensive publications (e.g. Curtin, 1985; National Research Council, 1989), this chapter draws particular attention to those studies which either measured nearwork directly, or used educational attainment, intellectual achievement, or other measures of intelligence or school achievement as a corollary for nearwork.

The significance of nearwork as it relates to refractive error has also been estimated statistically in population studies of refraction and related variables. Angle and Wissmann (1978) analysed data from Cycle III of the US Public Health Service Health Examination Survey of adolescents between 12 and 17 years of age (conducted between 1966 and 1970). Of the original random sample of 7514 people, 1219 subjects either had no data, no ocular data, or vision problems uncorrectable with lenses. These subjects were excluded from the analysis. The authors then doubled the available data by including both eyes rather than just one eye or the mean of the two eyes. This represents an inefficient sampling procedure because the two eyes are not independent, and little new information is gained for the amount of effort required to assess the second eye (Ederer, 1973). Of 12 590 eyes, 4341 (34.5 per cent) were classified as myopic (defined as either the eye required a corrective lens with a negative spherical equivalent, had uncorrected distance acuity worse than 6/6 or distance acuity that could be improved with a negative spherical lens, and additionally, that the eye did not have an uncorrectable vision problem). The amount of myopia was measured by the survey dentist as the spherical equivalent of either the glasses worn by the subject or a combination of distance acuity and trial lens powers.

The authors then performed a regression analysis on the estimated amount of myopia as a function of age from birth, age from menarche (for females), and years in school. Chronological age was used to test whether refractive error onset represents a biological correlate. Age from menarche was used to test whether myopia was associated with puberty, while years in school was the authors' measure of the effects of nearwork. The coefficient of the age term in the model was significant, as might be expected, indicating less hyperopia and more myopia with time. The additional age from menarche term was not significant when added to the model, indicating that time from the onset of puberty is not related to myopia for adolescent females. Their third model contained the age term and one for the number of years in school, with the following coefficients:

$$\text{Myopia} = -2.314 + 0.009 \times \text{months from birth} - 0.220 \times \text{highest grade in school}$$

Both coefficients were significant, but the R^2 value was only 0.023, while the R^2 value for the model containing age alone was 0.008. The positive sign for the age coefficient is of interest as it indicates that the predicted trend is for the eye to become less myopic with age, contrary to the more typical clinical finding that changes in refraction with age are overwhelmingly towards more myopia. The explanation suggested by their model is that the effects of age are outweighed by those of schooling, represented by the negative coefficient and greater magnitude of the latter term. The conclusion of the authors that this analysis 'explains all the tendency of myopia to appear and progress with age among 12–17-year-olds' seems overstated. First, the reported effect of age by Angle and Wissmann (1978) is not supported by their findings in a later analysis (Angle and Wissmann, 1980). The coefficient for age in a similar model in the later paper is not significant. Secondly, the measure of nearwork adopted by Angle and Wissmann (1978) may be flawed. If all subjects stayed in school until after graduation (18 years of age in the United States), then the nearwork term is essentially the same as the age term. This co-linearity should create high standard errors for the coefficients and reduce significance. Since both coefficients were significant, they were probably not identical terms because of other factors related to why schooling was not completed. One such factor might be lower intelligence or poorer reading ability in individuals dropping out of school, which many studies have shown are associated with more hyperopia and less myopia (Hirsch, 1959; Young, 1963; Grosvenor, 1970; Angle and Wissmann, 1980; Rosner and Belkin, 1987; Rosner and Rosner, 1989). Another factor might be that children of lower socio-economic status might be overrepresented in school drop-outs. Lower socioeconomic status is also associated with a higher prevalence of hyperopia and a lower prevalence of myopia (Angle and Wissmann, 1980; Sperduto *et al.*, 1983). The statistical estimate of the effect of nearwork in Angle and Wissmann's study (1978) is only as accurate as their measurement of this parameter. Even if it is assumed to be valid, only 2 per cent of the variance in refractive error was accounted for by nearwork in their model.

Angle and Wissmann (1980) again attempted to estimate the importance of nearwork in myopia using the same data set as in their earlier study, but including the additional variables of number of minutes spent reading per day and the score on the reading portion of the Wide Range Achievement Test (Guidance Associates, Inc., Delaware, USA) (Buros, 1972). They reported significant coefficients in several separate models examining refractive error with a single 'social' variable, either age, sex, race, family income, or region of origin. Their analysis showed the confounding effects on these factors when nearwork measures (level of school completed, minutes per day spent reading, and reading test scores) were taken together and added to the models. Thus these environmental variables representing the effects of nearwork were more related to myopia than were the social variables. The gender and region of origin terms were not confounded, meaning that the higher prevalence of myopia in girls and lower prevalence of myopia in the Southern USA could not be explained by the nearwork measures.

A problem with the analysis of Angle and Wissmann (1980) is that their measurements of nearwork estimate more than just this factor alone. Use of the number of minutes spent reading is a straightforward attempt to assess the exposure to nearwork. Level of school completed, however, is a flawed indicator of nearwork because of the factors discussed above, namely its similarity to age and its contamination by intelligence and socioeconomic status. The score on the reading test may be the poorest variable in the model. The Wide Range Achievement Test is not highly regarded due to incomplete standardization and questionable validity (Buros, 1972). Additionally, it is uncertain whether the test actually measures achievement, intelligence, personality, or a combination of these factors (Buros, 1972). The authors are testing the importance of nearwork and an environmental theory of myopia, therefore, with a set of variables which contain both environmental and potentially hereditary factors. Rather than adding terms one at a time to the model to analyse the effects of each variable separately, they use all three variables at once. Without assessing the separate effect of each variable, no conclusions can be drawn on the relative importance of nearwork compared with heredity, nor which variable is responsible for confounding the relationship between refractive error, age, and race. Even if one assumes that nearwork is adequately estimated, the proportion of variance explained is still low, at approximately 6 per cent.

The third major study that statistically analysed the amount of myopia attributable to nearwork was that of Richler and Bear (1980). Non-cycloplegic retinoscopy was performed on the right eyes of 971 individuals over 5 years of age. This represents around 80 per cent of the total population of three Newfoundland communities. Persons with greater than 6.00 D of myopia or amblyopia were excluded from the study ($n = 14$). Exposure to nearwork was estimated by the subject as the number of hours per day spent reading, sewing, or engaging in any near activity closer than 50 cm. Education was coded as the last grade completed. Compulsory education came to the area in 1949, meaning those individuals over 30 years of age received less formal education. On average, only those over the age of 50 years had left school earlier than approximately 13–14 years of age.

Adult subjects aged 15–59 years were divided into three groups (representing every 15 years of age). Children aged 9–14 years were placed in a fourth group, and any adults over 59 years formed a fifth group. Refractive error was significantly correlated with both education and nearwork in each age group, with the exception of the group over 60 years of age. Not surprisingly, education and nearwork were correlated in all age groups. In order to address the main question on the effect of nearwork, the authors calculated the partial correlation between refractive error and nearwork, correcting for the effects of education as well as age and gender. These partial correlations were also significant for each age group, except for the group over 60 years of age, suggesting that nearwork, separate from its relation to education, age, and gender, may play a role in the aetiology of myopia. The proportion of variance in refractive error explained by nearwork after correction for age, gender, and education ranged from 4 per cent to 12 per cent across age groups; i.e., slightly higher estimates than those reported by Angle and Wissmann (1978, 1980).

While this conclusion is in agreement with the studies of Angle and Wissmann, the measure of nearwork used by Richler and Bear (1980) may also be of limited value. Counting only the number of hours per day undertaking close work may be simpler and less contaminated by other factors than the measurements of Angle and Wissmann (1978, 1980), but the Angle and Wissmann studies assessed the effects of this exposure at a time when the outcome, refractive error, was developing, that is, between 12 and 17 years of age. In contrast,

Table 2.1 Prevalence of myopia by geographical location

Study	Location/race	Age (yr)	Prevalence of myopia (%)
Abiose *et al.*, 1980	Nigeria/African	12–20	<2.0
Hymans *et al.*, 1977	Israel/Jewish	>40	11.6
Shapiro *et al.*, 1982	Israel/Jewish	18–25	13.0
Sperduto *et al.*, 1983	USA/Caucasian	12–54	26.3
Sperduto *et al.*, 1983	USA/African–American	12–54	13.0
Taylor, 1980	Australia/Aborigine	20–30	4.8
Taylor, 1980	Australia/European origin	20–30	13.5
van Rens and Arkell, 1991	Alaska/Eskimo	5–80+	44.7
Wick and Crane, 1976	USA/Native American	6–10	13.0
Zadnik *et al.*, 1994	USA/Caucasian	6–14	7.5

Richler and Bear (1980) considered associations between the current level of nearwork and refractive error at ages that were considerably beyond the time when the eye was likely to have ceased normal growth.

Richler and Bear (1980) failed to explain why the behaviour related to onset and progression of myopia as a child persisted into adulthood. What factors made the myopic adult continue to do more close work and the hyperopic adult less? Their answer was that the amount of reading is habitual. Another possibility is that it reflects the level of intelligence, a factor associated with myopia in many studies (Hirsch, 1959; Young, 1963; Grosvenor, 1970; Angle and Wissmann, 1980; Rosner and Belkin, 1987; Rosner and Rosner, 1989). Another possible explanation is that ametropia might influence directly the amount of reading undertaken. Although Richler and Bear (1980) stated that people do not adjust their nearwork to their refractive error, it is a common clinical impression that reading is more convenient, and therefore may actually be more likely to occur for the myope than for the hyperope.

A cautionary note when interpreting the results of this study is that Richler and Bear (1980) included all refractive errors in their analysis, except high myopia. Therefore, when they interpreted negative correlations as associations with myopia, they were including not only more myopia, but also less hyperopia. They made the assumption that factors related to the decrease in hyperopia were also related to the progression of myopia, an assumption that has not been validated. However, Angle and Wissmann (1978, 1980)

restricted their analyses to only myopes. Since these analyses (Angle and Wissmann, 1978, 1980; Richler and Bear, 1980) were based upon linear regression, nearwork was modelled as a risk factor that displays some linear, dose–response behaviour. One unit of nearwork was related by some linear factor to an amount of myopia. This made a similar reasonable, but untested, assumption that the same factor which produced the onset of myopia was also related to its progression.

Thus much of our epidemiological knowledge concerning the relationship between nearwork and myopia is derived from the three studies cited above (Angle and Wissmann, 1978, 1980; Richler and Bear, 1980). They suffer uniformly, however, from issues such as uncertainty in assessing the amount of nearwork, confounding factors, and an inability to explain anything beyond a very small proportion of the variability in refractive error.

2.2   Demographic factors

2.2.1   Geography

The prevalence of myopia differs by geographical location (Table 2.1), but the data are contaminated by a variety of other factors that also differ with geography, such as culture, degree of Asian genetic influence, ethnicity, socio-economic status, degree of nearwork performed and ocular anatomy. Reports of associations between nearwork and myopia have come from all over the world. Table 2.2 summarizes these reports, focusing on the magnitude of the association. It is clear from Table 2.2 that the observed associations between myopia

Table 2.2 Representative studies showing associations among nearwork, education and/or myopia (direct and indirect) across geographical locations

Study	Source of patients	No. of patients	Result	Comments
Adams and McBrien, 1992	Clinical biomicroscopists (UK)	251 patients	No difference in adult myopia progression by amount of microscopy done (in hours per week)	Many adult onset (or progression) myopes
Angle and Wissmann, 1980	Health Examination Survey (USA)	4341 eyes (assuming independence between eyes in a patient)	Education explains 'all of' myopic progression	Problems with selection from data set
Angle and Wissmann, 1978	Health Examination Survey (USA)	3957 eyes (assuming independence between eyes in a patient)	Number of minutes spent reading per day help explain a small amount of the variance in degree of myopia	Problems with selection from data set
Ashton, 1985b	Hawaiian children	923 children	No relationship between myopia progression and nearwork, association between myopia and nearwork after adjustment for achievement	Across races: children with American–Japanese and American–European ancestry
Au Eong *et al.*, 1993a,b	Singaporean men undergoing compulsory medical examination	110 236 young men	Increasing prevalence of myopia and severe myopia with increasing education	Across races: Chinese, Malay, Indian and Eurasian; increase over a decade with increasing education
Hirsch, 1951	Schoolchildren (Puente, California)	840 schoolchildren	Less myopic shift in refractive error during the summer	
Morgan *et al.*, 1975	Inuit Eskimos (Canadian Arctic)	298 patients	Prevalence of myopia greater in children than parents	Hypothesized as caused by advent of Western education
Nadell *et al.*, 1957	Junior high school students (California)	409 students	No relationship between reading (in hours per day) and refractive error group	Small sample sizes in subgroups
Richler and Bear, 1980	Newfoundland communities	971 subjects	Correlation between nearwork and myopia; strength of association decreases with increasing age	Highly inbred communities
Young *et al.*, 1969	Eskimos (Barrow, Alaska)	197 patients	Prevalence of myopia greater in children than parents	Hypothesized as caused by advent of Western education
Zadnik *et al.*, 1994	Schoolchildren (Orinda, California)	716 schoolchildren	Association between nearwork and myopia, overshadowed by association between parental history of myopia and refractive error	Many young children who have yet to develop their myopia

and nearwork, or between myopia and education as a corollary for nearwork, occur across geographical locations. Differences in the magnitude of the association across geographical locations are difficult to compare, as various methods of measurement and analysis have been used. Whether in Singaporean young men (Au Eong *et al.*, 1993a, 1993b) or Inuit Eskimos (Morgan *et al.*, 1975), westernized education is frequently considered to exacerbate myopia.

Only in a study of junior high school students in California in the 1950s (Nadell and Weymouth, 1957) was this association not reported amongst the studies detailed in Table 2.1. Likewise, although the amount of microscopy performed per day did not correlate with adult progression of existing myopia (hours of microscopy per week ranged from 2 to 34 hours), these investigators (Adams and McBrien, 1992; McBrien and Adams, 1997) presumably chose to study microscopists because of the profession's high prevalence of myopic members. The lowest prevalence estimate in these primarily adult samples was found in aboriginal Australians (4.8 per cent), and should be contrasted with a value of triple this amount in Australians of European descent (13.5 per cent) (Taylor, 1980).

Oft-cited high prevalences amongst Singapore medical students (Chow *et al.*, 1990) parallel those of British biomicroscopists (Adams and McBrien, 1992; McBrien and Adams, 1997), American optometry students (Septon, 1984), and Norwegian medical students (Midelfart *et al.*, 1992), all of whom were predominantly Caucasian samples. Given the association between myopia and intelligence, the educational level is likely to inflate the prevalence of myopia in these samples (Tay *et al.*, 1992). Population-based surveys may give a more accurate picture. In Taiwan, a national examination of 13 818 children using cycloplegic retinoscopy and autorefraction demonstrated that the prevalence of myopia increases with age to high levels in all regions of the country. By the age of 15 years, the prevalence of myopia (which was not defined) had reached 71.2 per cent in the metropolitan areas and 58.9 per cent in the provinces (Lin *et al.*, 1986).

2.2.2   Degree of urbanization

A number of studies have reported markedly lower prevalences of myopia among more rural populations in eyes of distinctly different size and shape, i.e., eyes with thicker crystalline lenses of higher power (Garner *et al.*, 1988, 1990), especially when

Table 2.3 Prevalence of myopia by occupation in Danish studies 100 years apart

	Tscherning (1882) %	Goldschmidt (1968) %
Mainly university students	32.4	30.1
Mainly clerks	15.8	11.8
'Good' (not university) education	13.3	13.9
Fine work craftsmen	11.7	9.1
Heavy work craftsmen	5.3	4.3
Farm and unskilled laborers	2.5	2.9

From Rosenfield, 1994

compared with United States-based prevalences (Sperduto *et al.*, 1983; Zadnik *et al.*, 1994). These studies have been cited as evidence of the environmental aetiology of myopia. The relations between the evolutionary advantages of inheriting emmetropia in rural settings and the possible evolutionary advantage of myopia in urban settings are not discernible from studies conducted to date. Nevertheless, the associations among environmental indices for accommodative effort have been reported across cultures, races and around the world.

2.2.3   Occupation

The issue of occupation and its effect on the genesis of refractive error has intrigued eye care practitioners, vision researchers, ergonomists, and industrial safety officers alike (Tables 2.3 and 2.4). The effect of the change from workplaces with predominantly distance-vision demands to the computer-based workplace of the late 1990s with significantly increased near-vision demands is difficult to evaluate. One population-based study demonstrated an association between a higher prevalence of myopia with increasing family income (Sperduto *et al.*, 1983). Certainly, many optometrists would give anecdotal accounts of the patients who began using computers and whose myopia progressed during adulthood. They would also describe patients developing myopia or progressing in degree of myopia well into their late 30s and 40s. Additionally, recent cross-sectional studies show a decreasing prevalence of myopia with increasing age in subjects aged 40–70 years. In the Beaver Dam Eye Study, the prevalence of

Table 2.4 Prevalence of myopia by occupation

Study	Source	No. of patients	Age range (yr)	Prevalence of myopia (%)
Midelfart *et al.*, 1992	Norwegian medical students	140	22–26 (presumably)	50.3
Zylbermann *et al.*, 1993	Jewish students	224 girls, general schools 278 girls, Orthodox schools 175 boys, general schools 193 boys, Orthodox schools	14–18	31.7 36.2 27.4 81.3
Adams and McBrien, 1992	Clinical microscopists	251	21–63	71.0

myopia in 40–49-year-olds was 43 per cent, decreasing to 14 per cent in the 70–79-year-olds (Wang *et al.*, 1994). In the Baltimore Eye Survey, similar trends were found in both Caucasian and African-American groups (Katz *et al.*, 1997). These trends may either be interpreted as a dramatic shift in the prevalence of myopia over 30 years of age or an individual shift with age away from myopia and towards hyperopia.

Table 2.3, collated by Rosenfield (1994), shows the effect of both occupation and time. It indicates the prevalence of myopia in Danish studies 100 years apart, demonstrating remarkable stability in the prevalence of myopia across the century in a given occupational category.

The Working Group Report on Myopia Prevalence and Progression (National Research Council, 1989) provided a concise summary of progression of myopia during adulthood associated with occupations requiring intensive nearwork:

Longitudinal studies of the effect of length of time spent in a targeted activity range from 1 to 17 years' duration beginning with young adults ... Data suggest that the total amount of myopia that develops among those who were emmetropes or low hyperopes before entering environments associated with risk seldom exceeds 1.00 D, and that when myopia progresses in these environments, the [amount of myopia] progression is seldom as much as 2.00 D.

This would indicate that the myopia progression occurring during adulthood that is most associated with nearwork is of relatively low magnitude.

Much of the occupational data quoted in the Working Group's Report (National Research Council, 1989) is from military staff. Comparison of Air Force pilots with navigators showed that more navigators become myopic when followed from one to 20 years (Provines *et al.*, 1983). In fact, as many as 25 per cent of the navigators became myopic 16–20 years after study entry compared with only 18 per cent of the pilots. Others found similar rates of myopia development and progression in approximately 25 per cent of pilots and naval officers (Diamond, 1957; Kent, 1963). Other occupations reported to demonstrate a propensity for myopic development include Navy submarine crew members (Kinney *et al.*, 1980) and servicemen confined within ballistic missile sites (Greene, 1970). Both groups tended toward myopic changes with time in adulthood.

Recently, a longitudinal study has examined clinical microscopists in Great Britain (Adams and McBrien, 1992; McBrien and Adams, 1997). Sixty-six per cent of the eyes were myopic at the beginning of the 2-year study, 39 per cent of emmetropic eyes shifted from emmetropia to myopia and 48 per cent of initially myopic eyes progressed further in myopia. Myopic shifts were associated with axial length elongation. No association between myopic shift and either tonic accommodation or the number of hours each day spent at the microscope was found initially (Adams and McBrien, 1992).

As one might imagine, attempting to clarify the relations between occupation, education, degree of urbanization, age, gender, race, geography and socio-economic status in terms of their associations with myopia is extremely difficult. Table 2.4 summarizes studies where the sample population was relatively homogeneous in terms of the occupation represented, or where the investigators categorized the sample's occupation status well. One study of refractive error, intelligence and occupation indicated that occupation showed no inherent effect. Rather, the associations were dependent on

Table 2.5 Prevalence of myopia in (Causcasian) children

Study	n	Method of refraction	Age (yr)	Prevalence of myopia (%)
Laatikainen and Erkkilä, 1980	162	Retinoscopy after 1% cyclopentolate	7–8	1.9
	218		9–10	6.4
	222		11–12	7.2
	220		14–15	21.8
Sperduto et al., 1983	N/A	Health survey review (USA)	12–17	23.9
Blum et al., 1959	1163	Non-cycloplegic retinoscopy	5	2
			6	2.25
			7	2.5
			8	4
			9	5.5
			10	8
			11	10.5
			12	12.25
			13	13.25
			14	14.5
			15	15
Hirsch, 1964	605	Non-cycloplegic retinoscopy	13–14	15.2
Kempf et al., 1928	333	Retinoscopy after homatropine	6–8	1.2
	495		9–11	3.4
	1001		≥12	4.8
Zadnik et al., 1994	791	Cycloplegic retinoscopy (1% tropicamide)	6–14	7.5

the effects of IQ and socio-economic status (Young, 1955).

With the advent of the electronic display in the modern office, many practitioners believe that computer use is associated with adult onset or progression of myopia. Our review of the literature found a high prevalence of asthenopic symptoms among computer users but found no compelling evidence of association with myopia progression (Mutti and Zadnik, 1996). A recent study to investigate the possibility of an association between computer use and myopia onset and progression suffered from losses to follow-up, and from subjects switching between computer use groups during the study (Cole et al., 1996). The computer users were significantly more myopic than the control group (mean difference = 0.35 D, standard deviation not provided), but the authors did not feel that the difference was clinically significant. Rather, they considered that the difference in refractive error may have resulted from the selection of the sample population, i.e., that myopes

either tend to select, or alternatively are selected for, occupations involving video display terminals (Cole et al., 1996).

2.2.4 Age and time

Table 2.5 shows the prevalence of myopia by age in school-aged children (Kempf et al., 1928; Blum, et al., 1959; Hirsch, 1961; Laatikainen and Erkkila, 1980; Sperduto et al., 1983; Zadnik et al., 1993). These results document the increasing prevalence of myopia (and simultaneous decreasing prevalence of hyperopia) with increasing school age. Between 14 and 18 years of age, refractive error is thought to be stable (Goss and Winkler, 1983). Those who enter high school myopic tend to remain so, and the amount of myopia in a given individual does not change appreciably during the high school years (Roberts and Rowland, 1978; Sperduto et al., 1983).

The Working Group on Myopia Prevalence and Progression (National Research Council, 1989) analysed secular trends in the prevalence of myopia in college-based samples. They did not document any difference between the prevalence of myopia in the 1920s (Brown and Kronfeld, 1929; Jackson, 1932; Tassman, 1932) and the modern National Health and Nutrition Examination Survey data, despite the increased percentage of the general population enrolled in college in the 1980s. However, the Beaver Dam Eye Study (Wang *et al.*, 1994) did report a decrease in the prevalence of myopia in older age groups from 43 per cent in 40-year-olds to 14 per cent in 70-year-olds. This decline is similar to that found in earlier Alaskan (Young *et al.*, 1969) and Canadian (Morgan *et al.*, 1975) Eskimo samples.

Young *et al.* (1969) also pursued a nearwork or environmental theory for myopia in clinical research in an Eskimo population in Barrow, Alaska. Eskimos volunteered in family groups on a non-random basis. Investigators measured cycloplegic refractive error, ocular components, and selected psychometric variables. The proportion of the population with 0.25 D or more myopia in the younger group was 43.4 per cent compared with only 13.8 per cent in the older group. Only two out of the 131 subjects (1.5 per cent) over 45 years of age had this degree of myopia. Young *et al.* (1969) cited the increase in the population of Barrow in the early 1940s and concurrent increase in the number of children attending school with its intensive nearwork demands as the reason for the higher prevalence of myopia in these children. Additionally, the switch to a Western diet has also been suggested as a causative factor.

A similar pattern of increased myopia prevalence amongst younger individuals was reported by Morgan and Munro (1973) in a survey of refractive error of 2833 Eskimos in the Yukon and Northwest Territories. The prevalence of myopia peaked around 15 years of age at about 34 per cent, whereas for subjects above 25 years of age, the prevalence did not exceed 6 per cent. In a separate study of 298 Inuit Eskimos from the Canadian Arctic, Morgan *et al.* (1975) reported a prevalence of myopia (defined as visual acuity of 6/12 or worse, with improvement when viewing through a pinhole) of 31 per cent in those between 15 and 29 years of age, but of only 4 per cent in those of 30 years and older.

In contrast, myopia is reported to be quite common in West Greenland Eskimos across all ages. Alsbirk (1979) measured the average refractive error of both eyes in 483 residents of Umanaq by non-cycloplegic retinoscopy. Myopia, defined as any minus power spherical equivalent, was observed in 36 per cent of those individuals between 15 and 39 years of age, and in 37 per cent of subjects 40 years of age and older. The prevalence of myopia greater than 2.00 D for individuals between 15 and 39 years of age and 40 years of age and older was 5 per cent and 6 per cent, respectively. The quality of life of the Eskimo is quite different in Greenland when compared with Alaska and northern Canada. Alsbirk (1979) stated that 250 years of Danish administration and 100 years of a written Eskimo language have spared the Greenland communities of hunters and fishermen the 'violent changes' which took place in other Western countries. As an aside, the author also contended that the general population 'does not read much,' an interesting observation considering the high prevalence of myopia.

In Alaska, Eskimos led more rural, isolated and harsh lives as hunters and fishermen until a relatively more modern, settled lifestyle began to take hold in the 1940s. This raises the issue of selective survival as a reason for the lower prevalence of myopia (assuming adult myopia remained uncorrected) among adult Eskimos in Alaska compared with Greenland, as well as the difference between Alaskan and Canadian Eskimo adults and children. This and other related factors were catalogued by Morgan and Munro (1973), namely:

1 Selective survival or earlier mortality for myopes leading to their under-representation in the older populations of Alaska.
2 Poorer marriage prospects for the myopic Alaskan male due to reduced hunting capability and therefore fewer myopic children were produced before the arrival of Westernized civilization.
3 An influx of Danish myopic genes into the Greenland gene pool.
4 Dietary differences.
5 Spontaneous recovery from myopia for Alaskan Eskimos, and possibly also older residents of Beaver Dam, Wisconsin (Wang *et al.*, 1994).

2.2.5 Gender

Significant variations in myopia prevalence with gender have not been clearly demonstrated, and may also be confounded by age. A study examining a large sample of children from the United Kingdom showed no significant difference in prevalence between boys and girls (Peckham *et al.*, 1977). Hirsch (1952) observed a more myopic mean refractive error in 5–6-year-old boys when compared with girls of the same age, but the girls demonstrated more myopia by 14 years of age (Hirsch, 1952). A similar age-related gender-dependent trend has been reported in adults (Alsbirk, 1979). Additionally, Danish schoolgirls show a higher prevalence of myopia compared with boys (Goldschmidt, 1968). Many investigators raise the influence of puberty and the earlier maturation seen in girls as accounting for different rates of myopia progression (Goss and Winkler, 1983), and it is possible that some of these effects are due to bias in sample selection wherein girls are more likely to participate in these studies than boys (National Research Council, 1989).

2.2.6 Education

Ware (1813) is credited with making the first report in modern times of an association between the level of education and myopia. He noted that only 12 out of 10 000 recruits for military service over the previous 20 years had been discharged for myopia. At a military school in Chelsea, only three schoolchildren out of 1300 enrollees had myopia. These two groups were meant to indicate the prevalence of myopia amongst the lower, less educated classes. At Oxford, however, 32 out of 127 students were myopic. Details on examination techniques or criteria for defining myopia are absent, a common omission in the early myopia literature (National Research Council, 1989). Donders (1864) also noted that myopia was more prevalent in his wealthier, private patients and town dwellers than in his hospital patients or those who lived in the country. His explanation of this pattern provides an early statement of the nearwork theory of myopia. Donders's writings formed the medical and physiological framework for Cohn (1886), whose influential treatise examined the visual environment to which students were exposed during childhood in German schools.

Cohn observed that myopia was quite common in the town schools and more rigorous gymnasia but rare in the village schools. Out of 240 village schoolchildren between the ages of 6 and 13 years examined under atropine cycloplegia, only 1 per cent were myopic. Cross-sectionally, the prevalence of myopia in a Breslau gymnasium of 361 students increased from 13 per cent in the youngest class to 60 per cent in the oldest. In one of the earliest longitudinal studies of refraction, Cohn examined 138 of these same Breslau students 18 months later. Examination methods were unclear,

but Cohn found that 16 per cent of the emmetropes had become myopic during that time, and that 52 per cent of the myopes had progressed. No regressions in myopia were reported. Cohn interpreted these findings as evidence that schoolwork was responsible for the high prevalence of myopia.

Within a trial of bifocal lenses and beta-blockers for the control of myopia, Jensen (1991) evaluated time spent performing nearwork. She did not observe any significant difference in hours of nearwork undertaken per week when comparing groups of slowly and rapidly progressing myopic children (Jensen, 1991).

Many studies have reported a higher prevalence of myopia associated with increased education (Sperduto *et al.*, 1983), and others have reported a high prevalence of myopia in students (Septon, 1984; Bullimore *et al.*, 1989; Chow *et al.*, 1990; Midelfart *et al.*, 1992; Au Eong *et al.*, 1993a, 1993b), generally without comparing the students to other groups.

One study investigated students educated by different techniques, with more intensive nearwork being a characteristic of one method (Zylbermann *et al.*, 1993). Schoolchildren enrolled in Orthodox schools were compared with children enrolled in secular Jewish schools, and a higher prevalence and degree of myopia were found in boys enrolled in the Orthodox schools (typically involved in 16 hours a day of nearwork by 13 years of age). Of the boys in the Orthodox schools, 81.3 per cent were myopic by at least 0.50 D compared with only 27.4 per cent of the boys in the secular schools, 31.7 per cent of girls in the secular schools, and 36.2 per cent of girls in the Orthodox schools. The prevalence of myopia was marked in boys from the Orthodox schools, with 43.3 per cent having more than 4.00 D of myopia, compared with only 10.5 per cent of boys in the secular schools, 25.3 per cent of girls in the secular schools, and 21.4 per cent of girls in the Orthodox schools having this degree of ametropia. The authors stated that the nearwork demands are approximately equal for the teenagers (14–18 years of age) in secular schools and the girls in the Orthodox schools: a 6 hour school day and about 3 hours of homework after school hours. In contrast, the boys in Orthodox schools engage in an extraordinary amount of reading and scholarship: 16 hours per day for boys older than 13 years of age. Additionally, their reading is characterized by a rocking back and forth of the upper body, creating a varying accommodative and convergence demand during this prolonged nearwork. Zylbermann *et al.* claim that genetic heritages are 'evenly distributed in both systems'. The authors conclude that given the similar genetic backgrounds, the high prevalence and degree of myopia among Orthodox boys is due to their heavy and unique nearwork activity.

Zylbermann *et al.* may be correct in this conclusion, but there are several interesting points to consider in this study. One is that the amount of nearwork performed by boys in Orthodox schools is extremely high. Results from this intense exposure may not be generalizable to more ordinary levels of exposure to reading. The second is the authors' assumption of genetic similarity between groups. If there is a clear division between the education of Orthodox and more secular-minded Jews, it seems likely that marriage is not random, but rather that it also follows religious tradition. It seems very likely that genetic effects might be found in one community and not another. One possibility that should be explored is whether high myopia is a sex-linked trait in the Orthodox community (Worth, 1906). It is also interesting that boys in the secular school are less myopic than girls in the secular school. In order to examine the consistency of the authors' conclusions and the implications of the study, it would be valuable to know whether boys in secular schools do less nearwork than girls.

2.2.7 Intelligence

Numerous studies have documented associations between intelligence, school achievement and myopia. Myopes tend to have higher scores on tests of intelligence and cognitive ability (Hirsch, 1959; Young, 1963; Grosvenor, 1970; Young *et al.*, 1970; Rosner and Belkin, 1987; Cohn *et al.*, 1988; Williams *et al.*, 1988) and better grades in school (Ashton, 1985b) than other refractive error groups. However, investigations into the relationship between intelligence and myopia provide mixed results. For example, Young reported small but statistically significant correlations between myopia and both IQ and nearwork that increased with age (Young, 1955). Further, Hirsch (1959) observed an association between IQ testing and whether a child was a myope or non-myope. In general, relationships are stronger when achievement tests emphasize reading or language skills more than non-verbal skills (Baldwin, 1981).

Despite the substantial documentation of an association between myopia and nearwork, the relationship between these factors and intelligence has not been adequately investigated. Only one investigator has attempted to analyse all three factors in the same children, obtaining uncertain results. Ashton (1985b) examined self-reported grades in school, and results from cognitive tests used in the Hawaii Family Study of Cognition as measures of aptitude and achievement. Numbers of books and magazines read, hours spent doing homework and watching television, and years of education served as measures of nearwork. Unlike Angle and Wissmann (1980), who placed nearwork and achievement data together in their model of myopia without examining their separate effects, Ashton (1985b) first adjusted the nearwork variables for variation in achievement, and vice versa, i.e., he altered the aptitude variable for the amount of nearwork. Ashton then examined the relation between refractive error, achievement corrected values of nearwork, and nearwork-corrected values of achievement. Higher amounts of adjusted nearwork and achievement were associated with less hyperopia, or more myopia. Achievement and nearwork did not have the same effect on the progression of myopia with age. While high achievement was related to the progression of myopia, nearwork was not. This finding suggests that achievement may have the stronger relationship with myopia, independent of nearwork. The important question of whether aptitude or nearwork is more closely related to myopia, as well as the confounding effect one variable might have on another, deserves examination in greater detail.

Any association between myopia and an inherited variable would support a genetic basis for myopia. There is considerable evidence from analysis of over 100 studies that perhaps 50 per cent of the variance in performance on tests of intelligence can be explained by hereditary factors (Bouchard and McGue, 1981). One study in the IQ literature has examined the relation between intelligence and myopia, that is, asking whether intelligence and myopia are inherited together (Cohn *et al.*, 1988). The authors studied 60 sibling pairs, where one of the pair was a participant in the Center for Talented Youth at The Johns Hopkins University, a programme involving children whose scores for psychometrically measured reasoning ability were in the top 3 per cent for their age group. The second member of the pair was a sibling of either gender outside the programme, and presumably less gifted. The Raven Standard Progressive Matrices and Advanced Progressive Matrices, both so-called non-verbal tests of reasoning ability, were administered, along with measurement of refractive error by the automated SR-IV Pro-grammed Subjective Refractor (American Optical), and a survey of time spent reading and studying. Gifted children were more myopic and had higher IQ scores, and not surprisingly read more hours per day.

Cohn *et al.* (1988) used what they described as non-verbal tests, so the confounding effects resulting from the superior reading ability of myopes on IQ test scores (Young, 1963) should not be a factor. Cohn and co-workers also claimed that there is no evidence that reading can raise IQ scores by as much as one standard deviation, thus the higher scores of myopes are not likely to be due to their more frequent reading. He argues that either myopia is inherited in association with intelligence or it is caused by nearwork.

A different conclusion was reached by Rosner and Belkin (1987), who studied myopia, intelligence and level of education in 157 748 Israeli male military recruits between 17 and 19 years of age. Years of education was again used as an estimate of the cumulative exposure to nearwork. Refractions were performed by optometrists or ophthalmologists if distance acuity was poorer than 6/7.5, but the criteria for the definition of myopia were not given. The intelligence test was a combination of the verbal Otis test and a version of a non-verbal matrix test. They found that the prevalence of myopia was lowest (7.1 per cent) for those who had completed the fewest years of schooling (<8 years) and had the lowest IQ scores (≤80). The prevalence of myopia was highest (27.6 per cent) for those with the most schooling (≥12 years) and the highest IQ (≥128). Unfortunately, Rosner and Belkin (1987) did not analyse the impact of each variable separately in order to examine confounding factors. They reported that in a logistic regression with the natural log of the odds of myopia as the dependent variable, both years of education and IQ score were significant at a nearly equal level. Confounding would have occurred if either term alone had a larger coefficient than in the model containing both. However, neither these separate coefficients, nor their standard errors or probability values were presented for such an analysis. Their conclusions seem justified, namely that each term is associated with an increase in the prevalence of myopia, but the question of whether these two terms measure similar features remains unanswered. When years of education is supposed to represent the amount of reading done, as in Angle and Wissmann (1978, 1980) and Rosner and Belkin (1987), factors other than

intelligence related to dropping out of school, such as reading skill, should also be considered. Poor reading skill or other perceptual anomalies associated with hyperopia (Young, 1963; Angle and Wissmann, 1980; Rosner and Rosner, 1989), or asthenopia resulting from uncorrected hyperopia may cause poor performance in school, resulting in hyperopes being overrepresented among the recruits who completed the fewest number of years of education. Thus the relationship between myopia and number of years of education may not represent the effects of actually performing nearwork but rather the effect of an inability to perform nearwork. This issue of the relationship between nearwork and myopia and the potential for confounding by intelligence and other cognitive factors remain important, unresolved issues requiring further study.

The literature on the role of environment and heredity in the aetiology of myopia seems to provide few clear answers. Nearwork appears to explain only a small portion of the variance in refractive error in human studies, and the proposed mechanism is uncertain. Surprisingly, although twin studies and analysis of the components suggest a strong genetic influence, refractive error has a low heritability. One of the difficulties in finding a cause for myopia is that studies in humans are restricted to observation and lack the inferential power of controlled experimentation. An important development in the study of myopia is the utility of animal models for myopia which make such experimentation possible.

If one ascribes to theories that include both genetic (Young, 1955; Sorsby *et al.*, 1962, 1966; Alsbirk, 1979; Basu and Jundal, 1983; Ashton, 1985a; Goss *et al.*, 1988; Teikari *et al.*, 1991, 1992; Gwiazda *et al.*, 1993; Zadnik *et al.*, 1994) and environmental (Angle and Wissmann 1978, 1980; Richler and Bear, 1980; Zylbermann *et al.*, 1993) components in the aetiology of myopia, then it is possible to devise a simple explanation for the association between nearwork and myopia as reflected by the association between intelligence or school achievement and myopia. Perhaps myopia and intelligence are both inherited via nearby alleles or genes, and thus intelligent, achieving children and adults tend to read more. This would result in the patterns previously described.

2.2.8   Military cadets

Principally owing to their accessibility and homogenity, samples comprising military cadets have often been examined with regard to the nature of their refractive error. In fact, the report Myopia: Prevalence and Progression (National Research Council, 1989) was commissioned by the US Air Force School of Aerospace Medicine with the statement:

> The impact of both juvenile and young adult myopia on the recruitment and retention of Air Force Academy students is substantial and has enormous economic and social consequences. Qualifications for military pilots currently specify no refractive error greater than 0.25 D of myopia in any meridian – although waivers may be granted for myopia up to 1.25 D. A high prevalence of myopia in the applicant pool necessarily places constraints on recruitment. Students who are either qualified at entry or have a waiver run the risk of losing their waivers for pilot qualification should they develop myopia greater than 1.25 D by the time they complete four years of study. This poses a real problem for the US Air Force, not to mention for students' career plans.

Accordingly, the military may spend considerable time and money educating a future pilot, only to find that his potentially nearwork-induced adult onset myopia puts him or her outside the uncorrected visual acuity requirement range. The entrance restriction of only minimal myopia may also restrict the intellectual ability of applicants, given the association of intelligence and/or academic achievement with myopia.

When the various studies of military cadets are looked at as a whole, the best estimate of myopia onset and/or progression is that 20 per cent of emmetropes and low hyperopes entering such an intense academic setting become low myopes, and that more than half of entering myopes show myopia progression (National Research Council, 1989). The US Air Force Academy Class of 1985 was studied intensively across their enrolment period (O'Neal and Connon, 1987). At least a 0.50 D myopic shift was seen in 21 per cent, 25 per cent and 55 per cent of eyes initially classified as hyperopic, emmetropic and myopic, respectively.

Others workers have reported similar patterns of myopia onset and progression to that observed by O'Neal and Connon (1987). For example, Sutton and Ditmars (1970) observed that 15 per cent of West Point army cadets who were not myopic on entry had become myopic by graduation. Additionally, a mean myopic increase of 0.66 D was reported in a sample of 418 West Point cadets between entrance and graduation (National Research Council, 1989).

These military cadet data are often cited as evidence of the ability of intensive nearwork environments to cause myopia or to cause existing myopia to progress. As pointed out in the 1989 Progression and Prevalence of Myopia Working Group Report:

> Unfortunately, the military academy studies are often subject to additional biases that make interpretation of progression data difficult. For example, prior to entry into military academies, candidates receive refractive examinations from family [eye] doctors, some of whom might be expected to empathize with applicants and underestimate the presence of myopia. Candidates with hyperopia are also more likely to be identified as emmetropic, since cycloplegic refractions are not routine prior to entry into the academies. To the extent that this is true, myopic shifts would be underestimated in hyperopia and overestimated for myopia.

2.3   Statistical aspects of relationships between nearwork, myopia, education and intelligence

A major difficulty when investigating these associations is that the variables of interest are interrelated. Education and intelligence are obviously associated, and bright children may either like to read or are encouraged to do so by their parents. Most studies have concentrated on carefully assessing only one or two of the pertinent variables, leaving the others to casual assessment that is subject to criticism. Population-based studies, for example, rarely measure refractive error directly (Sperduto et al., 1983), whereas work in the field of education often does not assess refractive error or nearwork.

The Orinda Longitudinal Study of Myopia (Zadnik et al., 1993) is attempting to assess these variables in a comprehensive way in a large sample of children. Refractive error is assessed with cycloplegic autorefraction because it is the most repeatable measurement in the context of a longitudinal study (Zadnik et al., 1992). Nearwork is quantified with a questionnaire administered annually to parents and children (Figure 2.1). Achievement test scores for each child is available as testing occurs on the campuses of the Orinda Union School District, and the principal investigators have access to the childrens' school folders in order to gather their Iowa Tests of Basic Skills achievement data, administered in the Orinda Union School District from the third grade (around 9 years of age

How often does this child read for pleasure (outside of school)?

1 Never
2 Rarely
3 Sometimes
4 Often
5 Child doesn't read yet

During the school year, how many hours per week (outside of school) would you estimate this child:

Studies or reads for school assignments	_____ hours
Reads for pleasure	_____ hours
Watches television	_____ hours
Plays video/computer games	_____ hours
Engages in outdoor/ sports activities	_____ hours

Figure 2.1 Nearwork questionnaire from the parental survey used in the Orinda Longitudinal Study of Myopia (Zadnik *et al.*, 1994)

onwards). It is hoped that this data set will eventually shed light on these associations and their interrelated intricacies in a way that previous data sets have been unable to do.

2.4   Orinda longitudinal study of myopia data

What follows are preliminary analyses of nearwork in a sample of 791 children enrolled in the Orinda Longitudinal Study of Myopia (Zadnik *et al.*, 1993) and examined in the 1994–5 academic year. Parents are asked to report individually the number of hours per week their child spends studying outside of school, reading for pleasure, watching television, playing video games and engaging in sports or outdoor activities.

Table 2.6 shows the number of hours per week reported by the parents for these various activities by age group. Age is a statistically significant variable only for hours spent studying and hours spent reading for pleasure. The nearwork composite variable, dioptre-hours (Zadnik *et al.*, 1994), also differs significantly with age. Table 2.7 shows the nearwork profile by refractive error group (defined by the cycloplegic autorefraction value in the vertical meridian, *see* Harris, 1988). Myopes spend significantly more time reading for pleasure and studying, and significantly less time engaged in sports activities.

These data suggest that the questionnaire provides a valid assessment of nearwork. Other studies have reported associations of nearwork with myopia (Angle and Wissmann, 1978, 1980; Richler and Bear, 1980), and the fact that the Orinda study has observed similar findings would indicate that nearwork is being measured in a meaningful way. Similarly, one would expect that nearwork, especially that concerned with reading, would show an effect with age, and this is indeed the case (Table 2.6). This also supports the validity of the measurement.

This study has previously tested the predictive ability of nearwork for myopia, and found that nearwork made a statistically significant contribution to a logistic regression model with myopia

Table 2.6 Nearwork data (mean, SD) from the Orinda Longitudinal Study of Myopia by age group

Age at last birthday (yr)	Time spent studying (hr/wk)	Time spent reading for pleasure (hr/wk)	Time spent watching television (hr/wk)	Time spent playing video games (hr/wk)	Time spent in sports activities (hr/wk)	Dioptre-hours
6–7	2.18 ± 2.00	3.48 ± 3.17	8.75 ± 6.07	2.44 ± 2.60	11.08 ± 7.51	30.62 ± 14.99
8–9	4.25 ± 2.94	3.74 ± 3.47	7.82 ± 5.45	2.53 ± 2.70	10.83 ± 7.10	36.89 ± 17.64
10–11	6.34 ± 3.82	4.22 ± 4.25	7.79 ± 5.29	2.39 ± 2.68	10.35 ± 6.47	45.08 ± 20.65
≥12	9.65 ± 5.22	4.48 ± 4.24	8.50 ± 6.49	2.44 ± 3.75	10.29 ± 7.14	55.73 ± 24.79

$n = 791$ children tested in the 1994–5 academic year. There is a statistically significant effect of age for studying and reading for pleasure (one-way analysis of variance, $P = 0.0001$ and $P = 0.046$ respectively). Dioptre-hours = $3 \times$ (hours spent reading + hours spent studying) + $2 \times$ (hours spent playing video games + hours spent watching television). The number of dioptre-hours differs with age (one-way analysis of variance, $P = 0.0001$).

Table 2.7 Nearwork data (mean, SD) from the Orinda Longitudinal Study of Myopia by refractive error group

Refractive error group (vertical meridian)	Time spent studying (hr/wk)	Time spent reading for pleasure (hr/wk)	Time spent watching television (hr/wk)	Time spent playing video games (hr/wk)	Time spent in sports activities (hr/wk)	Dioptre-hours
Myopes (0.75 D or more myopia)	8.77 ± 5.59	5.55 ± 3.97	9.06 ± 6.74	2.29 ± 2.71	8.19 ± 5.83	58.35 ± 25.22
Emmetropes (between −0.75 D myopia and 1.00 D hyperopia)	5.54 ± 4.43	3.84 ± 3.87	8.06 ± 5.89	2.47 ± 3.07	10.87 ± 7.13	41.13 ± 21.41
Hyperopes (1.00 D or more)	4.75 ± 4.38	3.72 ± 3.26	8.43 ± 5.17	2.51 ± 2.83	10.96 ± 7.26	38.85 ± 19.27

$n = 791$ children tested in the 1994–5 academic year. There is statistically significant effect of refractive error for studying and reading for pleasure (one-way analysis of variance, $P = 0.0001$ and $P = 0.0015$ respectively), with myopes doing more reading in both cases. There is a statistically significant effect of refractive error for sports activities (one-way analysis of variance, $P = 0.0010$), with myopes doing fewer hours of these activities on average. Dioptre-hours = 3 × (hours spent reading + hours spent studying) + 2 × (hours spent playing video games + hours spent watching television). The number of dioptre-hours differs with refractive error group (one-way analysis of variance, $P = 0.0001$).

(0.75 D in both meridia) classified as either present or absent, but that its effect is far outweighed by parental history of myopia (Zadnik *et al.*, 1994).

2.5   Future studies

At present there is no widely accepted survey for exposure to nearwork. It is difficult to evaluate the importance of nearwork without a precise estimate of the actual cumulative amount of nearwork to which children are exposed. It would seem that the methods used to develop dietary questionnaires would also lend themselves to categorizing human visual activities. For example, if a person can be expected to report his or her dietary intake reliably from 10 years earlier (Wang *et al.*, 1994), then parents might be expected to describe their children's daily visual activities. Some laboratories have advocated the use of diaries completed by the children. However, we do not expect that this will prove to be a reliable way of measuring nearwork, especially in younger children. For example, the survey shown in Figure 2.1, administered with verbal instruction from an investigator, cannot be used in children younger than 9 or 10 years of age.

The issue of the influence of nearwork on the development of refractive error still warrants investigation. The issue of causation will be difficult to assess because it does not appear that the effect of nearwork on myopia is as striking, for example, as the relationship between cigarette smoking and lung cancer. More subtle causations are, by definition, difficult to identify and quantify in epidemiological studies. A randomized clinical trial where children were randomized either to nearwork or no nearwork groups would be unethical. The field needs continued, carefully designed studies, assessing nearwork, refractive error, achievement, intelligence and other related factors in reliable ways in order to continue to move forward. The identification of risk factors for myopia remains a field of great interest and debate.

References

Abiose, A., Bhar, I. S. and Allanson, M. A. (1980) The ocular health status of postprimary school children in Kaduna, Nigeria: report of a survey. *J. Ped. Ophthalmol. Strab.* **17**, 337–340.

Adams, D. W. and McBrien, N. A. (1992) Prevalence of myopia and myopic progression in a population of clinical microscopists. *Optom. Vis. Sci.* **69**, 467–473.

Alsbirk, P. H. (1979) Refraction in adult West Greenland Eskimos. A population study of spherical refractive errors, including oculometric and familial correlations. *Acta Ophthalmol.* **57**, 84–95.

Angle, J. and Wissmann, D. A. (1978) Age, reading, and myopia. *Am. J. Optom. Physiol. Opt.* **55**, 302–308.

Angle, J. and Wissmann, D. A. (1980) The epidemiology of myopia. *Am. J. Epidemiol.* **111**, 220–228.

Ashton, G. C. (1985a) Segregation analysis of ocular refraction and myopia. *Hum. Hered.* **35**, 232–239.

Ashton, G. C. (1985b) Nearwork, school achievement and myopia. *J. Biosoc. Sci.* **17**, 223–233.

Au Eong, K. G., Tay, T. H. and Lim, M. K. (1993a) Education and myopia in 110 236 young Singaporean males. *Sing. Med. J.* **34**, 489–492.

Au Eong, K. G., Tay, T. H. and Lim, M. K. (1993b) Race, culture and myopia in 110 236 young Singaporean males. *Sing. Med. J.* **34**, 29–32.

Baldwin, W. R. (1981) A review of statistical studies of relations between myopia and ethnic, behavioral, and physiological characteristics. *Am. J. Optom. Physiol. Opt.* **58**, 516–527.

Basu, S. K. and Jundal, A. (1983) Genetic aspects of myopia along the Shia Muslin Danoodi Bahnas of Udaiper, Rajnsthan. *Hum. Hered.* **33**, 163–169.

Blum, H. L., Peters, H. B. and Bettman, J. W. (1959) *Vision Screening for Elementary Schools: The Orinda Study.* University of California Press.

Bouchard, T. J. and McGue, M. (1981) Familial studies of intelligence: a review. *Science* **212**, 1055–1059.

Brown, E. V. L. and Kronfeld, P. (1929) The refraction curve in the US with special reference to the first two decades. *Proc. 13th Int. Cong. Ophthalmol.* **13**, 87–98.

Bullimore, M. A., Conway, R. and Nakash, A. (1989) Myopia in optometry students: family history, age of onset and personality. *Ophthal. Physiol. Opt.* **9**, 284–288.

Buros, O. K. (1972) In *The Seventh Mental Measurements Yearbook*, The Gryphon Press, pp. 65–68.

Chow, Y. C., Dhillon, B., Chew, P. T. *et al.* (1990) Refractive errors in Singapore medical students. *Sing. Med. J.* **31**, 472–473.

Cohn, H. (1886) *The Hygiene of the Eye in Schools* (English translation by W. P. Turnbull). Simpkin, Marshall & Co.

Cohn, S. J., Cohn, C. M. G. and Jensen, A. R. (1988) Myopia and intelligence: a pleiotropic relationship? *Hum. Genet.* **80**, 53–58.

Cole, B. L., Maddocks, J. D. and Sharpe, K. (1996) Effect of VDUs on the eyes: report of a 6-year epidemiological study. *Optom. Vis. Sci.* **73**, 512–528.

Curtin, B. C. (1985) *The Myopias. Basic Science and Clinical Management.* Harper & Row.

Diamond, S. (1957) Acquired myopia in airline pilots. *J. Aviat. Med.* **28**, 559–568.

Donders, F. C. (1864) *On the Anomalies of Accommodation and Refraction of the Eye.* The New Sydenham Society.

Ederer, F. (1973) Shall we count numbers of eyes or numbers of subjects? *Arch. Ophthalmol.* **89**, 1–2.

Garner, L. F., Kinnear, R. F., McKellar, M. *et al.* (1988) Refraction and its components in Melanesian schoolchildren in Vanuatu. *Am. J. Optom. Physiol. Opt.* **65**, 182–189.

Garner, L. F., Meng, C. K., Grosvenor, T. P. *et al.* (1990) Ocular dimensions and refractive power in Malay and Melanesian children. *Ophthal. Physiol. Opt.* **10**, 234–238.

Goldschmidt, E. (1968) On the etiology of myopia. An epidemiological study. *Acta Ophthalmol.* Suppl. **98**, 1–172.

Goss, D. A., Hampton, M. J. and Wickham, M. G. (1988) Selected review on genetic factors in myopia. *J. Am. Optom. Assoc.* **59**, 875–884.

Goss, D. A. and Winkler, R. L. (1983) Progression of myopia in youth: age of cessation. *Am. J. Optom. Physiol. Opt.* **60**, 651–658.

Greene, M. R. (1970) Submarine myopia in the Minutemen. *J. Am. Optom. Assoc.* **41**, 1012–1016.

Grosvenor, T. (1970) Refractive state, intelligence test scores, and academic ability. *Am. J. Optom. Arch. Am. Acad. Optom.* **64**, 482–498.

Gwiazda, J., Thorn, F., Bauer, J. *et al.* (1993) Emmetropization and the progression of manifest refraction in children followed from infancy to puberty. *Clin. Vis. Sci.* **8**, 337–344.

Harris, W. F. (1988) Algebra of sphero-cylinders and refractive errors, and their means, variance, and standard deviation. *Am. J. Optom. Physiol. Opt.* **65**, 794–802.

Hirsch, M. J. (1951) Effect of school experience on refraction of children. *Am. J. Optom. Arch. Am. Acad. Optom.* **28**, 445–454.

Hirsch, M. J. (1952) The changes in refraction between the ages of 5 and 14, theoretical and practical considerations. *Am. J. Optom. Arch. Am. Acad. Optom.* **29**, 445–459.

Hirsch, M. J. (1959) The relationship between refractive state of the eye and intelligence test scores. *Am. J. Optom. Arch. Am. Acad. Optom.* **36**, 12–21.

Hirsch, M. J. (1961) A longitudinal study of refractive state of children during the first six years of school. *Am. J. Optom. Arch. Am. Acad. Optom.* **38**, 564–571.

Hyams, S. W., Pokotilo, E. and Shkurko, G. (1977) Prevalence of refractive errors in adults over 40: a survey of 8102 eyes. *Br. J. Ophthalmol.* **61**, 428–432.

Jackson, E. (1932) Norms of refraction. *J. Am. Med. Assoc.* **98**, 761–767.

Jensen, H. (1991) Myopia progression in young school children. A prospective study of myopia progression and the effect of a trial with bifocal lenses and beta blocker eye drops. *Acta Ophthalmol.* Suppl. **200**, 1–55.

Katz, J., Tielsch, J. M. and Sommer, A. (1997) Prevalence and risk factors for refractive errors in an adult inner city population. *Int. Ophthalmol. Clin.* **38**, 334–340.

Kempf, G. A., Collins, S. D. and Jarman, B. L. (1928) *Refractive Errors in Eyes of Children as Determined by Retinoscopic Examination with Cycloplegia.* US Public Health Service.

Kent, P. R. (1963) Acquired myopia of maturity. *Am. J. Optom. Arch. Am. Acad. Optom.* **40**, 247–256.

Kinney, J. A. S., Luria, S. M., Ryan, A. P. *et al.* (1980) The vision of submariners and National Guardsmen: a longitudinal study. *Am. J. Optom. Physiol. Opt.* **57**, 469–478.

Laatikainen, L. and Erkkila, H. (1980) Refractive errors and other ocular findings in school children. *Acta Ophthalmol.* **58**, 129–136.

Lin, L. L.-K., Chen, C.-J., Hung, P.-T. *et al.* (1986) Nation-wide survey of myopia among schoolchildren in Taiwan, 1986. *Acta Ophthalmol.* Suppl. **185**, 29–33.

McBrien, N. A. and Adams, D. W. (1997) A longitudinal investigation of adult-onset and adult-progression of myopia in an occupational group. Refractive and biometric findings. *Invest. Ophthalmol. Vis. Sci.* **38**, 321–333.

McBrien, N. A. and Barnes, D. A. (1984) A review and evaluation of theories of refractive error development. *Ophthal. Physiol. Opt.* **4**, 201–213.

Midelfart, A., Aamo, B., Sjøhaug, K. A. *et al.* (1992) Myopia among medical students in Norway. *Acta Ophthalmol.* **70**, 317–322.

Morgan, R. W., Speakman, J. S. and Grimshaw, S. E. (1975) Inuit myopia: an environmentally induced 'epidemic'? *Canad. Med. Assoc. J.* **112**, 575–577.

Morgan, R.W. and Munro, M. (1973) Refractive problems in northern natives. *Can. J. Ophthalmol.* **8**, 226–228.

Mutti, D. O. and Zadnik, K. (1996) Is computer use a risk factor for myopia? *J. Am. Optom. Assoc.* **67**, 521–530.

Nadell, M. C. and Weymouth, F. W. (1957) The relationship of frequency of use of the eyes in close work to the distribution of refractive error in a selected sample. *Am. J. Optom. Arch. Am. Acad. Optom.* **34**, 523–536.

National Research Council (1989) *Myopia: Prevalence and Progression.* National Academy Press (Washington DC).

O'Neal, M. R. and Connon, T. R. (1987) Refractive error change at the United States Air Force Academy Class of 1985. *Am. J. Optom. Physiol. Opt.* **64**, 344–354.

Peckham, C. S., Gardiner, P. A. and Goldstein, H. (1977) Acquired myopia in 11-year-old children. *Br. Med. J.* **1**, 542–545.

Provines, W. F., Woessner, W. M., Rahe, A. J. *et al.* (1983) The incidence of refractive anomalies in the USAF rated population. *Aviat. Space Environ. Med.* **54**, 622–627.

Richler, A. and Bear, J. C. (1980) Refraction, nearwork and education. A population study in Newfoundland. *Acta Ophthalmol.* **58**, 468–478.

Roberts, J. and Rowland, M. (1978) Refraction status and motility defects of persons 4–74, United States, 1971–1972. US Department of Health, Education and Welfare.

Rosenfield, M. (1994) Accommodation and myopia. Are they really related? *J. Behav. Optom.* **5**, 3–25.

Rosner, J. and Rosner, J. (1989) Relation between tonic accommodation and visual perceptual skills development in 6- to 12-year-old children. *Optom. Vis. Sci.* **66**, 526–529.

Rosner, M. and Belkin, M. (1987) Intelligence, education, and myopia in males. *Arch. Ophthalmol.* **105**, 1508–1511.

Septon, R. D. (1984) Myopia among optometry students. *Am. J. Optom. Physiol. Opt.* **61**, 745–751.

Shapiro, A., Stollman, E. B. and Merin, S. (1982) Do sex, ethnic origin or environment affect myopia? *Acta Ophthalmol.* **60**, 803–808.

Sorsby, A., Leary, G. A. and Fraser, G. R. (1966) Family studies on ocular refraction and its components. *J. Med. Genet.* **3**, 269–273.

Sorsby, A., Sheridan, M. and Leary, G. A. (1962) *Refraction and Its Components in Twins.* Medical Research Council Special Reports Series No. 303. HMSO.

Sperduto, R. D., Siegel, D., Roberts J. *et al.* (1983) Prevalence of myopia in the United States. *Arch. Ophthalmol.* **101**, 405–407.

Sutton, M. R. and Ditmars, D. L. (1970) Vision problems at West Point. *J. Am. Optom. Assoc.* **41**, 263–265.

Tassman, I. S. (1932) Frequency of the various kinds of refractive errors. *Am. J. Ophthalmol.* **15**, 1044–1053.

Tay, M. T. H., Au Eong, K. G., Ng, C. Y. *et al.* (1992) Myopia and educational attainment in 421 116 young Singaporean males. *Ann. Acad. Med.* **21**, 785–791.

Taylor, H. R. (1980) Racial variations in vision. *Am. J. Epidemiol.* **115**, 139–142.

Teikari, J. M., Kaprio, J., Koskenvuo, M. *et al.* (1992) Heritability of defects of far vision in young adults–a twin study. *Scand. J. Soc. Med.* **20**, 73–78.

Teikari, J. M., O'Donnell, J., Kaprio, J. *et al.* (1991) Impact of heredity in myopia. *Hum. Hered.* **41**, 151–156.

van Rens, G. H. M. B. and Arkell, S. M. (1991) Refractive errors and axial length among Alaskan Eskimos. *Acta Ophthalmol.* **69**, 27–32.

Wang, Q., Klein, B. E. K., Klein, R. *et al.* (1994) Refractive status in the Beaver Dam Eye Study. *Invest. Ophthalmol. Vis. Sci.* **35**, 4344–4347.

Ware, J. (1813) Observations relative to the near and distant sight of different persons. *Phil. Trans. R. Soc. Lon.* **103**, 31–50.

Wick, B. and Crane, S. (1976) A vision profile of American Indian children. *Am. J. Optom. Physiol. Opt.* **53**, 34–40.

Williams, S. M., Sanderson, G. F., Share, D. L. *et al.* (1988) Refractive error, IQ and reading ability: a longitudinal study from age seven to 11. *Develop. Med. Child Neurol.* **30**, 735–742.

Worth, C. (1906) Hereditary influence in myopia. *Trans. Ophthalmol. Soc. UK* **26**, 141–144.

Young, F. A. (1955) Myopes versus non myopes–a comparison. *Am. J. Optom. Arch. Am. Acad. Optom.* **32**, 180–191.

Young, F. A. (1963) Reading, measures of intelligence and refractive errors. *Am. J. Optom. Arch. Am. Acad. Optom.* **40**, 257–264.

Young, F. A., Leary, G. A., Baldwin, W. R. *et al.* (1970) Refractive errors, reading performance, and school achievement among Eskimo children. *Am. J. Optom. Arch. Am. Acad. Optom.* **47**, 384–390.

Young, F. A., Leary, G. A., Baldwin, W. R. *et al.* (1969) The transmission of refractive errors within Eskimo families. *Am. J. Optom. Arch. Am. Acad. Optom.* **46**, 676–685.

Zadnik, K., Mutti, D. O. and Adams, A. J. (1992) The repeatability of measurement of the ocular components. *Invest. Ophthalmol. Vis. Sci.* **33**, 2325–2333.

Zadnik, K., Mutti, D. O., Friedman, N. E. *et al.* (1993) Initial cross-sectional results from the Orinda Longitudinal Study of Myopia. *Optom. Vis. Sci.* **70**, 750–758.

Zadnik, K., Satariano, W. A., Mutti, D. O. *et al.* (1994) The effect of parental history of myopia on children's eye size. *J. Am. Med. Assoc.* **271**, 1323–1327.

Zylbermann, R., Landau, D. and Berson, D. (1993) The influence of study habits on myopia in Jewish teenagers. *J. Ped. Ophthalmol. Strab.* **30**, 319–322.

3

Structural correlates of myopia

Christine F. Wildsoet

Myopia occurs when the axial length of the eye becomes too long for its refractive power. The resulting ametropia may be corrected by either standard optical means such as spectacles or contact lenses, or by a growing number of surgical procedures. However, these methods of correction will not alter the progression of myopia, which may be accompanied by potentially serious ocular complications such as glaucoma and retinal detachment, both of which may ultimately lead to blindness. While there is a growing body of evidence suggesting an association between nearwork and the development of myopia, it is of some concern that little is understood regarding the mechanisms underlying the development of myopia and, more generally, of how eye growth is regulated. Such information is fundamental to the development of an effective treatment for this condition. Recent research involving animal models of myopia has provided valuable information in this area. This chapter reviews the main features of human myopia against the background of these animal data. By way of introduction, the chapter first provides an overview of the various classification systems that have been used to describe human myopia, with the implication that there may be several fundamentally different forms of human myopia.

3.1 Myopia–some classification systems

Before any discussion of how myopia develops, one must ask how many discrete types of myopia

exist. Several alternative classification systems have been proposed, with emphases on either the optical, developmental or pathological aspects of the condition as described below. However, it should be noted that none provides an unambiguous classification of myopia. These systems of classification are also reviewed in a slightly different context in Chapter 1, and a more comprehensive historical overview was provided by Grosvenor (1987).

3.1.1 Classification based upon refractive error

The simplest and least ambiguous classification system is one based upon the magnitude of the refractive error. Three main categories are generally used, namely low, moderate and high myopia. However, there is some disagreement as to what constitutes appropriate limits for each of the three categories, and their selection is essentially arbitrary. For example, while the upper cut-off figures of 2–3 D for low myopia and 6–7 D for moderate myopia are encountered in many studies (e.g. Weymouth and Hirsch, 1991), they are not standardized. Additionally, classification of individual subjects may vary according to whether cycloplegia was used to control accommodation during refractive assessments. More myopia or pseudomyopia (apparent myopia arising from a sustained accommodative response, *see* section 5.7) may be seen when testing without cycloplegia. These issues would be of relatively minor importance were it not for the fact that such categorizations are given important weight, both clinically and in research. For example, it is generally asserted that high myopia carries the greatest risk of complications from ocular disease, yet the targeting of only the high myopia subgroup in screening strategies to detect pathology is only appropriate if such conditions never occurred in other myopes and if all myopes could be uniquely classified. This is clearly not the case.

The degree of myopia was also the basis for the refractive error classification system developed by Hirsch (1950), who proposed that the overall distribution of ametropia could be described in terms of four component curves. Three of the four refractive subgroups generated, namely the alpha, beta and gamma subgroups, contained myopes. The gamma subgroup includes the high and rarer forms of myopia (e.g. high congenital, degenerative and Marfan's lenticular myopia) and stand apart from the other two subgroups which comprise lower levels of myopia. Of these, the alpha group is the larger and includes myopes up to 5 D (as well as emmetropic and low to moderate hyperopes) while the beta subgroup covers from emmetropia to 8 D of myopia (mean between 3 D and 5 D of myopia). However, classification of individual subjects using this scheme is problematic due to the overlapping distribution of the latter two subgroups.

3.1.2   Classification based upon pathology

The presence or absence of related retinal pathology has also provided the basis for myopia classification. For example, Duke-Elder and Abrams (1970) divided myopia into simple and degenerative (or malignant) forms. The latter represents the pathological group which is further subdivided into congenital axial myopia, associated myopia, developmental degenerative myopia and myopia acquired with disease. The simple myopia group included the remaining cases of acquired myopia, which are generally low to moderate in magnitude.

Curtin (1985) considered not only the presence of pathological changes, but also the degree of refractive error and the age of onset. He adopted the term pathological myopia in preference to degenerative myopia, and applied it strictly to cases where complications occurred as a direct consequence of excessive elongation of the globe. Although this definition identifies a discrete group, the other two categories used by Curtin, namely physiological and intermediate myopia, are less clear. These types of myopias are further subdivided into congenital (present at birth), childhood (developing between 5 and 12 years of age)

and late myopia (occurring during adult life), and are limited to eyes without pathology. The feature used for initial categorization is whether ocular axial elongation is normal or excessive. This begs the question of what constitutes normal ocular growth, an issue which is re-examined later in this review.

3.1.3   Classification based upon age of onset or presumed aetiology

While the classification systems described above do not identify individual cases unambiguously, other schemes based upon assumptions concerning the origin or age of myopia onset have their own limitations. One example, albeit rarely used, is a three-way classification system comprising congenital, hereditary and acquired myopia (Weymouth and Hirsch, 1991). The first category encompasses cases of myopia that are presumed to be present at birth (although measurements are rarely made at that time), while the second category encompasses myopia accompanied by a positive family history of this condition, whether congenital or late-onset. The remaining cases are presumed to fall in the third category, namely acquired myopia. The value of this system must be questioned in terms of two inherent assumptions, firstly that hereditary trends can be easily identified, and secondly that hereditary myopia and acquired myopia are separate entities.

The difficulties raised in respect to classification systems are avoided when myopia is categorized on the basis of age of onset. Grosvenor (1987) recognized four groups, namely congenital, youth-onset, early adult-onset and late adult-onset. The first of these categories covers those cases where myopia is present at birth and persists through infancy, with high myopia being the general rule. The remaining categories are demarcated by age of onset. Thus, youth-onset myopia becomes manifest during the early childhood or teenage years, early adult-onset between 20 and 40 years of age, and late adult-onset myopia after 40 years of age. Although this approach requires an accurate refractive history to be established, it is less problematic than related systems which further subdivide youth-onset myopia into childhood (juvenile-onset) myopia and late-onset myopia based on the time during the teenage years when the myopia becomes clinically manifest. Apart from the difficulty in defining the age of onset accurately, there is little agreement on the age demarcation between the latter two categories, being variously set at 15 years or later (McBrien and Millodot, 1987; Grosvenor and Scott, 1991; Bullimore *et al.*, 1992).

3.1.4 Classification based upon presumed optical basis

Various workers have attempted to classify myopia based on its presumed optical basis. Thus Sorsby *et al.* (1957) grouped low refractive errors ranging from 4 D myopia to 4 D hyperopia on the basis that the dimensions of the individual biometric parameters were similar to emmetropic eyes. These refractive errors were therefore considered to be a consequence of a mismatching (or miscorrelation) of apparently normal ocular parameters. Refractive errors outside this range could generally be attributed to at least one abnormal ocular component, for example, axial length, and these eyes are categorized separately. Borish (1970) formalized this classification system with the terms correlation and component myopia. However, the weight of evidence from other studies described in detail in section 3.3 argues that all human myopia is axial in nature, casting doubt on whether these concepts of correlation myopia and component myopia have real significance.

Prompted by insights from animal studies concerning the regulation of refractive error, this chapter will adopt two categories of myopia, namely congenital and developmental myopia. Congenital myopia describes myopia which is present at birth and is of sufficient magnitude that it persists throughout life. Developmental myopia has multiple aetiologies and a variable time course of development. Thus, while neonatal refractive errors normally shift towards a near emmetropic state during early childhood, this may eventually give way to myopia (either during later childhood or adulthood). The argument will be presented that developmental myopia is due to one ocular component, namely axial length. Evidence from recent animal studies indicates that eyes can regulate their ametropia, and that refractive changes are largely accomplished through adjustments in axial length. These studies are briefly reviewed in the following section, and are covered in more detail in Chapter 4.

3.2 Animal models of myopia–what do they tell us?

Form deprivation, most commonly created by the introduction of diffusers or lid suture, has been used to induce myopia, most commonly in the

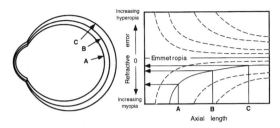

Figure 3.1 Global expansion of an eye to involve both the anterior corneal segment and posterior vitreous segment will cause all refractive errors, whether they be hyperopic or myopic in nature, to drift towards emmetropia. The graph on the right illustrates this passive emmetropization process: the hypothetical curves linking axial length and refractive error represent eyes with different starting refractive errors and ocular dimensions. As a specific example, the drawing on the left provides three snapshots of the same growing eye (A, B, C); the solid curve in the right-hand diagram describes the relationship between axial length and refractive error for this eye and the superimposed arrows identify the refractive errors corresponding to the three different eye sizes

chick, tree shrew and monkey (Sherman *et al.*, 1977; Wiesel and Raviola, 1977; Wallman *et al.*, 1978; Yinon, 1980). Although species differ in relation to their susceptibility as a function of age, axial myopia is the inevitable result. Specifically, myopia occurs through ocular elongation, with the changes being restricted largely to the posterior wall of the eye (Hodos and Kuenzel, 1984; Raviola and Wiesel, 1985; Marsh-Tootle and Norton, 1989). In contrast, the anterior ocular segment is minimally involved. If only part of the visual field is deprived, then the axial elongation is localized to the corresponding deprived segment, thereby implying a localized visual basis for this phenomenon (Wallman *et al.*, 1987; Norton and Siegwart, 1991).

In normal visual development, refractive errors tend to drift naturally toward emmetropia (Figure 3.1), irrespective of their starting point. This emmetropization process, while seemingly dependent upon normal visual experience (since it is disrupted by form deprivation), is at least in part an optical consequence of proportional growth, and thus passive in nature (Hofstetter, 1967; Wallman and Adams, 1987). This notion was referred to as the 'inflatable globe' by Koretz *et al.* (1995). However, the possibility that active processes are also involved was raised by experiments showing recovery from induced refractive errors, as well as the ability of eyes to compensate for retinal defocus imposed by lenses. This work demonstrating active emmetropization (as opposed to passive mechanisms) is potentially of great interest and significance in relation to the development of myopia in humans, and is summarized below.

Recovery from form deprivation myopia, representing the first line of evidence for active emmetropization, has been demonstrated in both chick and tree shrew (Wallman and Adams, 1987; Norton, 1990; McBrien and Norton, 1992), although the time constraints are shorter for the tree shrew. Nevertheless, in both species, the vitreous chamber elongation ceases when deprivation is terminated, and in a young animal continued normal growth restores both the normal proportions of the eye and emmetropia. Recovery from form deprivation myopia has yet to be demonstrated in the monkey, although recovery from the retinal defocus induced by contact lenses has been reported (Smith *et al.*, 1994).

The second line of evidence for active emmetropization relates to compensation for spectacle lens-induced focusing errors. This has been demonstrated in the three animal species named above (Hung *et al.*, 1995; Schaeffel *et al.*, 1988; Siegwart and Norton, 1993) and guinea pigs (McFadden and Wallman, 1995). The response following the introduction of negative lenses is increased axial elongation, which reduces the imposed refractive error (hyperopia in this case) over time. As with form deprivation, these compensatory changes are largely restricted to the vitreous chamber. Therefore, when the lenses are removed, these eyes are myopic. Again, species differ in their capacity to respond to induced refractive errors. Young chicks are able to compensate completely for lenses up to –10 D, when applied at hatching, in a little over one week (Irving *et al.*, 1992). Positive lenses are equally effective in inducing hyperopia (Irving *et al.* 1992; Wildsoet and Wallman, 1995). The response rates are slower in both tree shrews (Siegwart and Norton, 1993) and monkeys (Hung *et al.*, 1995).

These data present a strong argument in favour of an active emmetropization process. That compensation can occur in response to both positive and negative lenses demonstrates the bi-directionality of the emmetropization process and implies that the sign of imposed focusing errors can be distinguished. Precisely how the eye is able to detect and analyse ametropia is unresolved, but these mechanisms may be important to our understanding of how myopia develops. At the same time, these findings raise the question of how myopia can develop in a system that has the capacity to correct for it.

Any discussion of emmetropization would be incomplete without comment on the biological significance of the term. An optical definition for an emmetropic eye is one in which parallel rays of light from a distant object of regard are brought to a focus on the retina under conditions of minimal accommodation. However, this state of focus seems to be rarely achieved in nature. For example, early in life, many eyes appear to have idiosyncratic refractive set-points which are the target of active emmetropization. For example in the chick, when refractive errors were perturbed experimentally prior to lens wear, eyes made hyperopic to varying degrees by either continuous light or optic nerve section returned to these same refractive states after compensating for the imposed defocus (Bartmann *et al.*, 1994; Wildsoet, 1997). The significance of this concept of preferred refractive states or set-points for human myopia and its correction will be taken up toward the end of section 3.2.1 in relation to the work of Medina and Fariza (1987, 1993).

3.2.1   Myopia in humans–form deprivation versus anomalous emmetropization

Animal studies have documented two different visual manipulations that produce myopia. Firstly, form deprivation potently drives ocular elongation and myopia; secondly, the emmetropization process, responding to imposed hyperopic defocus, also leads to refractive changes. Could human myopia be the result of form deprivation or of anomalous emmetropization, rather than simply being a consequence of one's specific genetic make-up? The evidence for the first two options is presented below.

Form deprivation myopia exists in humans. Congenital and early developmental anomalies resulting in retinal image degradation are associated with myopia and increased axial elongation. Corneal opacities, cataracts and ptosis are three such conditions that have been well studied (Robb, 1970; Fledelius, 1976; O'Leary and Millodot, 1979; Hoyt *et al.*, 1981; Rabin *et al.*, 1981; von Noorden and Lewis, 1987; Shih and Lin, 1989; Twomey *et al.*, 1990), and associations of myopia with retrolental fibroplasia (Fledelius, 1976; Yamamoto *et al.*, 1979; Gunn *et al.*, 1980; Rabin *et al.*, 1981) and prolonged occlusion therapy (Muñoz and Capó, 1995) have also been noted. Additionally, there is an association between myopia and myelination of the retinal nerve fibre layer, albeit variable (Holland and Anderson, 1976; Shih and Lin, 1989; Summers *et al.*, 1991), perhaps reflecting the more localized nature of the deficit in many eyes and the failure of measurement protocols to detect related local growth changes.

The cases of myopia described above were associated with identifiable pathology and are relatively rare. A more important question is whether the more commonly encountered form of human myopia can likewise be attributed to form deprivation. This possibility was the subject of speculation by Wallman *et al.* (1987) who, as an explanation for the apparent association of myopia with reading, proposed that printed text, because of its bias towards high spatial frequencies, might impose a deprivation state for all but the high acuity central retina. Unfortunately, it is impossible to test this hypothesis directly in humans, although the close link between the level of education achieved and the prevalence of myopia represents a major piece of evidence for an association between nearwork and myopia (*see* reviews by Curtin, 1985; Bear, 1991; *see also* Chapter 2).

The alternative hypothesis that human myopia represents an anomalous emmetropization response is supported by the lens studies in animals. To complete this analogy, it is necessary to invoke a mechanism by which a hyperopic error signal would be imposed, as is the case when negative lenses are used in the animal studies. The most likely source of hyperopic errors is accommodation. Following a period of distance fixation, the introduction of a near object of regard will create hyperopic retinal defocus. An increased accommodative response will reduce this defocus, but when a lag of accommodation exists (i.e., the accommodative response is less then the dioptric stimulus), then some hyperopic retinal defocus will remain. Furthermore, these lags of accommodation are likely to be greater in cases of accommodative dysfunction, which may be associated with developing myopia (Jones, 1990; Gwiazda *et al.*, 1993, 1995; *see* Chapter 5). Accordingly, this hypothesis predicts that elimination of these focusing errors would halt the progression of myopia. This is a difficult prediction to test in humans, since one cannot require that they only view objects at the distance for which they are corrected. However, a number of observations support the plausibility of this view. For example, one might predict that children with esophoria at near would generally underaccommodate in order to avoid diplopia arising from excessive convergence; the resulting hyperopic defocus might subsequently lead to the development of myopia. Accordingly in these children, the wearing of bifocals (which presumably reduces the degree of retinal defocus) retards myopic progression (Goss, 1994; Goss and Uyesugi, 1995; *see* Chapter 7). Furthermore, an association has also been reported between high clinical measures of accommodative lag (using the binocular dynamic cross-cylinder test) and lower myopia progression rates in bifocal wearers (Goss and Uyesugi, 1995). Finally, Medina and Fariza (1987, 1993) argued that the traditional correction of myopia with negative lenses reintroduces the error that initially stimulated its development, and therefore is likely to accelerate its progression. This conclusion is also compatible with the notion that individual eyes have preferred refractive set-points to which they return after being corrected, as discussed earlier in relation to compensation for imposed refractive errors in chick.

These various issues in relation to the aetiology of human myopia are taken up in other chapters in this book. It will be clear from the preceding discussion that human myopia may not reflect solely an individual's genetic profile. Furthermore, both of the analogies drawn from animal models would predict that developmental myopia is axial in nature. This issue constitutes the major focus of the next section.

3.3 Myopia–a problem of an excessively long eye?

In this section it will be argued that it is of limited value to think of common myopias as resulting from the combination of ocular components having normal ocular dimensions (i.e., correlation ametropia). Rather, the existing correlational studies of both juvenile-onset and adult-onset myopia suggest that myopia results from excessive elongation of the eye. Of course, it is difficult to infer causation from correlation. For example, consider Figure 3.2. Figure 3.2A shows a high negative correlation between corneal radius of curvature and refractive error, indicating that more myopic eyes have flatter corneas. This is the opposite finding to that which would be required if the cornea was to contribute to the refractive error. However,

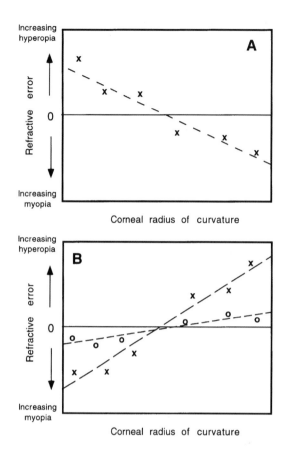

Figure 3.2 High correlations between the corneal radius of curvature and refractive error do not necessarily mean that a cause and effect relationship exists. For example, the negative correlation between these parameters shown in (A) indicates that myopic eyes have flatter corneas, the opposite of what is expected if the cornea were to contribute to the refractive state. The converse situation is depicted by the two sets of data (from different hypothetical patients) in (B), although the slopes of their hypothetical regression lines are significantly different (albeit positive), indicating different contributions of the cornea to the refractive state

even where correlation and directionality constraints are met, as in Figure 3.2B, it is clear that the extent to which corneal curvature differences account for the refractive change is dependent upon the magnitude of the slope of the fitted regression line. Unfortunately such slope data are frequently not provided. When more than one parameter is involved, as in the case at hand, it is possible that the variability in one parameter may partly obscure the influence of another in simple regression analyses. The latter problem may be avoided by the use of partial correlation analyses

(this allows one or more variables to be fixed and so the variable of interest to be identified) yet such analyses are seldom encountered. On the other hand, longitudinal studies in relation to myopia are limited in number and quality because of the problems associated with tracking large numbers of subjects over time. Nonetheless, such studies do allow the specific investigation of the ocular changes underlying the development of myopia. Data from both types of studies have been used in reconstructing, for the human myopic eye, a cohesive picture which is developed progressively over the following sections.

3.3.1   Classic population studies

One of the most frequently cited studies in relation to the optical basis of myopia was a cross-sectional study of young adults (20–35 years) by Stenström (1948). Based upon correlation analyses, Stenström concluded that axial length was the main determinant of refractive error, because these two parameters exhibited a strong linear correlation. Similar analyses were carried out on subgroups with and without conus (a characteristic fundus feature of high myopia), with a similar outcome. That the conus group had longer eyes is also consistent with the clinical interpretation of conus as a sign of excessive eye growth. A moderate negative correlation was also observed between refractive error and anterior chamber depth (myopes having deeper anterior chambers), and in this case the regression function was non-linear. These data have been subsequently re-analysed many times by other workers. For example, Hirsch and Weymouth (1947) derived first order and some second order partial correlations (i.e., one or two variables held fixed, respectively) from these data as a way of measuring the relative contributions of various ocular components to the refractive state. They concluded that 50 per cent of the variability in refractive error was due to differences in axial length, while 25 per cent and 20 per cent of the variability were due to the cornea and crystalline lens, respectively.

Van Alphen (1961) undertook more extensive analyses of Stenström's data and derived partial (first, second and third order) and multiple correlation coefficients. These data, as well as correlation data from Stenström's original study and that of Hirsch and Weymouth, are compared in Table 3.1. Van Alphen depicted a myopic eye as one with longer than normal axial length and/or increased corneal curvature with a flatter (and thus less powerful) crystalline lens. It should be noted that the corneal and lenticular differences will have oppo-

Table 3.1 The contribution of various ocular components to refractive error: a comparison of zero order and first and second partial correlation coefficients derived by van Alphen (1961) from data of Stenström (1948)*

Compared parameters	Zero order correlation coefficients	First order partial correlation coefficients	Second order partial correlation coefficients
Refractive errors vs axial length	−0.76	−0.87	−0.87
Refractive error vs corneal radius	+0.18	−0.67	+0.70
Refractive error vs anterior chamber depth	−0.34	+0.33	+0.25
Axial length vs corneal radius	+0.31	+0.70	+0.93
Axial lenth vs anterior chamber depth	+0.44	+0.50	+0.46
Corneal radius vs anterior chamber depth	−0.10	−0.28	−0.37

* The latter two coefficents are subject to variation, according to which variable is fixed; the data presented represent the highest values reached in these analyses.

site effects upon the refractive error and thus tend to neutralize one other. That axial length is the major determinant of the refractive state is further reinforced by these correlation data in which the highest correlations are found in the refractive error: axial length comparisons. These parameters also have similar distribution profiles, being both leptokurtic and skewed (Tron, 1940; Stenström, 1948). Further analyses of Stenström's data by Carroll (1981, 1982) found a nearly perfect linear relationship between refractive error and axial length, with the slope of this relationship (−0.37 mm/D) indicating that axial length accounted almost entirely for the refractive differences.

Other analyses undertaken by Stenström provide an important perspective on eye shape (Table 3.1). Specifically, examination of the correlations between individual ocular components indicated that axial length and corneal radius of curvature were positively correlated (+0.31), whereas axial length and lens power were negatively correlated (−0.36). In other words, larger eyes tended to have flatter corneas and less powerful crystalline lenses. These relationships imply that the cornea and crystalline lens are influenced by ocular growth as part of the passive emmetropization process alluded to earlier. However, the observation that some eyes

become myopic instead of remaining emmetropic indicates that this coupling is not always consistent, a point discussed later in relation to the work of Scott and Grosvenor (1993).

The data described above are consistent with the proposal that all myopia is axial in origin. However, other workers have not supported this hypothesis. Among its strongest opponents were Sorsby *et al.* (1957, 1961, 1962; Sorsby and Leary, 1970) who undertook their own population studies. They argued that low refractive errors cannot be attributed to any one structural component but rather result from a mismatching of these components. This conclusion was based upon cross-sectional data indicating that low myopes (and also low hyperopes) had similar ocular dimensions to emmetropes. Accordingly, they introduced the terms correlation ametropia (apparently equivalent to Tron's (1940) term, combination ametropia), to describe the low refractive error group (4 D hyperopia to 4 D myopia), and component ametropia to describe higher refractive errors in which one component, typically axial length, lay outside the normal range observed in emmetropic individuals. This latter group comprised less than 3 per cent of the total population.

Using an alternative approach, Scott and Grosvenor (1993) sought to develop structural models for both emmetropic and myopic eyes by applying a multiple sample analysis technique to data from 42 eyes in each of these two refractive groups (ages 17–26 years; emmetropes: mean refractive error = +0.32, [range +1.50 to −0.50 D]; myopes: mean refractive error = −5.9 D [range −5.00 to −7.00 D]). This analysis identified parameters that distinguish between the two refractive groups. Scott and Grosvenor concluded that their emmetropic and myopic groups belonged to two separate populations exhibiting different relationships between anterior and vitreous chamber depths. More importantly, they concluded that all refractive components except anterior chamber depth contributed to myopia, with corneal radius of curvature and vitreous chamber depth being the main determinants (standardized regression coefficients being +0.96 and −0.96 for corneal radius of curvature and vitreous chamber depth respectively). The result in relation to corneal curvature is at odds with the conclusions of Stenström, who found this parameter to be only weakly correlated with refractive error for the population as a whole. This difference highlights an important issue in relation to these studies, namely that the method of analysis adopted may alter the outcome significantly. Scott and Grosvenor also noted that myopic eyes had steeper corneas than emmetropic eyes, a result consistent with Van Alphen's model of myopia (Van Alphen, 1961). This result is also seemingly paradoxical in that corneal radius of curvature and vitreous chamber depth were highly correlated (+0.79), implying that flatter corneas were generally coupled with longer vitreous chamber depths, yet the latter were also likely to be associated with increasing myopia. Scott and Grosvenor, in an explanation of this paradox, hypothesized that different processes may underlie the elongation of myopic and emmetropic eyes, an issue which will be returned to section 3.5. Firstly, the data relative to age of onset will be examined with respect to the ocular components underlying myopia, and the possibility that childhood myopia is different from myopia of later onset will be explored. Inter-racial differences that might imply that different forms of myopia exist will also be considered.

3.3.2   Childhood and late-onset myopia

Childhood myopia is clearly axial in nature. This conclusion appears to be the general consensus across both cross-sectional and longitudinal studies (Larsen, 1971a–d; McBrien and Millodot 1987;

Fledelius, 1988, 1995; Goss et al., 1990; Grosvenor and Scott, 1991, 1993; Jensen, 1991; Bullimore et al., 1992). One example of a longitudinal study in this category was that of Fledelius (1988), who compared refractive changes between 10 and 18 years of age with changes in the various ocular components for a group of 67 subjects. Significant changes in both refractive error (1.17 D) and axial length (0.62 mm) were observed, and these axial changes were of sufficient magnitude and in the appropriate direction to account for the refractive shifts. Similar results were reported in the shorter term and/or smaller scale longitudinal studies of Jensen (1991), and Grosvenor and Scott (1993). Goss and Winkler (1983) noted that childhood myopia progression (and presumably axial elongation as the underlying cause), generally ceased, along with that of overall body growth, i.e., somewhere between 15 and 17 years of age, although slightly earlier in females. The argument that childhood myopia is axial in nature also implies that neither the lens nor cornea play a role in the development of childhood myopia. This evidence will be considered further.

During childhood, the crystalline lens decreases its refractive power and this dioptric reduction will oppose the development of myopia. For example, Zadnik et al. (1995) reported lens thinning between 6 and 10 years of age. This change, equivalent to a 3.33 D hyperopic shift, serves to attenuate at least part of the expected drift toward myopia with the continuing growth of the eye during childhood (and puberty for some individuals; Fledelius, 1988). Interestingly, Zadnik et al. (1995) also reported that in myopic eyes, the crystalline lenses showed greater thinning, and other studies have reported either similar trends (Garner et al., 1992; Fledelius, 1995) or no significant difference in lens power amongst various refractive subgroups (Larsen, 1971c; McBrien and Millodot, 1987; Grosvenor and Scott, 1991; Jensen, 1991; Bullimore et al., 1992). The involvement of the anterior ciliary region in the ocular enlargement process would explain these crystalline lens thickness changes, assuming that the lens does not enlarge at the same rate; thus a larger myopic eye would have an enlarged ciliary body ring, leading to increased stretch and thus thinning of the lens to which it is attached. This may be considered as yet another example of passive emmetropization, which is of insufficient magnitude in the case of myopic eyes to maintain the emmetropic state.

The cornea appears to play a minimal role in the development of childhood myopia, although the supporting evidence for this statement is less clear cut than is the case for the crystalline lens. It is often claimed that the cornea undergoes almost no growth or change in curvature after 2–3 years of age (Sorsby *et al.*, 1961; Duke-Elder and Abrams, 1970; Hirsch and Weymouth, 1991, p. 40). This suggests that the cornea can have little active part in any subsequent refractive changes. However, reports of steeper than normal corneas in some cross-sectional studies of myopic eyes suggest a corneal contribution to myopic development in childhood. For example, Grosvenor and Scott (1991) observed a mean difference in corneal power of +1.37 D between their myopic and emmetropic subgroups, and smaller differences in the same direction are evident in the data of McBrien and Millodot (1987) (mean difference = +0.27 D) and of Bullimore *et al.* (1992) (mean difference = +0.32 D). However, it is possible that these differences existed prior to the development of myopia, as suggested by longitudinal studies of childhood myopia. For example, Fledelius (1988) noted that changes in corneal radius exhibited a poor correlation with refractive changes; in addition, larger eyes tended to have flatter corneas. Likewise, Goss and Erickson (1987) noted that corneal changes up to 15 years of age were negligible, despite a mean rate of myopia progression of approximately 0.5 D per annum. Similar results were obtained in other longitudinal studies by Jensen (1991), Pärssinen and Lyyra (1993) and Grosvenor and Scott (1993). In summary, corneal steepening apparently does not underlie the development of childhood myopia, although corneal curvature may be inherently steeper in these myopic eyes.

In view of the finding that the axial changes underlying experimental myopia appear to be largely restricted to the vitreous chamber, it is of interest to examine whether anterior chamber growth has a role in the development of myopia during childhood. This question is not easy to address because thinning of the lens, as sometimes seen in childhood myopia, may also effect changes in anterior chamber depth, thereby complicating the interpretation of such data. Grosvenor and Scott (1993) found no significant correlation between changes in anterior chamber depth and refractive error over a three-year period, although baseline cross-sectional data indicated deeper anterior chambers in their 'youth-onset' myopes, when compared with emmetropes. Similar trends are evident in other cross-sectional data (McBrien and Millodot, 1987; Bullimore *et al.*, 1992). In contrast, Larsen (1971a) showed a significant negative correlation between anterior chamber depth and refractive error, albeit only for one subgroup of 12-year-old girls ($r = -0.885$). Also, because mean refractive data were not provided, the extent to which these anterior chamber differences could account for the observed refractive changes cannot be assessed.

Late-onset myopia or young-adult myopia refers to that myopia which first becomes manifest during the late teenage years, and there is strong evidence that this myopia has an axial basis despite the commonly held belief that eye growth is essentially completed by the end of puberty. For example, three cross-sectional studies by McBrien and Millodot (1987), Grosvenor and Scott (1991) and Bullimore *et al.* (1992) all indicated a strong association between refractive error and vitreous chamber length. In only one case, namely the study of McBrien and Millodot (1987), were significant changes in the anterior chamber and crystalline lens noted, and in this case these trends were similar to those reported in juvenile-onset myopia, i.e. deeper anterior chambers and thinner lenses. Grosvenor and Scott (1993), in their longitudinal study, also reported significant correlations between refractive changes and changes in both vitreous chamber depth and axial length. Together, these various data support an axial basis for late-onset myopia.

The above findings imply that the capacity of the eye to grow is retained beyond puberty. Other data have also demonstrated that axial elongation may occur well into adulthood. Indirect evidence is provided by Adams (1987), who described his own case history which included a myopic shift of approximately 3.5 D between 24 and 42 years of age. This change was assumed to be axial in origin because corneal changes over this 18-year period were negligible. However, an even more dramatic example of adult eye growth was provided by a longitudinal study of clinical microscopists by McBrien and Adams (1997). Here, the youngest subject at the start of this two-year study was 21 years, and the median age of the group was 29.7 years. Despite this, 39 per cent of the initially emmetropic subjects became myopic (mean increase = 0.58 D) and a further 48 per cent of the initially myopic subjects showed myopic progression (mean increase = 0.77 D). In both cases the changes were associated with elongation of the vitreous chamber (0.26 and 0.24 mm compared with 0.02 and 0.03 mm for equivalent non-progressing groups). Simensen and Thorud (1994) reported a similar axial basis to myopia observed in textile workers, 80 per cent of whom did not require a spectacle correction before 20 years of age, and hence were presumed to be late-developing myopes. An axial length difference of 1.54 mm (corresponding to 3.75 D of myopia), was observed between the myopic and emmetropic groups examined in this study.

The role of the cornea in the aetiology of late-onset myopia is somewhat unclear, as evidenced by the following two single case studies. Kent (1963) reported that corneal steepening accounted for over half of the refractive changes. In contrast, a case report by Jiang and Woessner (1996) observed that refractive shifts were significantly correlated with changes in vitreous chamber depth but not with corneal changes. In support of Kent's findings, Goss and Erickson (1987) also noted concurrent corneal steepening in a group of progressing myopes; furthermore, the rates of change in these parameters were significantly correlated. Jiang and Woessner pointed out that the corneal changes alone accounted for less than half of the observed myopia progression in the study of Goss and Erickson, and the weight of other evidence also argued against a significant corneal contribution. Thus, while Grosvenor and Scott (1991) reported steeper than normal corneas in a cross-sectional study of early adult-onset myopes, the same workers, in a subsequent longitudinal study (Grosvenor and Scott, 1993), found no evidence of corneal steepening being associated with myopia progression. Finally, in two other cross-sectional studies by Bullimore *et al.* (1992) and McBrien and Millodot (1987), late-onset myopes and emmetropes were found to have similar corneal curvatures. These findings suggest that the cornea plays a negligible role in the development of late-onset myopia, although corneal differences may exist between myopes and emmetropes.

Later in life, it would appear that other ocular components predominate as aetiological causes of myopia. For example, in late-adult onset myopia (i.e., myopia first becoming manifest after 45 years of age), central (nuclear) lenticular changes represent the most likely structural correlate (Hirsch, 1958).

In summary, two or three potentially different forms of developmental myopia may exist, one first becoming evident during childhood, another occurring in the late teenage years and a third which first becomes evident after 45 years of age.

However, apart from the differences in age of onset, no significant differences appear to exist that could suggest the involvement of different mechanisms. Grosvenor and Scott (1991, 1993, 1994) concluded that both childhood and late-onset myopia (their youth-onset and early adult-onset myopia categories) are largely axial in origin. Nonetheless, they did not exclude the possibility of corneal involvement, and proposed that corneal steepening may occur very early in the development of myopia, possibly before the refractive changes can be detected at a clinical level (Grosvenor and Scott, 1993).

3.3.3 Corneal radius of curvature relative to axial length: the significance of this relationship for myopia

Grosvenor (1988) suggested that the ratio between axial length and corneal radius of curvature (AL:CR) may represent another way of exploring the role of the cornea in the development of myopia. He indicated that higher values of this ratio might constitute a risk factor for myopia. The implicit hypothesis, namely that myopes may have different ratios, is derived from the notion put forward by Van Alphen (1961) that ocular stretch may differentially affect the corneal and posterior (vitreous) segments of the eye. This hypothesis is also consistent with the axial model of myopia suggested in the preceding section. Specifically, it is predicted that myopic eyes have larger AL:CR ratios, simply as a consequence of their increased axial length. This is consistent with Grosvenor's findings when comparing AL:CR ratios in populations of emmetropes and myopes. For comparative purposes, AL:CR ratios data have been computed from a number of studies, and in all cases, the observed trends could be explained on the basis that axial elongation dominates over corneal changes as a determinant of myopia. Firstly, the ratio increases with the degree of myopia (Figure 3.3A), and secondly, childhood myopia is associated with higher AL:CR values than late-onset myopia (Figure 3.3B). The former trend was consistently found for presumed racially homogenous groups (Grosvenor, 1988; Fulk *et al.*, 1992; Pärssinen and Lyyra, 1993; Carney *et al.*, 1997). Finally analysis of data from Lin *et al.* (1996) indicated that this ratio increases concurrent with myopia development.

Could higher AL:CR ratios constitute a risk factor for myopia, as proposed by Grosvenor (1988)? His argument is based upon observed racial differ-

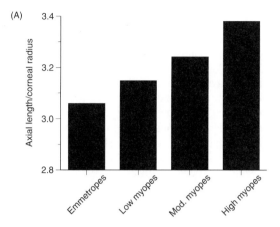

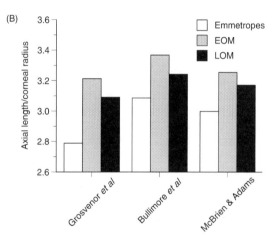

Figure 3.3 Ratios of axial length to corneal radius of curvature (AL:CR) for various refractive groups compared. (A) Data from Carney *et al.* (1997) show an increase in AL:CR ratio with increasing myopia. That early-onset myopes (EOM) have larger AL:CR ratios than age-matched late-onset myopes (LOM), with emmetropes having the smallest ratios of these three groups, are the consistent trends across three studies by Grosvenor and Scott (1991), Bullimore *et al.* (1992) and McBrien and Adams (1997), shown in (B)

ences in susceptibility to myopia, and corresponding variations in the AL:CR ratios. Goss and Jackson (1995) described significantly larger ratios in children who became myopic when compared with those who remained emmetropic, with the larger ratios being a consequence of the 'became myopic' group having steeper corneas. There was no significant difference in axial length between these two groups. Conceivably, early (pre-myopia) corneal steepening as hypothesized by Grosvenor and Scott (1993) could be involved. An alternative

hypothesis is that at least a subgroup of these eyes always had relatively steep corneas, and thus would need to undergo less elongation than the 'remained emmetropic' eyes before becoming myopic. The latter issue is revisited in a discussion of low birth weight infants where steeper than normal corneas appear to be the norm (Fledelius, 1976; Inagaki, 1986).

3.3.4   Vitreous chamber enlargement in myopia: is there an axial bias?

Eye shape is determined by underlying growth processes. Eye shape must also reflect the shape of the vitreous chamber where most of the myopic enlargement occurs. Accordingly, it is of interest to know whether eye shape changes during myopic development. Two studies using different examination techniques concluded that eye shape does not change significantly during the development of myopia, at least for moderate degrees of myopia (5–6.5 D on average). Using high resolution magnetic resonance imaging to compare myopic, emmetropic and hyperopic eyes, Cheng *et al.* (1992) found that while myopic eyes were larger than the other two refractive groups, all shared a similar spheroelliptical shape. Likewise, Meyer-Schwickerath and Gerke (1984), using A-scan ultrasonography, observed only minimal differences between equatorial and axial ocular dimensions. These results are also consistent with the observations of Weymouth and Hirsch (1950), based upon a compilation of data from three much earlier studies, of good correlations between axial and vertical eye diameters, with slopes near unity; that the myopia under consideration was axial in nature is also confirmed in their comment that myopia was characterized by big eyes. This suggests that the cornea did not share in this expansion process (i.e., passive emmetropization), although this issue was not specifically addressed. Together, these studies link myopia with a general expansion of the vitreous chamber, and the same appears to be true for deprivation myopia in the tree shrew and at least some monkeys (Raviola and Wiesel, 1985; Greene and Guyton, 1986; Phillips and McBrien, 1995). However, this may not be the case for higher amounts of myopia in humans. For example, a study of high myopes (mean = −12.9 D) by Meyer-Schwickerath and Gerke (1984) reported that axial dimensions exceeded equatorial dimensions by over 2 mm. Staphylomata, which are commonly encountered in high myopia, will also bias the axial dimensions because of their typical posterior location (Curtin *et al.*, 1979). Thus an axial bias in eye shape appears to be an indicator of high myopia. It may also be concluded that models based upon peripheral refraction data which represented myopic eyes as having near 'emmetropic' equatorial dimensions actually pertain to high myopia (Charman and Jennings, 1982; Dunne *et al.*, 1987; Logan *et al.*, 1995; Logan and Gilmartin, 1996). The latter work is described in more detail in section 3.4.

3.3.5 Racial differences and myopia

There are significant differences in the prevalence of myopia across races. One might also ask whether there are racial differences in the origin and/or nature of the presenting myopia? In the majority of studies cited, Caucasian and/or Northern European subjects have predominated. These populations have a myopia prevalence level similar to that reported for the United States population, i.e., around 25 per cent (Sperduto *et al.*, 1983). In contrast, much higher prevalence values have been reported for people of Chinese and Japanese backgrounds. For example, a study by Kozaki *et al.* (1969) of Japanese schoolchildren reported that 37 per cent of 6-year-olds were myopic, with the prevalence rising to 85 per cent for 12-year-old children. Hosaka (1988) gives a figure of 50.7 per cent for the average prevalence of myopia in urban Japanese primary school children. What are the implications of these data with respect to the aetiology of myopia?

For the Japanese population, there is considerable evidence that their myopia is axial in nature. Tokoro and Kabe (1964) followed the progression of juvenile myopia in 42 eyes and observed both increases in axial length and decreases in corneal and crystalline lens power between 7 and 15 years of age. However, both axial growth and myopic progression slowed after this time. Similar trends were reported in a longitudinal study by Tokoro and Suzuki (1968), and a cross-sectional one by Hosaka (1988), where increasing vitreous chamber length was found to be coupled with increasing myopia. In contrast, no significant correlation existed between refractive error and either anterior chamber depth or lens thickness. Similar trends were observed for data from three different age groups, i.e., 10–19, 20–29 and 30–39 years. The axial nature of even very low myopia (0.5–1.25 D) is implied by a correspondingly larger mean axial length when compared with that for an emmetropic group, although the statistical significance of this difference (0.33 mm) was not reported.

Axial myopia is also the general finding of studies examining Chinese populations. Lin *et al.* (1988) reached this conclusion for Taiwanese Chinese based upon two separate studies; a longitudinal study of school children between 13 and 15 years of age, and a cross-sectional study of teenagers between 16 and 19 years of age. The contribution of the cornea was specifically explored for the older group and found to play only a minor role. Similar conclusions may also be drawn from three other studies; two cross-sectional surveys of university students (Shih *et al.*, 1989; Lin *et al.*, 1991) and a five-year longitudinal study of medical students (Lin *et al.*, 1996). Low correlations between refractive error and corneal curvature were observed in the cross-sectional studies, while Lin *et al.* (1996) reported corneal flattening rather than the steepening that might have been predicted.

The nature of myopia in Taiwanese Chinese and Hong Kong Chinese appears to be similar. Accordingly, data pooled across ages from a cross-sectional study of children between 6 and 17 years of age (Lam and Goh, 1991a) revealed strong correlations between refractive error and both vitreous chamber depth and axial length but no significant correlation between refractive error and corneal radius of curvature. However, as in some of the previously cited studies, corneal radius of curvature was found to be positively correlated with axial length, indicating that larger eyes tended to have flatter corneas. Myopia prevalence figures from this study ranged from between 30 per cent (in 6–7 years olds) to 70 per cent (in 16–17 year-old males). Comparison of these data with a subsequent study of young adults between 19 and 39 years of age (Goh and Lam, 1994) confirmed that myopia continues to progress after 16–17 years of age, although its overall prevalence does not change. This myopia was also axial in nature. Indeed, vitreous chamber depth and axial length (these parameters are highly correlated) proved to be the only ocular parameters that correlated significantly with refractive error. An interesting incidental observation from these data is that while females recorded a slightly higher mean refractive error (−3.19 vs −2.99 D), the opposite finding would have been predicted from the values of vitreous chamber depth, which were shorter in females (17.16 vs 17.77 mm, i.e., equivalent to a 1.7 D difference in refractive error). This difference can be accounted for by the observation that the females tended to have steeper corneas than their male counterparts (7.62 vs 7.81 mm, equivalent to a 0.6 D difference in refractive error). Although myopia was less prevalent amongst older Hong Kong Chinese (29 per cent in those over 40 years of age), it was still axial in nature (Lam *et al.*, 1994).

Since the high prevalence of myopia seen in the Japanese and Chinese populations is not reproduced in all Asian populations, it would be of interest to know whether the ocular correlates of myopia varied with the frequency of myopia. A review of relevant studies suggests that this is not the case. In a cross-sectional study of Malay and Melanesian children, Garner *et al.* (1990) found a comparatively low prevalence of myopia in 15–16 year-old Malay children (25.6 per cent) and an even smaller prevalence (4.3 per cent) in Melanesian children of the same age. Nonetheless, for the Malay children, refractive error was still correlated strongly with axial length ($r = -0.66$), implying that axial elongation was the major cause of myopia. Melanesian children showed only a weak correlation between refractive error and axial length, but this presumably reflects the low prevalence of myopia and narrower refractive error distribution for this group. These studies supply other indirect evidence in support of an axial basis for the observed myopia in that longer eyes are associated with flatter, less powerful corneas and decreased crystalline lens power. These correlations, which were seen in both groups of children, are in the opposite direction to that which would be required for the cornea and lens to have contributing roles in the development of myopia.

Given the racial differences in the susceptibility to myopia, are there corresponding differences in AL:CR ratios? Values of this ratio for a number of studies are shown in Figure 3.4. Both Tibetan and Melanesian adolescents, who exhibited a low prevalence of myopia, also had the two lowest AL:CR values, with mean values of 2.99 (Garner *et al.*, 1995) and 2.95 (Garner *et al.*, 1990), respectively. In contrast, the highest values are from groups of Hong Kong and Taiwanese Chinese, with mean values of 3.22 (Goh and Lam, 1994) and 3.27 (Lin *et al.*, 1996), respectively (*see* Figure 3.4A). Values for Caucasian children of 2.99 (Zadnik *et al.*, 1994) and 3.05 (based upon Sorsby's data: ratio derived by Grosvenor, 1988), are similar to those obtained for the Melanesian and Tibetan populations. Thus, these data are in accordance with Grosvenor's hypothesis, although there are some exceptions. For example, the value of 3.16 for a

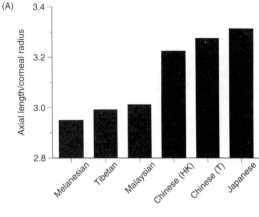

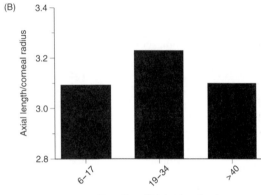

Figure 3.4 Derived ratios of axial length to corneal radius of curvature (AL:CR). Compared in (A) are six different Asian populations. The highest values were recorded for Hong Kong (HK) and Taiwanese (T) Chinese and Japanese populations; the values of the Melanesian, Tibetan and Malaysian populations were much lower and in accord with the lower prevalence of myopia in these groups (Garner *et al.*, 1990, 1995; Lam *et al.*, 1991; Lin *et al.*, 1996; Tokoro *et al.*, 1967). Among the Hong Kong Chinese groups shown in (B), the 19–34 year age group recorded the highest AL:CR ratio and was most myopic (−2.99 D); interestingly, the youngest and oldest groups had similar AL:CR ratios, although the younger group was more myopic (−1.59 D vs −0.28 D), indicating that the AL:CR ratio alone is not a predictor of myopia (Lam *et al.*, 1991a, 1994; Goh and Lam, 1994)

group of myopic Scandinavian children (Pärssinen and Lyyra, 1993) is surprisingly high when compared with that found in Chinese children (3.08) with a similar amount of myopia. That Chinese populations between 6 and 17 years and over 40 years of age have similar AL:CR ratios but significantly different mean refractive errors (Lam and Goh, 1991a; Lam *et al.*, 1994) represents a second example. This observation suggests that there is a fundamental difference in the shape of the Chinese eye when compared with the Caucasian eye, which may act as a predisposing factor in accord with Grosvenor's hypothesis, but need not be linked with myopic development. Since the older Chinese group did not demonstrate significant degrees of myopia, one might suggest that additional factors, presumably environmental, determined whether or not these eyes became myopic.

3.3.6   Congenital myopia–a separate entity?

Congenital myopia is myopia that is present at birth and persists throughout life; hence it might be argued that this myopia should be categorized separately. This myopia comprises approximately 2 per cent of all myopia (Grosvenor, 1987) and some cases can be linked to premature birth and/or low birth weight. For example, Fletcher and Brandon (1955) reported a 100 per cent prevalence of myopia in 462 premature infants, with the lowest birth weight infants generally showing the highest myopia (between 10 and 20 D in those weighing less than 1250 g). Similar findings for premature infants have been reported more recently by Dobson *et al.* (1981), Grose and Harding (1990) and Quinn *et al.* (1992). This myopia appears to be refractive in nature, since these eyes tend to be undersized with highly curved corneas (Fledelius, 1976; Inagaki, 1986; Baldwin, 1990), a reflection of their relative immaturity. If these eyes retained their steeper corneal profiles during development, then this would place them at greater risk of developing myopia later in life, according to Grosvenor's hypothesis that a high AL:CR ratio is a predisposing factor for myopia. It is unclear whether this is the case, since many of these eyes exhibit early emmetropization, as indicated by longitudinal studies showing a rapid decrease in myopia over the first 6–12 months of life (Scharf *et al.*, 1975, Dobson *et al.*, 1981; Grose and Harding, 1990; Ehrlich *et al.*, 1995). Indeed, only approximately 2 per cent of such cases retain their myopia, thereby meeting the definition of congenital myopia. The failure of these eyes to emmetropize may be due to the neonatal refractive error being too high, and/or the cornea being too steep. However, the picture is likely to be more complex since retinopathy of prematurity (ROP) has also been associated with high neonatal myopia and/or myopia which increases after birth (Shapiro *et al.*,

Table 3.2 Systemic disorders commonly associated with myopia

Condition	Typical amount of myopia
Marfan's syndrome*	Frequently high
Stickler syndrome	Moderate to high
Kneist syndrome	High
Pierre Robin syndrome	High
Noonan's syndrome	Unspecified
De Lange syndrome*	High
Homocystinuria*	Unspecified
Down's syndrome	Frequently high
Albinism	May be high

* Prevalence of myopia generally greater than 50%. From Curtin, 1985.

1980; Quinn *et al.*, 1992; Lue *et al.*, 1995). Even relatively mild cases of ROP may show such trends (Lue *et al.*, 1995). One might presume that in these cases, retinal function is sufficiently abnormal to preclude normal emmetropization.

3.3.7   Myopia as part of a syndrome

In addition to developmental and congenital myopia, there are uncommon cases in which myopia presents as one feature of a general body syndrome. Table 3.2 lists some of these conditions, which have been comprehensively reviewed by Curtin (1985). No consistent trends appear to exist within this group in relation to the type of myopia. For example, the high myopia commonly encountered in Marfan's syndrome may be due, in part, to abnormalities within the ciliary zonular system which leave the lens in a partly accommodated state (and sometimes also dislocated from its normal position, a condition known as ectopia lentis). On the other hand, progressive ocular enlargement appears to be an almost consistent feature of this syndrome (Allen *et al.*, 1967; Curtin, 1985). This may reflect the direct involvement of the sclera in the disease process, as both qualitative and quantitative defects in fibrillin, a glycoprotein associated with elastin, have been noted in this connective tissue disorder (Kumar *et al.*, 1992). It is also possible that, at least in some cases, anterior segment changes produce significant retinal image distortion, leading to form deprivation myopia.

3.4 Aberrations and excessive axial growth

It was speculated earlier that the more common, developmental form of myopia might represent an inappropriate emmetropization response, for example, to an accommodative focusing error. An alternative possibility, not necessarily incompatible with the first, is that myopic eyes have excessive optical aberrations which, by reducing retinal image quality, could impair accommodation or emmetropization. The available data, summarized in this section, are equivocal in relation to this hypothesis.

On-axis optical aberrations, both chromatic and monochromatic, are measurable in the human eye, and inter-subject variations in aberrations undoubtably occur. However, Wildsoet *et al.* (1993) found no significant difference in chromatic aberration between young myopes and emmetropes. On the other hand, in a related study of monochromatic aberrations (Collins *et al.*, 1995), myopes were found to have lower fourth order aberrations (this includes spherical aberration), and during accommodation their longitudinal spherical aberration became significantly negative compared with the low positive values seen in the emmetropic group. Further optical differences between myopic and emmetropic eyes were suggested by the more frequently encountered distortions in recorded aberroscope grid patterns in the myopic group that were so excessive as to preclude their analysis. Thirty-six per cent of myopes compared with only 7 per cent of emmetropic patterns fell into this category. It is tempting to speculate, based upon these data, that myopia may originate from increased aberrations, and furthermore, that the amount of myopia is causally related to the magnitude of these aberrations. The latter prediction is not borne out by the data although this does not rule out a causal link if a valid analogy can be made to the findings in chicks that the rate of compensation to imposed refractive errors is not directly related to the magnitude of imposed defocus (Wildsoet and Wallman, 1997).

If monochromatic aberrations do vary with refractive state, then the cornea would seem the most likely candidate since it is the most powerful refracting surface within the eye. It is therefore of particular interest that Carney *et al.* (1997) reported corneal shape variations in relation to the degree of myopia. Specifically, these workers reported a tendency of the cornea to flatten less rapidly in the periphery with increasing myopia; accordingly, Q values used to describe corneal asphericity became progressively less negative. These results contrast with a previous report of no significant differences in corneal shape between myopic, emmetropic and hyperopic refractive groups (Sheridan and Douthwaite, 1989), although variations in measurement technique may have contributed to these different results. Carney *et al.* also reported that although there was an overall trend toward flatter corneas in larger eyes (as previously described), their high myopia group had significantly steeper corneas than the emmetropic or low myopic groups. In light of previous speculation concerning a possible link between premature birth and steeper than normal corneas, one is tempted to suggest that at least some of the high myopes in this study might have been born prematurely. Furthermore, Pärssinen (1993) has described a temporal to nasal shift in the position of the corneal apex during myopia progression in children, with the likely implication that ocular aberrations also change during myopia development.

Astigmatism may also play a role in the development of myopia because of its potential to degrade the retinal image. It occurs as a peripheral aberration in all eyes, and may also be a component of the on-axis refractive errors in some eyes. Fulton *et al.* (1982) reported an association between on-axis astigmatism and myopia in children. Here, astigmatic eyes ($\geq$1 DC) exhibited both greater degrees of myopia and more myopic progression than non-astigmatic eyes. In addition, eyes with oblique astigmatism had significantly higher amounts of myopia (almost double) than eyes with non-oblique astigmatism. In an earlier study, Hirsch (1963) concluded that against-the-rule astigmatism was a risk factor for myopia on the basis of a predominance of this type of astigmatism among myopes. Similarly, young monkeys with against-the-rule astigmatism were less hyperopic than those exhibiting with-the-rule astigmatism (Huang *et al.*, 1996). Nonetheless, myopia *per se* was not seen. In contrast, Grosvenor *et al.* (1987) reported greater progression rates in myopic children having with-the-rule astigmatism when compared with those with either against-the-rule astigmatism or no astigmatism. Thus no definite conclusions can be drawn from these data.

Are there any other data providing different perspectives concerning on-axis astigmatism that could imply a role in the development of myopia?

The possibility that racial differences in susceptibility to myopia might reflect variations in astigmatism is not borne out by available data. For example, the more susceptible Chinese eyes do not have higher astigmatism. More specifically, similar patterns of astigmatism, i.e. mainly with-the-rule astigmatism of relatively low magnitude, have been reported in both Chinese (Lam and Goh, 1991b) and Caucasian (Hirsch, 1963) children. Finally, although an apparent association between astigmatism and myopia is evident in data for very young children (up to 38.5 months of age; Ehrlich *et al.*, 1995), a number of other human studies have reported developmental decreases in astigmatism (Atkinson and French, 1980; Gwiazda *et al.*, 1984; Howland and Sayle, 1984; Abrahamsson *et al.*, 1988). This raises the alternative possibility that rather than being a cause of myopia, astigmatism might serve as a cue to emmetropization (Wallman, 1993).

The notion that deprivation of the peripheral retina in humans may result in myopia was discussed earlier with regard to the hypothesis put forward by Wallman *et al.* (1987) for the apparent link between excessive reading and myopia. In a similar context, off-axis aberrations are also of potential interest because of their impact on image quality at more peripheral retinal locations. The earliest study of peripheral astigmatism was by Ferree *et al.* (1931), which has been followed by a number of subsequent investigations, for example by Rempt *et al.* (1971) and Millodot (1981). The general consensus is that the type of peripheral astigmatism varies with the on-axis refractive error. Thus myopes most commonly show compound myopic astigmatism (both meridians are myopic), whereas emmetropes demonstrate mixed astigmatism (one meridian is myopic and the other hyperopic) and hyperopes exhibit compound hyperopic astigmatism (both meridians are hyperopic). Furthermore, Millodot (1981) indicated that the relative amount of astigmatism did not vary between the refractive groups. Charman and Jennings (1982) also noted that the refractive errors of these three refractive groups tended to converge at large peripheral angles, corresponding to the retinal equator. These data are consistent with the model for retinal shape proposed by Dunne *et al.* (1987) which represented its surface by an ellipsoid of constant equatorial radius, and assumed an axial bias to ocular growth. Peripheral astigmatism measurements in anisomyopes (i.e., subjects with different amounts of myopia in their two eyes) are also consistent with this model (Logan *et al.*, 1995;

Logan and Gilmartin, 1996). Taken together, these various observations suggest that differences in peripheral astigmatism are more likely to be a product of myopic growth than its cause.

3.5   What drives elongation of the myopic eye?

Are myopic eyes longer because normal ocular growth is accelerated or prolonged in the case of myopia, or does myopia represent an abnormality of normal growth processes? As noted previously, it is a widely held belief that normal ocular growth is completed towards the end of puberty (e.g. Weymouth and Hirsch, 1950; Sorsby *et al.*, 1961; Sorsby and Leary, 1970; Larsen, 1971d; Goss *et al.*, 1990). Does the post-puberty development or progression of myopia imply abnormal growth? Additionally, is scleral stretching (possibly because of scleral weakness) important in myopia (e.g. Van Alphen, 1961; Curtin, 1985)? This section reviews ocular structural changes in myopia, and also discusses scleral biochemical and biomechanical data as well as IOP findings which provide some insight into the mechanisms underlying ocular elongation in myopia.

3.5.1   Scleral changes in myopia and implications for underlying growth mechanisms

If myopic eyes expand, then the sclera must either accommodate to, or produce this expansion. Some progress towards an understanding of the processes involved has been made through studies of the scleral changes found in experimentally induced myopia in animals. The more limited data covering human myopia is reviewed against this background.

As the eye enlarges, the sclera must expand its surface area. Either new tissue must be added or existing tissue remodelled. Although the chick sclera has been extensively studied in this context, the human sclera is comprised of fibrous connective tissue while only the outer layer of the chick sclera is fibrous. However, like human sclera, the tree shrew sclera is fibrous in nature, and as it has been more widely studied than human sclera, it is the main focus of the following discussion. A variety of biochemical assays, including measurement of hydroxyproline levels, which reflect collagen content, and sulphated glycosoaminoglycans (GAGs), which provide an index of extracellular matrix proteoglycans (labelling studies measure their level of glycosylation), have been used.

Results of biochemical and histological studies are generally consistent with active remodelling of the sclera during myopic growth. For example, Norton and Rada (1995) observed no change in DNA levels but decreased sulphated GAGs and hydroxyproline levels in deprived myopic eyes when compared with control (untreated) eyes. The latter changes were restricted to the posterior pole, which was also thinner than normal (Kang and Norton, 1993; Phillips and McBrien, 1995). An interesting aside here is that the outer fibrous layer of chick sclera, which is most like mammalian sclera, also shows both thinning (Gottlieb *et al.*, 1990) and decreased GAG synthesis (Marzani and Wallman, 1997). Indirect evidence for scleral remodelling in the tree shrew comes from the observation of no significant difference between the wet weights of the scleras from control and deprived myopic eyes (Kang and Norton, 1993; Phillips and McBrien, 1995), while the dry weights show a decrease with form deprivation (Reeder and McBrien, 1993). Accordingly, these data tend to rule out active tissue addition. While the extent to which sclera remodelling contributes to normal ocular growth is not specifically addressed by these studies, it is clear that myopic growth is different from normal ocular growth (at least where normal and myopic eyes of the same animal are compared), and this difference involves scleral remodelling. The latter conclusion is also reinforced by three further observations. Firstly, treatments which block collagen cross-linking increase the response to form deprivation but have no effect on normal ocular development (McBrien and Norton, 1994). Secondly, collagen fibril diameters are reduced in the scleras of myopic eyes (Cornell and McBrien, 1994). Thirdly, activity of some gelatinase members of the matrix metalloproteinase family of enzymes, is increased in myopic eyes (Rada and Brenza, 1995; Guggenheim and McBrien, 1996).

Greater scleral creep (or extensibility) could conceivably underlie the development of myopia, and is also a potential outcome of increased scleral remodelling. Data reported by Siegwart and Norton (1994) for the tree shrew support this hypothesis. However, Phillips and McBrien (1995), in noting similar extensibility differences between myopic and normal scleras showed that they could be entirely explained by the differences in scleral thickness (myopic scleras being thinner). Similar observations of scleral thinning (Raviola and Wiesel, 1985) and decreased collagen fibre size have been reported following the induction of experimental myopia in monkeys (Funata and Tokoro, 1990).

In humans, similar differences between myopic and emmetropic scleras have been noted to those outlined for the tree shrew, suggesting that similar mechanisms are involved. However, studies of human sclera have been mainly limited to highly myopic, and often older eyes. Nonetheless, scleral thinning has been noted, not only in highly myopic eyes (Curtin, 1958; Curtin *et al.* 1979) but in association with low to moderate amounts of myopia (Avetisov *et al.*, 1984; Cheng *et al.*, 1992). This scleral thinning appears to be more exaggerated at the posterior pole. The scleras of highly myopic eyes also exhibit altered collagen architecture (fibrils with altered striations and star-shaped configurations) and collagen fibres are generally smaller than normal overall, resulting in a loss of the usual size gradient evident in normal scleras (Garzino, 1956; Curtin *et al.*, 1979; Liu *et al.*, 1986; Sellheyer and Spitznas, 1988). Curtin *et al.* (1979) also noted that these scleras had an abnormal amount of interfibrillary substance which led them to speculate that there might be an underlying derangement in the chemical composition of the proteoglycan component of this interfibrillary substance. Avetisov *et al.* (1984) reported decreased total collagen (oxyproline levels) and glycoaminoglycan-containing proteoglycans (hexosamine levels), even with moderate myopia. On the other hand, there was a relative increase in the levels of the soluble collagen fractions. The latter trend is more characteristic of younger eyes, and might indicate a slowing of the normal maturation processes, although conceivably, increased scleral remodelling might result in a similar outcome.

As in tree shrew sclera, human myopic sclera was mechanically weaker. Specifically, Avetisov *et al.* (1984) observed that tensile strength was decreased in myopic eyes, with the change being greatest at the posterior pole, where the sclera is thinnest. A parallel may also be drawn with the *in vivo* finding of reduced scleral rigidity, as measured by tonometry in myopic teenagers (Castrén and Pohjola, 1961a, 1961b), although Perkins (1981a) suggested that the latter trend could be an artifact of the larger volumes of myopic eyes. Avetisov *et al.* (1984) also noted that some young, apparently normal (non-myopic) human eyes shared some of the characteristics of the myopic eyes studied, including a decrease in mechanical strength. In an explanation of these results, the authors raised the possibility of an inborn structural deficiency, which could also represent a risk factor for myopia. However, a similar result might be expected if these eyes were previously normal and had only recently adopted a myopic mode of growth, and therefore had not yet changed their refractive state. The data do not allow these two alternatives to be distinguished.

Do the scleral differences between myopic and normal eyes represent causative processes unique to myopic growth, or are they simply a consequence of the greater rate of growth in myopic eyes? In animal studies, it is usual to compare myopic and normal eyes from the same animal, and therefore some of the observed differences may be an artifact of the difference in eye size. For example, the myopic eyes may be equivalent to more mature normal eyes of similar size. On the other hand, some of the human data reported by Avetisov *et al.* (1984) suggest that myopic eyes may either maintain, or revert back to, a more juvenile mode of growth. It is also likely that similar growth signals might have various outcomes at different times during development, because levels of circulating hormones change dramatically over this course (Curtin *et al.*, 1979; Balacco-Gabrieli, 1983). However, whatever the mechanism, in humans at least, the predilection of the posterior sclera to expand most in high myopia may reflect inherent differences between the posterior pole and the rest of the sclera, even in normal eyes.

The relative immaturity of the posterior portion of the eye, which matures anteroposteriorly (Sellheyer and Spitznas, 1988), may underlie some of the observed spatial differences which include relatively more collagen (including soluble collagen; Avetisov *et al.*, 1984), chondroitin sulphate and uronic acid at the posterior region of the eye (Trier *et al.*, 1990). From a biomechanical perspective, the delayed maturation of the posterior sclera also renders it weaker than the more anterior scleral regions (Avetisov *et al.*, 1984). If the maturation process is delayed even more in myopic eyes, then this might account for the apparent reversion to a more juvenile mode of growth described by Avetisov *et al.* (1984) for myopic eyes. Also, if sufficiently delayed, a predicted outcome would be an overall axial bias to eye growth, as has been described in highly myopic eyes. As a final aside to these growth issues, a possible explanation for corneal steepening being a potential feature of myopia development (Kent, 1963; Goss and Erickson, 1987; Grosvenor and Scott, 1991) might be that the cornea can come under the influence of the same factors that trigger the remodelling processes in the sclera.

3.5.2   IOP, glaucoma and myopia

Whatever the role of the biochemical and biomechanical properties of the sclera in the ocular expansion of myopia, it is also necessary to consider the role of intraocular pressure (IOP). From a mechanical perspective, the eye can be viewed as a balloon, with IOP providing an inflationary force that effects changes in eye size. The capacity of the sclera to resist IOP (acting tangentially at the sclera) is largely dependent upon its inherent compliance (stretchability), although the forces experienced by the sclera also increase with eye size (Friedman, 1966). For an eye to enlarge more than normal, as in myopia, one could envisage either scleral compliance being normal and IOP being raised, or alternatively, scleral compliance being abnormal and IOP being normal. In accord with the latter alternative, there is at least some evidence that myopic scleras are more compliant (possibly due to remodelling), as discussed in the previous section. However, there are also indications that myopic eyes have higher IOP. Of course, these two alternatives need not be mutually exclusive, and indeed, IOP may modulate scleral remodelling, and thus indirectly, its compliance (Nickla *et al.*, 1998). An overview of the relevant literature is provided here; a comprehensive review of the issues involved is available in Pruett (1988).

The ability of excessively high IOP in humans to produce ocular expansion ultimately leading to buphthalmos is well demonstrated in cases of congenital glaucoma (Donaldson, 1966; Toulemont *et al.*, 1995). However, there is no clear answer as to whether increased IOP plays a role in the ocular enlargement of myopia. In children, higher levels of IOP have been recorded in myopic compared with non-myopic groups (Abdalla and Hamdi, 1970; Ziobrowski and Zygulska-Mach, 1981; Edwards and Brown, 1993; Quinn *et al.*, 1995), and associations between IOP and both myopia progression rate (Pärssinen, 1990; Jensen, 1992) and refractive error (Pärssinen, 1990) have been made. Similar associations have been described for adult populations (Tomlinson and Phillips, 1970; David *et al.*, 1985; Tovena *et al.*, 1989), and strong associations also exist between myopia and both ocular hypertension (Perkins and Phelps, 1982; Seddon *et al.*, 1983) and glaucoma (Goldwyn *et al.*, 1970; Daubs and Crick, 1981; Perkins and Phelps, 1982; Lotufo *et al.*, 1989). In addition to the clinical ramifications for glaucoma screening protocols, these results suggest that increased IOP may play a fundamental role in myopic growth. However, other interpretations of these data may be valid. For example, myopia and glaucoma may represent different expressions of the same connective tissue disorder involving the sclera and trabecular meshwork, respectively (Curtin *et al.*, 1979; Fong *et al.*, 1990). Furthermore, the higher IOP in myopic eyes may be a consequence of, rather than the cause of myopia. This would be consistent with a longitudinal study of refractive error development in children, which recorded increased IOP only after the appearance of myopia (Edwards and Brown, 1996). Finally, other studies have failed to observe a relationship between IOP and refractive error/axial length (e.g. Daubs and Crick, 1981; Bonomi *et al.*, 1982). Thus the case for a role of IOP in myopia development remains equivocal.

The force of IOP is not exerted directly on the sclera because of the intervening retinal and choroidal layers. Van Alphen (1961, 1986) has speculated that the choroid may play an important role in ocular growth by modulating the influence of IOP on the sclera (*see* Chapter 6). In chicks, choroidal thickening and thinning are associated with decreased and increased ocular growth, respectively (Wildsoet and Wallman, 1995). This result is consistent with thinner choroids having reduced pressure-buffering capacity. It is of interest that choroidal thinning is a frequently reported feature of highly myopic human eyes (Curtin, 1985), and similar trends have also been observed using high resolution magnetic resonance imaging at the posterior pole of eyes having moderate amounts of myopia (mean = 6.5 D; Cheng *et al.*, 1992). Thus, myopic eyes in both human and chick have thinner choroids. However, whether a causal relation exists between choroidal thinning and increased ocular enlargement (rather than a consequential one) remains to be established.

3.5.3 Retinal and choroidal changes during myopia development: clinically relevant signs

Reference has been made to data indicating that myopic eyes have thinner scleras, but of potentially greater clinical interest is how the retina and choroid are affected in myopia. One might expect stretching and thinning of both tissues, because of their limited capacities to grow (i.e., add tissue), and thus to compensate for the surface area expansion that accompanies ocular enlargement. This prediction appears to be borne out, at least for high myopia, where clinical signs of stretch are described for both the retina and choroid.

In the case of the choroid, clinical signs of stretch include increased fundus tessellation (a stippled or striated appearance) and optic nerve crescents (conus). The former is consistent with the choroid becoming increasingly thin as the eye enlarges, while the latter would occur if, instead of stretching, the choroid became unanchored from its attachment site at the margin of the optic nerve head. The prevalence of optic nerve crescents is strongly correlated with axial length and/or refractive error (Curtin and Karlin, 1971; Shih *et al.*, 1989, 1996; Fulk *et al.*, 1992), and the level of fundus tessellation is similarly well correlated with axial length (Otsuka, 1967; Shih *et al.*, 1989). As noted previously, choroidal thinning has been measured directly with MRI imaging. In moderately myopic eyes there was a decrease of approximately 50 per cent in the thickness of the choroid at the posterior pole, with respect to emmetropic eyes (Cheng *et al.*, 1992). Because these thickness changes are more pronounced posteriorly, for both the choroid and sclera, this would imply a close association between these two tissues. This coupling could be mediated by blood vessels traversing the sclera en route to the choroid. These vessels, by acting as anchorage points, could thus ensure that the choroid expands its surface area in parallel with local scleral changes. Furthermore, co-culture experiments involving both choroidal and scleral tissue from chicks raise the possibility of biochemical interactions between these two tissues (Marzani and Wallman, 1997). Finally, ocular pulse, another measure of choroidal function, has been found to be lower than normal in myopic eyes (Perkins, 1981b; To'mey *et al.*, 1981; Shih *et al.*, 1991). This difference is likely to reflect, at least in part, the larger volume of myopic eyes, but has also been interpreted as evidence of altered ocular circulation (To'mey *et al.*, 1981; Shih *et al.*, 1991).

The retina has almost its full complement of cells at birth, and must become thinner during normal development in order to maintain coverage of the scleral shell. Myopic eyes, being larger than normal, show evidence of increased retinal stretch and thinning. Visual function tests are one source of evidence of retinal stretch, although in the absence of overt pathology, these changes are subtle. For example, impaired blue colour discrimination and dark adaptation (Mäntyjärvi and Tuppurainen, 1995) have been observed in myopes. However, Comerford *et al.* (1987) found no significant difference between high myopes (mean = −7.3 D) who were free from degenerative changes, and an age-matched control group, in either static or dynamic spatial contrast sensitivity, or temporal modulation sensitivity, whether measured at photopic, mesopic or scotopic levels. The spatial contrast sensitivity result has also been corroborated by Collins and Carney (1990). These results imply that as the retina expands its surface area and retinal neurones become increasingly separated, they are able to maintain coverage of the changing surface. This has been demonstrated directly in the chick, specifically for retinal amacrine and ganglion cells that rearrange their dendritic trees to this end (Teakle *et al.*, 1993; Troilo *et al.*, 1996). The presumed increase in receptive field sizes that would result from this expansion is also consistent with speculations of Winn and others (Bradley *et al.*, 1983; Winn *et al.*, 1988) to explain an apparent mismatch between calculated retinal image size and perceived image size for human anisometropes.

Apart from the psychophysical data described above, there is also clinical evidence of retinal stretch. For example, increased retinal stretching is indicated by the straighter course of retinal blood vessels in myopic eyes (Bradley *et al.*, 1983) and there is evidence, at least in the chick, that retinal pigment epithelial cells also undergo stretching (Lin *et al.*, 1993). There are also a variety of retinal pathologies which may be interpreted as evidence of retinal thinning, for example, lattice, pavingstone and pigmentary degeneration, and white with/without pressure, although some of these conditions may represent secondary sequelae to pathological changes in the choroid or pigment epithelium. These lesions predominantly affect the already thin retinal periphery and their presence is well correlated with axial length (Pierro *et al.*, 1992). Other common findings include retinal tears, holes or detachments, lacquer cracks and Fuch's spot, a central lesion. These various pathologies are well described by Curtin (1985), who links these changes with abnormal ocular elongation (leading to posterior staphylomata). These cases are specifically categorized as pathological myopia by Curtin, although it is not clear where the dividing line between normal and abnormal elongation should be drawn. A tentative range of 25.5–26.5 mm (approximately equivalent to between 5 and 7.5 D of myopia) has been proposed (Curtin, 1985; Grossniklaus and Green, 1992).

3.6   Conclusion

This overview of the literature leaves little doubt that human myopia, as most commonly encountered, is a consequence of having an eye whose axial length is too long for its refractive power, with potentially serious implications. Indeed, pathological myopia represents the seventh leading cause of blindness in the United States (Hotchkiss and Fine, 1981). Importantly, animal models of myopia show the same axial overgrowth. Although the underlying growth mechanisms, and precise stimuli for myopia development in humans are not yet fully understood, it is likely that these mysteries will ultimately be solved by the combined efforts of experimental and clinical researchers. Further investigation of the apparent association between nearwork and the development of myopia is but one avenue for researchers to follow. Finally, it is in the interest of the myopic patient that appropriate distillation of the new knowledge and ideas that come from such research occurs, and it is to be hoped that this present review contributes to that goal.

Acknowledgements

I wish to thank Professor Josh Wallman and Dr Debora Nickla for their invaluable input into this chapter, and also Dr David Troilo and Professor Richard Held, who provided additional feedback.

References

Abdalla, M. I. and Hamdi, M. (1970) Applanation ocular tension in myopia and emmetropia. *Br. J. Ophthalmol.* **54**, 122–125.

Abrahamsson, M., Fabian, G. and Sjöstrand, J. (1988) Changes in astigmatism between the ages of 1 and 4 years: a longitudinal study. *Br. J. Ophthalmol.* **72**, 145–149.

Adams, A. (1987) Axial length elongation, not corneal curvature, as a basis of adult onset myopia. *Am. J. Optom. Physiol. Opt.* **64**, 150–152.

Allen, R. A., Straatsma, B. R., Apt, L. and Hall, M. O. (1967) Ocular manifestations of the Marfan Syndrome. *Trans. Am. Acad. Ophthalmol. Otolaryngol.* **71**, 18–38.

Atkinson, J., Braddick, O. and French, J. (1980) Infant astigmatism: its disappearance with age. *Vision Res.* **20**, 891–893.

Avetisov, E. S., Savitskaya, N. F., Vinetskaya, M. I. and Iomdina, E. N. (1984) A study of biochemical and biomechanical qualities of normal and myopic eye sclera in humans of different age groups. *Metab. Pediatr. Syst. Ophthalmol.* **7**, 183–188.

Balacco-Gabrieli, C. (1983) The etiopathogenesis of degenerative myopia. *Ann. Ophthalmol.* **15**, 312–314.

Baldwin, W. R. (1990) Refractive status of infants and children. In: *Principles and Practice of Pediatric Optometry* (A. A. Rosenbloom and M. W. Morgan, eds). Lippincott.

Bartmann, M., Schaeffel, F., Hagel, G. and Zrenner, E. (1994) Constant light affects retinal dopamine levels and blocks deprivation myopia but not lens-induced refractive errors in chickens. *Vis. Neurosci.* **11**, 199–208.

Bear, J. C. (1991) Epidemiology and genetics of refractive anomalies. In: *Refractive Anomalies: Research and Clinical Applications* (T. A. Grosvenor and M. C. Flom, eds). Butterworth–Heinemann, pp. 57–80.

Bonomi, L., Mecca, E. and Massa, F. (1982) Intraocular pressure in myopic anisometropia. *Int. Ophthalmol.* **5**, 145–148.

Borish, I. M. (1970) Clinical Refraction, vol. 1, 3rd edn. Professional Press, pp. 89–90.

Bradley, A., Rabin, J. and Freeman, R. D. (1983) Non-optical determinants of aniseikonia. *Invest. Ophthalmol. Vis. Sci.* **24**, 507–512.

Bullimore, M. A., Gilmartin, B. and Royston, J. M. (1992) Steady-state accommodation and ocular biometry in late-onset myopia. *Doc. Ophthalmol.* **80**, 143–155.

Carney, L. G., Mainstone, J. C. and Henderson, B. A. (1997) Corneal topography and myopia. *Invest. Ophthalmol. Vis. Sci.* **38**, 311–320.

Carroll, J. P. (1981) Regression curves for the optical parameters of the eye. *Am. J. Optom. Physiol. Opt.* **58**, 314–323.

Carroll, J. P. (1982) Component and correlation ametropia. *Am. J. Optom. Physiol. Opt.* **59**, 28–33.

Castrén, J. A. and Pohjola, S. (1961a) Refraction and scleral rigidity. *Acta Ophthalmol.* **39**, 1011–1014.

Castrén, J. A. and Pohjola, S. (1961b) Scleral rigidity at puberty. *Acta Ophthalmol.* **39**, 1015–1019.

Charman, W. N. and Jennings, J. A. M. (1982) Ametropia and peripheral refraction. *Am. J. Optom. Physiol. Opt.* **59**, 922–923.

Cheng, H. -M., Omah S. S and Kwong, K. K. (1992) Shape of the myopic eye as seen with high-resolution magnetic resonance imaging. *Optom. Vis. Sci.* **69**, 698–701.

Collins, J. W. and Carney, L. G. (1990) Visual performance in high myopia. *Curr. Eye Res.* **9**, 217–223.

Collins, M. J., Wildsoet, C. F. and Atchison, D. A. (1995) Monochromatic aberrations and myopia. *Vision Res.* **35**, 1157–1163.

Comerford, J. P., Thorn, F. and Corwin, T. R. (1987) Effect of luminance level on contrast sensitivity in myopia. *Am. J. Optom. Physiol. Opt.* **64**, 810–814.

Cornell, L. M. and McBrien, N. A. (1994) Alterations in collagen fibril diameter in the sclera of experimentally myopic tree shrew eyes. *Invest. Ophthalmol. Vis. Sci.* **35** (ARVO Suppl.), 2068.

Curtin, B. J. (1958) Scleral changes in pathological myopia. *Trans. Am. Acad. Ophthalmol. Otolaryngol.* **62**, 777–790.

Curtin, B. J. (1985) *The Myopias: Basic Science and Clinical Management.* Harper & Row.

Curtin, B. J. and Karlin, D. B. (1971) Axial length measurements and fundus changes of the myopic eye. *Am. J. Ophthalmol.* **71**, 42–53.

Curtin, B. J., Iwamoto, T. and Renaldo, D. P. (1979) Normal and staphylomatous sclera of high myopia. *Arch. Ophthalmol.* **97**, 912–921.

Daubs, J. G. and Crick, R. P. (1981) Effect of refractive error on the risk of ocular hypertension and open angle glaucoma. *Trans. Ophthalmol. Soc. UK* **101**, 121–126.

David, R., Zangwill, L. M., Tessler, Z. and Yassur, Y. (1985) The correlation between intraocular pressure and refractive status. *Arch. Ophthalmol.* **103**, 1812–1815.

Dobson, V., Fulton, A., Manning, K., Salem, D. and Peterson, R. (1981) Cycloplegic refractions of premature infants. *Am. J. Ophthalmol.* **91**, 490–495.

Donaldson, D. D (1966). *Atlas of External Diseases of the Eye*, vol. 1. *Congenital Anomalies and Systemic Diseases.* C. V. Mosby, pp. 44–46.

Duke-Elder, S. and Abrams, D. (1970) *System of Ophthalmology*, vol V: *Ophthalmic Optics and Refraction* (S. Duke-Elder, ed.). C. V. Mosby, pp. 207–362.

Dunne, M. C. M., Barnes, D. A. and Clement, R. A. (1987) A model for retinal shape changes in ametropia. *Ophthal. Physiol. Opt.* **7**, 159–160.

Edwards, M. H. and Brown, B. (1993) Intraocular pressure in a selected sample of myopic and non-myopic Chinese children. *Optom. Vis. Sci.* **70**, 15–17.

Edwards, M. H. and Brown, B. (1996) IOP in myopic children: the relationship between increases in IOP and the development of myopia. *Ophthal. Physiol. Opt.* **16**, 243–246.

Ehrlich, D. L., Atkinson, J., Braddick, O., Bobier, W. and Durden, K. (1995) Reduction of infant myopia: A longitudinal cycloplegic study. *Vision Res.* **35**, 1313–1324.

Ferree, C. E., Rand, G. and Hardy, C. (1931) Refraction for the peripheral field of vision. *Arch. Ophthalmol.* **5**, 717–731.

Fledelius, H. C. (1976) Prematurity and the eye. *Acta Ophthalmol.* Suppl. 128, 1–245.

Fledelius, H. C. (1988) Corneal curvature radius – oculometric considerations with reference to age and refractive change. *Acta Ophthalmol.* Suppl. 185, 74–77.

Fledelius, H. C. (1995) Adult onset myopia-oculometric features. *Acta Ophthalmol* **73**, 397–401.

Fletcher, M. C. and Brandon, S. (1955) Myopia of prematurity. *Am. J. Ophthalmol.* **40**, 474–481.

Fong, D. S., Epstein, D. L. and Allingham, R. R. (1990) Glaucoma and myopia: are they related? *Int. Ophthalmol. Clin.* **30**, 215–218.

Friedman, B. (1966) Stress upon the ocular coats: effects of scleral curvature, scleral thickness, and intra-ocular pressure. *Eye Ear Nose Throat Monthly*, **45**, 59–65.

Fulk, G. W., Goss, D. A., Christensen, M. T., Cline, K. B. and Herrin-Lawson, G. A. (1992) Optic nerve crescents and refractive error. *Optom. Vis. Sci.* **69**, 208–213.

Fulton, A. B., Hansen, R. M. and Petersen, R. A. (1982) The relation of myopia and astigmatism in developing eyes. *Ophthalmology* **89**, 298–302.

Funata, M. and Tokoro, T. (1990) Scleral change in experimentally myopic monkeys. *Graefe's Arch. Clin. Exp. Ophthalmol* **228**, 174–179.

Garner, L. F., Meng., C. K., Grosvenor, T. P. and Mohidin, N. (1990) Ocular dimension and refractive power in Malay and Melanesian children. *Ophthal. Physiol. Opt.* **10**, 234–238.

Garner, L. F., Yap, M. K. and Scott, R. (1992) Crystalline lens power in myopia. *Optom. Vis. Sci.* **69**, 863–865.

Garner, L. F., Yap, M. K. H., Kinnear, R. F. and Frith, M. J. (1995) Ocular dimensions and refraction in Tibetan children. *Optom. Vis. Sci.* **72**, 266–271.

Garzino, D. A. (1956) Modificazioni del collagene sclerale nella miopia maligna. *Rassegna Italiana D'Ottalmologia* **25**, 241–244.

Goh, W. S. and Lam, C. S. (1994) Changes in refractive trends and optical components in Hong Kong Chinese aged 19–39 years. *Ophthal. Physiol. Opt.* **14**, 378–382.

Goldwyn, R., Waltman, S. R. and Becker, B. (1970) Primary open-angle glaucoma in adolescents and young adults. *Arch. Ophthalmol.* **84**, 579–582.

Goss, D. A. (1994) Effect of spectacle correction on the progression of myopia in children–a literature review. *J. Am. Optom. Assoc.* **65**, 117–128.

Goss, D. A. and Erickson, P. (1987) Meridional corneal components of myopia progression in young adults and children. *Am. J. Optom. Physiol. Opt.* **64**, 475–481.

Goss, D. A. and Jackson, T. W. (1995) Clinical findings before the onset of myopia in youth. I. Ocular optical components. *Optom. Vis. Sci.* **72**, 870–878.

Goss, D. A. and Uyesugi, E. F. (1995) Effectiveness of bifocal control of childhood myopia progression as a function of near point phoria and binocular cross-cylinder. *J. Optom. Vis. Develop.* **26**, 12–17.

Goss, D. A. and Winkler, R. L. (1983) Progression of myopia in youth: age of cessation. *Am J. Optom. Physiol. Opt.* **60**, 651–658.

Goss, D. A., Cox, V. D., Herrin-Lawson, G. A., Nielson, E. D. and Dolton, W. A. (1990) Refractive error, axial length, height as a function of age in young myopes. *Optom. Vis. Sci.* **67**, 332–338.

Gottlieb, M. D., Joshi, H. B. and Nickla, D. L. (1990) Scleral changes in chicks with form-deprivation myopia. *Curr. Eye Res.* **9**, 1157–1165.

Greene, P. R. and Guyton, D. L. (1986) Time course of rhesus lid–suture myopia. *Exp. Eye Res.* **42**, 529–534.

Grose, J. and Harding, G. (1990) The development of refractive error and pattern visually evoked potentials in preterm infants. *Clin. Vis. Sci.* **5**, 375–382.

Grossniklaus, H. E. and Green, W. R. (1992) Pathologic findings in pathologic myopia. *Retina* **12**, 127–133.

Grosvenor, T. (1987) A review and a suggested classification system for myopia on the basis of age-related prevalence and age of onset. *Am. J. Optom. Physiol.* **64**, 545–554.

Grosvenor, T. (1988) High axial length/corneal radius as a risk factor in the development of myopia. *Am. J. Optom. Physiol. Opt.* **65**, 689–696.

Grosvenor, T. and Scott, R. (1991) Comparison of refractive components in youth-onset and early adult-onset myopia. *Optom. Vis. Sci.* **68**, 204–209.

Grosvenor, T. and Scott, R. (1993) Three-year changes in refraction and its components in youth-onset and early adult-onset myopia. *Optom. Vis. Sci.* **70**, 677–683.

Grosvenor, T. and Scott, R. (1994) Role of the axial length/corneal radius ration in determining the refractive state of the eye. *Optom. Vis. Sci.* **71**, 573–579.

Grosvenor, T., Perrigin, D. M., Perrigin, J. and Maslovitz, B. (1987) Houston Myopia Control Study; a randomized clinical trial. Part II. Final report by the patient care team. *Am. J. Optom. Physiol. Opt.* **64**, 482–498.

Guggenheim, J. A. and McBrien, N. A. (1996) Form-deprivation myopia induces activation of scleral matrix metalloproteinase–2 in tree shrew. *Invest. Ophthalmol. Vis. Sci.* **37**, 1380–1395.

Gunn, T. R., Easdown, J., Outerbridge, E. W. and Aranda, J. V. (1980) Risk factors in retrolental fibroplasia. *Pediatrics* **65**, 1096–1100.

Gwiazda, J., Bauer, J., Thorn, F. and Held, R. (1995) A dynamic relationship between myopia and blur-driven accommodation in school-aged children. *Vis. Res.* **35**, 1299–1304.

Gwiazda, J., Scheiman, M., Mohindra, I. and Held, R. (1984) Astigmatism in children: changes in axis and amount from birth to six years. *Invest. Ophthalmol. Vis. Sci.* **25**, 88–92.

Gwiazda, J., Thorn, F., Bauer, J. and Held, R. (1993) Myopic children show insufficient accommodative response to blur. *Invest. Ophthalmol. Vis. Sci.* **34**, 690–694.

Hirsch, M. J. (1950) An analysis of inhomogeneity of myopia in adults. *Am. J. Optom. Arch. Am. Acad. Optom.* **27**, 562–571.

Hirsch, M. J. (1958) Changes in refractive state after the age of forty-five. *Am. J. Optom. Arch. Am. Acad. Optom.* **35**, 229–237.

Hirsch, M. J. (1963) Changes in astigmatism during first eight years of school–an interim report from the Ojai Longitudinal Study. *Am. J. Optom. Arch. Am. Acad. Optom.* **40**, 127–132.

Hirsch, M. J. and Weymouth, F. W. (1947) Notes on ametropia–a further analysis of Stenström's data. *Am. J. Optom. Arch. Am. Acad. Optom.* **24**, 601–608.

Hirsch, M. J. and Weymouth, F. W. (1991) Changes in optical elements: hypothesis for the genesis of refractive anomalies. In: *Refractive Anomalies: Research and Clinical Applications* (T. Grosvenor and M. C. Flom, eds). Butterworth–Heinemann, pp. 39–56.

Hodos, W. and Kuenzel, W. J. (1984) Retinal-image degradation produces ocular enlargement in chicks. *Invest. Ophthalmol. Vis. Sci.* **25**, 652–659.

Hofstetter, H. W. (1967) Emmetropization–biological process or mathematical artifact? *Am. J. Optom. Arch. Am. Acad. Optom.* **46**, 447–450.

Holland, P. M. and Anderson, B. (1976) Myelinated nerve fibers and severe myopia. *Am. J. Ophthalmol.* **81**, 597–599.

Hosaka, A. (1988) The growth of the eye and its components. *Acta Ophthalmol.* Suppl. 185, 65–68.

Hotchkiss, M. L. and Fine, S. L. (1981) Pathologic myopia and choroidal neovascularization. *Am. J. Ophthalmol.* **91**, 177–183.

Howland, H. C. and Sayle, N. (1984) Photorefractive measurements of astigmatism in infants and young children. *Invest. Ophthalmol. Vis. Sci.* **25**, 93–102.

Hoyt, C., Stone, R. D. and Fromer, C. (1981) Monocular axial myopia associated with neonatal eyelid closure in human infants. *Am. J. Ophthalmol.* **91**, 197–200.

Huang, J., Hung, L.-F. and Smith III, E. L. (1996) Effects of optically induced astigmatism on refractive development of infant monkeys. *Invest. Ophthalmol. Vis. Sci.* **37** (ARVO Suppl.), S1000.

Hung, L.-F., Crawford, M. L. J. and Smith III, E. L. (1995) Spectacles lenses alter eye growth and refractive status of young monkeys. *Nature Medicine* **1**, 761–765.

Inagaki, Y. (1986) The rapid change of corneal curvature in the neonatal period and infancy. *Arch. Ophthalmol.* **104**, 1026–1027.

Irving, E. L., Sivak, J. G. and Callender, M. G. (1992) Refractive plasticity of the developing chick eye. *Ophthal. Physiol. Opt.* **12**, 448–456.

Jensen, H. (1991) Myopia progression in young school children. A prospective study of myopia progression and the effect of trial with bifocal lenses and beta blocker eye drops. *Acta Ophthalmol.* Suppl. 200, 3–79.

Jensen, H. (1992) Myopia progression in young school children and intraocular pressure. *Doc. Ophthalmol.* **82**, 249–255.

Jiang, B. and Woessner, W. (1996) Vitreous chamber elongation is responsible for myopia development in a young adult. *Optom. Vis. Sci.* **73**, 231–234.

Jones, R. (1990) Accommodation and convergence control system parameters are abnormal in myopia. *Invest. Ophthalmol. Vis. Sci.* **31** (ARVO Suppl.), 81.

Kang, R. N. and Norton, T. T. (1993) Alteration of scleral morphology in tree shrews with induced myopia. *Invest. Ophthalmol. Vis. Sci.* **34** (ARVO Suppl.), 1209.

Kent, P. R. (1963) Acquired myopia of maturity. *Am. J. Optom. Arch. Am. Acad. Optom.* **40**, 247–255.

Koretz, J. F., Rogot, A. and Kaufman, P. L. (1995) Physiological strategies for emmetropia. *Trans. Am. Ophthalmol. Soc.* **93**, 105–122.

Kozaki, M., Nakayama, S. and Mizuno, N. (1969) On mass-examination with a visual screening car. *Folia Ophthalmol. Jpn.* **20**, 129–139.

Kumar, V., Cotran, R. S. and Robbins, S. L. (1992) *Basic Pathology.* W. B. Saunders, p. 86.

Lam, C. S. Y. and Goh, W. S. H. (1991b) Astigmatism among Chinese school children. *Clin. Exp. Optom.* **74**, 146–150.

Lam, C. S. Y. and Goh, W. S. H. (1991a) The incidence of refractive errors among school children in Hong Kong and its relationship with optical components. *Clin. Exp. Optom.* **74**, 97–103.

Lam, C. S. Y., Goh, W. S. H., Tang. Y. K., Tsui, K. K., Wong, W. C. and Man, T. C. (1994) Changes in refractive trends and optical components of Hong Kong Chinese aged over 40 years. *Ophthal. Physiol. Opt.* **14**, 383–388.

Larsen, J. S. (1971a) The sagittal growth of the eye. I. Ultrasonic measurement of the depth of the anterior chamber from birth to puberty. *Acta Ophthalmol.* **49**, 239–262.

Larsen, J. S. (1971b) The sagittal growth of the eye. IV. Ultrasonic measurement of the axial length of the eye from birth to puberty. *Acta Ophthalmol* **49**, 873–886.

Larsen, J. S. (1971c) The sagittal growth of the eye. II. Ultrasonic measurement of the axial diameter of the lens and the anterior segment from birth to puberty. *Acta Ophthalmol.* **49**, 427–440.

Larsen, J. S. (1971d) The sagittal growth of the eye. III. Ultrasonic measurement of the posterior segment (axial length of the vitreous) from birth to puberty. *Acta Ophthalmol.* **49**, 441–453.

Lin, T., Grimes, P. A. and Stone, R. A. (1993) Expansion of the retinal pigment epithelium in experimental myopia. *Vision Res.* **33**, 1881–1885.

Lin, L. L.-K., Hung, L.-F., Shih, Y.-F., Hung, P.-T. and Ko, L.-S. (1988) Correlation of optical components with ocular refraction among teen-agers in Taipei. *Acta Ophthalmol.* Suppl. 185, 69–73.

Lin, L. L.-K., Shih, Y.-F., Lee, Y., Hung, P.-T. and Hou, P.-K. (1996) Changes in ocular refraction and its components among medical students–a 5 year longitudinal study. *Optom. Vis. Sci.* **73**, 495–498.

Lin, L. L.-K., Wang., T.-H., Jan, J.-H., Shih, Y.-F, Ko, L.-S. and Hou, P.-K. (1991) Survey of the ocular refraction with its optical components among freshmen in National Taiwan University. *Trans. Ophthalmol. Soc. Repub. China* **30**, 597–604.

Liu, K.-R., Chen, M.-S. and Ko, L.-S. (1986) Electron microscopic studies of the scleral collagen fiber in excessively high myopia. *J. Formosan Med. Assoc.* **85**, 1032–1038.

Logan, N. S. and Gilmartin, B. (1996) Optic disc size and disc-to-fovea distance in ametropia. *Invest. Ophthalmol. Vis. Sci.* **37** (ARVO Suppl.), S476.

Logan, N. S., Gilmartin, B., Wildsoet, C. F., Dunne, M. C. M. and, Malingré, R. (1995) Asymmetry of schematic retinal contours in anisomyopia. *Invest. Ophthalmol. Vis. Sci.* **36** (ARVO Suppl.), S949.

Lotufo, D., Ritch, R., Szmyd, L. and Burris, J. (1989) Juvenile glaucoma, race, and refraction. *J. Am. Med. Assoc.* **261**, 249–252.

Lue, C. L., Hansen, R. M., Reisner, D. S., Findl, O., Petersen, R. A. and Fulton, A. B. (1995) The course of myopia in children with mild retinopathy of prematurity. *Vision Res.* **35**, 1329–1335.

Mäntyjärvi, M. and Tuppurainen, K. (1995) Colour vision and dark adaptation in high myopia without central retinal degeneration. *Br. J. Ophthalmol.* **79**, 105–108.

Marsh-Tootle, W. L. and Norton, T. T. (1989) Refractive and structural measures of lid-sutured myopia in tree shrew. *Invest. Ophthalmol. Vis. Sci.* **30**, 2245–2257.

Marzani, D. and Wallman, J. (1997) Growth of the two layers of the chick sclera is modulated reciprocally by visual conditions. *Invest. Ophthalmol. Vis. Sci.* **38**, 1726–1739.

McBrien, N. A. and Norton, T. T. (1992) The development of experimental myopia and ocular component dimensions in monocularly lid-sutured tree-shrews (*Tupaia belangeri*). *Vision Res.* **32**, 843–852.

McBrien, N. A. and Adams, D. W. (1997) A longitudinal investigation of adult-onset and adult progression of myopia in an occupational group. *Invest. Ophthalmol. Vis. Sci.* **38**, 321–333.

McBrien, N. A. and Norton, T. T. (1994) Prevention of collagen increases form-deprivation myopia in tree shrew. *Exp. Eye Res.* **59**, 475–486.

McBrien, N. A. and Millodot, M. (1987) A biometric investigation of late onset myopic eyes. *Acta Ophthalmol.* **65**, 461–468.

McFadden, S. and Wallman, J. (1995) Guinea pig eye growth compensates for spectacle lenses. *Invest. Ophthalmol. Vis. Sci.* **36** (ARVO Suppl.), S758.

Medina, A. (1987) A model for emmetropization: The effects of correcting lenses. *Acta Ophthalmol.* **65**, 565–571.

Medina, A. and Fariza, E. (1993) Emmetropization as a first-order feedback system. *Vision Res.* **33**, 21–26.

Meyer-Schwickerath, G. and Gerke, E. (1984) Biometric studies of the eyeball and retinal detachment. *Br. J. Ophthalmol.* **68**, 29–31.

Millodot, M. (1981) Effect of ametropia on peripheral refraction. *Am. J. Optom. Physiol. Opt.* **58**, 691–695.

Muñoz, M. and Capó, H. (1995) High myopia following excessive occlusion therapy in the first year (Letter). *Br. J. Ophthalmol.* **79**, 297.

Nickla, D. L., Wildsoet, C. and Wallman, J. (1998) The circadian rhythm in intraocular pressure and its relation to diurnal ocular growth changes in chicks. *Exp. Eye Res.* **66**, 183–193.

Norton, T. (1990) Experimental myopia in tree shrews. In: *Myopia and the Control of Eye Growth*. Ciba Foundation Symposium 155 (G. R. Bock and K. Widdows, eds). Wiley, pp. 178–199.

Norton, T. T. and Rada, J. A. (1995) Reduced extracellular matrix in mammalian sclera with induced myopia. *Vision Res.* **35**, 1271–1281.

Norton, T. T. and Siegwart, J. T. (1991) Local myopia produced by partial visual-field deprivation in tree-shrew. *Soc. Neurosci. Abstr.* **17**, 558.

O'Leary, D. J. and Millodot, M. (1979) Eyelid closure causes myopia in humans. *Experientia* **35**, 1478–1479.

Otsuka, J. (1967) Research on the etiology and treatment of myopia. *Acta Soc. Ophthalmol. Jpn* **71** (Suppl.), 1–8.

Pärssinen, O. (1990) Intraocular pressure in school myopia. *Acta Ophthalmol.* **68**, 559–563.

Pärssinen, T. O. (1993) Corneal refraction and topography in school myopia. *C. L. A. O. J.* **19**, 69–72.

Pärssinen, O. and Lyyra, A. L. (1993) Myopia and myopic progression among schoolchildren: a three-year follow-up study. *Invest. Ophthalmol. Vis. Sci.* **34**, 2794–2802.

Perkins, E. S. (1981a) Ocular volume and ocular rigidity. *Exp. Eye Res.* **33**, 141–145.

Perkins, E. S. (1981b) The ocular pulse. *Curr. Eye Res.* **1**, 19–23.

Perkins, E. S. and Phelps, C. D. (1982) Open-angle glaucoma, ocular hypertension, low-tension glaucoma, and refraction. *Arch. Ophthalmol.* **100**, 1464–1467.

Phillips, J. R. and McBrien, N. A. (1995) Form deprivation myopia: elastic properties of sclera. *Ophthal. Physiol. Opt.* **15**, 357–362.

Pierro, L., Camesasca, F. I., Mischi, M. and Brancato, R. (1992) Peripheral retinal changes and axial myopia. *Retina* 12(1), 12–17.

Pruett, R. C. (1988) Progressive myopia and intraocular pressure, what is the linkage? A literature review. *Acta Ophthalmol.* Suppl. 185, 117–129.

Quinn, G. E., Berlin, J. A., Young, T. L., Ziylan, S. and Stone, R. A. (1995) Association of intraocular pressure and myopia in children. *Ophthalmology* **102**, 180–185.

Quinn, G. E., Dobson, V. and Repka, M. X. (1992) Development of myopia in infants with birth weights less than 1251 grams. The Cryotherapy for Retinopathy of Prematurity Cooperative Group. *Ophthalmology* **99**, 329–340.

Rabin, J., Van-Sluyters, R. C. and Malachi, R. (1981) Emmetropization: a vision-dependent phenomenon. *Invest. Ophthalmol. Vis. Sci.* **20**, 561–564.

Rada, J. A. and Brenza, H. L. (1995) Increased latent gelatinase activity in the sclera of visually deprived chicks. *Invest. Ophthalmol. Vis. Sci.* **36**, 1555–1565.

Raviola, E. and Wiesel, T. N. (1985) Animal model of myopia. *N. Engl. J. Med.* **312**, 1609.

Reeder, A. P. and McBrien, N. A. (1993) Biochemical changes in the sclera of tree shrews with high degrees of experimental myopia. *Ophthal. Physiol. Opt.* **13**, 105.

Rempt, F., Hoogerheide, J. and Hoogenboom, W. P. H. (1971) Peripheral retinoscopy and the skiagram. *Ophthalmologica* **162**, 1–10.

Robb, R. M. (1977) Refractive errors associated with hemangiomas of the eyelids and orbit in infancy. *Am. J. Ophthalmol.* **83**, 52–58.

Schaeffel, F., Glasser, A. and Howland, H. C. (1988) Accommodation, refractive error and eye growth in chickens. *Vision Res.* **28**, 639–657.

Scharf, J., Zonis, S. and Zeltzer, M. (1975) Refraction in Israeli premature babies. *J. Pediatric Ophthalmol. Strab.* **12**, 193–196.

Scott, R. and Grosvenor, T. (1993) Structural model for emmetropic and myopic eyes. *Ophthal. Physiol. Opt.* **13**, 41–47.

Seddon, J. M., Schwartz, B. and Flowerdew, G. (1983) Case-control study of ocular hypertension. *Arch. Ophthalmol.* **101**, 891–894.

Sellheyer, K. and Spitznas, M. (1988) Development of the human sclera–a morphological study. *Graefe's Arch. Clin. Exp. Ophthalmol.* **226**, 89–100.

Shapiro, A., Yanko, L., Nawratzki, I. and Merin, S. (1980) Refractive power of premature children at infancy and early childhood. *Am. J. Ophthalmol.* **90**, 234–238.

Sheridan, M. and Douthwaite, W. A. (1989) Corneal asphericity and refractive error. *Ophthal. Physiol. Opt.* **9**, 235–238.

Sherman, S. M., Norton, T. T. and Casagrande, V. A. (1977) Myopia in the lid-sutured tree shrew (*Tupaia glis*). *Brain Res.* **124**, 154–157.

Shih, Y.-F. and Lin, L. L.-K. (1989) Clinical observations on occlusion myopia. *J. Formosan Med. Assoc.* **88**, 164–168.

Shih, Y.-F., Lin, Y.-C., Wang, T.-H., Lin, L. L.-K., Hwang, J.-K. and Hung, P.-T. (1996) The optic disc morphometric changes in high myopia. *Tzu Chi. Med. J.* **8**, 97–102.

Shih, Y.-F., Horng, I.-H., Yang, C.-H., Lin, L. L.-K., Peng, Y. and Hung, P.-T. (1991) Ocular pulse amplitude in myopia. *J. Oc. Pharmacol.* **7**, 83–87.

Shih, Y.-F., Wang, A.-H. and Ko, L.-S. (1989) Refractive status of medical students in National Taiwan University. *Trans. Ophthalmol Soc. Repub. China* **28**, 53–58.

Siegwart, J. T. and Norton, T. T. (1993) Refractive and ocular changes in tree shrews raised with plus or minus lenses. *Invest. Ophthalmol. Vis. Sci.* **34** (ARVO Suppl.), 1208.

Siegwart, J. T. and Norton, T. T. (1994) Increased scleral creep in tree shrews with deprivation-induced myopia. *Invest. Ophthalmol. Vis. Sci.* **35** (ARVO Suppl.), 2068.

Simensen, B. and Thorud, L. O. (1994) Adult-onset myopia and occupation. *Acta Ophthalmol.* **72**, 469–471.

Smith III, E. L., Hung, L.-F. and Harwerth, R. S. (1994) Effects of optically induced blur on the refractive status of young monkeys. *Vision Res.* **34**, 293–301.

Sorsby, A. and Leary, G. A. (1970) *A Longitudinal Study of Refraction and Its Components During Growth.* Medical Research Council Special Report Series No. 309. HMSO.

Sorsby, A., Benjamin, D., Davey, J. B., Sheridan, M. and Tanner, J. M. (1957) *Emmetropia and Its Aberrations.* Medical Research Council Special Report. Series No. 293. HMSO.

Sorsby, A., Benjamin, B. and Sheridan, M. (1961) *Refraction and Its Components During the Growth of the Eye from the Age of Three.* Medical Research Council Special Report Series No. 301. HMSO.

Sorsby, A., Leary, G. A. and Richards, M. J. (1962) Correlation ametropia and component ametropia. *Vision Res.* **2**, 309–313.

Sperduto, R. D., Siegel, D., Roberts, J. and Rowland, M. (1983) Prevalence of myopia in the United States. *Arch. Ophthalmol.* **101**, 405–407.

Stenström, S. (1948) Investigation of the variation and the correlation of the optical elements of human eyes (trans. D. Woolf). *Am. J. Optom. Arch. Am. Acad. Optom.* **25**, 218–232, 286–299, 340–350, 388–397, 438–451, 496–505.

Summers, C. G., Romig, L. and Lavoie, J. D. (1991) Unexpected good results after therapy for anisometropic amblyopia associated with unilateral peripapillary myelinated nerve fibers. *J. Pediatr. Ophthalmol. Strab.* **28**, 134–136.

Teakle, E. M., Wildsoet, C. F. and Vaney, D. I. (1993) Spatial organization of dopaminergic amacrine cells in chick retina: consequences of myopia. *Vision Res.* **33**, 2383–2396.

To'mey, K. F., Faris, B. M., Jalkh, A. and Nasr, A. (1981) Ocular pulse in high myopia: a study of 40 eyes. *Ann. Ophthalmol.* (May), 569–571.

Tokoro, T. and Kabe, S. (1964) Relation between changes in the ocular refraction and refractive components and development of the myopias. *Acta Soc. Ophthalmol. Jpn* **68**, 1240–1253.

Tokoro, T. and Suzuki, K. (1968) Significance of changes of refractive components to development of myopia during seven years. *Acta Soc. Ophthalmol. Jpn* **72**, 264–269.

Tokoro, T., Nakao, H. and Otsuka, M. (1967) Progress of myopia and changes of refractive components–6 cases followed up to 5 years. *Acta Soc. Ophthalmol. Jpn* **71**, 30–38.

Tomlinson, A. and Phillips, C. I. (1970) Applanation tension and axial length of the eyeball. *Br. J. Ophthalmol.* **54**, 548–553.

Toulemont, P., Urvoy, M., Coscas, G., Lecallonnec, A. and Cuvilliers, A. F. (1995) Association of congenital microcornea with myopia and glaucoma. A study of 23 patients with congenital microcornea. *Ophthalmology* **102**, 193–198.

Tovena, G., Parisi, G., Bellucci, R. and Polinelli, G. P. (1989) Relations between refractive status and intra-ocular pressure in young males. *Bolenttino Di Oculistica* **68**, 705–711.

Trier, K., Olsen, E. B. and Ammitzboll, T. (1990) Regional glycosaminoglycans composition of the human sclera. *Acta Ophthalmol.* **68**, 304–306.

Troilo, D., Xiong, M., Crowley, J. C. and Finlay, B. L. (1996) Factors controlling the dendritic aborization of retinal ganglion cells. *Vis. Neurosci.* **13**, 721–733.

Tron, E. (1940) *Modern Trends in Ophthalmology.* Butterworth.

Twomey, J. M., Gilvarry, A. and Restori, M. (1990) Ocular enlargement following infantile corneal opacification. *Eye* **4**, 497–503.

Van Alphen, G. W. H. M. (1961) On emmetropia and ametropia. *Ophthalmologica* **142** (Suppl.), 1–92.

Van Alphen, G. W. H. M. (1986) Choroidal stress and emmetropization. *Vision Res.* **26**, 723–734.

Von Noorden, G. K. and Lewis, R. A. (1987) Ocular axial length in unilateral congenital cataracts and blepharoptosis. *Invest. Ophthalmol. Vis. Sci.* **28**, 750–752.

Wallman, J. (1993) Retinal control of eye growth and refraction. *Prog. Retinal Res.* **12**, 133–152.

Wallman, J. and Adams, J. I. (1987) Developmental aspects of experimental myopia in chicks: Susceptibility, recovery and relation to emmetropization. *Vision Res.* **27**, 1139–1163.

Wallman, J., Gottlieb, M. D. and Rajaram, V. (1987) Local retinal regions control local eye growth and myopia. *Science* **237**, 73–77.

Wallman, J., Turkel, J. and Trachtman, J. N. (1978) Extreme myopia produced by modest changes in early visual experience. *Science* **201**, 1249–1251.

Weymouth, F. W. and Hirsch, M. J. (1950) Relative growth of the eye. *Am. J. Opt. Arch. Am. Acad. Optom.* **27**, 317–328.

Weymouth, F. W. and Hirsch, M. J. (1991) Theories, definitions, and classifications of refractive errors. In: *Refractive Anomalies.* (T. Grosvenor and M. C. Flom, eds). Butterworth–Heinemann, pp. 1–14.

Wildsoet, C. F. (1997) Active emmetropization–evidence from chick and properties of the underlying mechanism. *Aust. NZ J. Ophthalmol.* **25** (Suppl.), A13.

Wildsoet, C. F. and Wallman, J. (1995) Choroidal and scleral mechanisms of compensation for spectacle lenses in chicks. *Vision Res.* **35**, 1175–1194.

Wildsoet, C. F. and Wallman, J. (1997) Is the rate of lens-compensation proportional to the degree of defocus? *Invest. Ophthalmol. Vis. Sci.* **38** (ARVO Suppl.), S461.

Wildsoet, C. F., Atchison, D. A. and Collins, M. J. (1993) Longitudinal chromatic aberration as a function of refractive error. *Clin. Exp. Optom.* **76**, 119–122.

Wiesel, T. N. and Raviola, E. (1977) Myopia and eye enlargement after neonatal lid fusion in monkeys. *Nature (Lond.)* **266**, 66–68.

Winn, B., Ackerley, R. G., Brown, C. A., Murray, F. K., Prias, J. and St John, M. F. (1988) Reduced aniseikonia in axial anisometropia with contact lens correction. *Ophthal. Physiol. Opt.* **8**, 341–344.

Yamamoto, M., Tatsuami, H. and Bun, J. (1979) A follow-up study of refractive errors in premature infants. *Jpn J. Ophthalmol.* **23**, 435–443.

Yinon, U. (1980) Myopia in the eye of developing chicks following monocular and binocular lid suture. *Vision Res.* **20**, 137–141.

Zadnik, K., Mutti, O. D. and Adams, A. J. (1995) Longitudinal evidence of crystalline lens thinning in children. *Invest. Ophthalmol. Vis. Sci.* **36**, 1581–1587.

Zadnik, K., Satariano, W. A., Mutti, D. O., Sholtz, R. and Adams, A. (1994) The effect of parental history of myopia on children's eye size. *J. Am. Med. Assoc.* **271**, 1323–1327.

Ziobrowski, S. and Zygulska-Mach, H. (1981) The study of ocular tension in myopic school-children and adolescents. *Doc. Proc. Series* (Third International Conference on Myopia) **28**, 367–374.

Environmentally induced refractive errors in animals

Earl L. Smith III

4.1 Introduction

The roots of the idea that the visual environment actively influences ocular growth and the refractive status of the eye can be traced back to the last century. In 1866, Cohn reported on the association between myopia and formal schooling, and is recognized as one of the first investigators to propose that nearwork, and especially reading caused myopia (Weymouth and Hirsch, 1991). Although myopia and near visual environments have been linked in numerous subsequent studies of human subjects, these investigations have not been able to identify conclusively the extent to which the visual environment impacts refractive development, to isolate convincingly the critical aspects of nearwork that potentially induce ocular changes, or to determine confidently the physiological mechanisms which would mediate environmental influences on the eye's refractive status. However, recent work with animal subjects has begun to provide answers to many fundamental questions on the role of vision in refractive development.

This chapter reviews the evidence from animal investigations that vision-dependent mechanisms actively influence the eye's refractive state. A wide variety of animal species have been employed in these studies, with the chicken being the most common animal used in refractive error research. However, to facilitate comparisons with the human condition, this review concentrates, where possible, on results obtained in studies that employed macaque monkeys as subjects. A number of excellent papers that review much of the literature from subprimate species are available to the interested reader (Goss and Criswell, 1981; Yinon, 1984; Wallman; 1993).

Overall, studies of the refractive status of laboratory and feral animals provide strong support for the concept that ocular growth is regulated by visual experience. For purposes of discussion, these studies can be segregated into two broad lines of research. One line focuses primarily on the influence of viewing distance on the eye's refractive status. In some cases, alterations in viewing distance have been experimentally imposed on laboratory animals. While in others, investigators have tried to take advantage of natural or more global environmental differences in viewing distance. The impetus for this research grew from the well-established association between myopia and nearwork visual environments found in the human population. The results of these studies have frequently been interpreted along the lines of the 'use–abuse' theory of myopia. The second research line is centred on the influence of the quality and/or nature of the retinal image on the eye's refractive status. Although the initial findings that launched much of this research were discovered fortuitously, this line of investigation has provided the clearest evidence that visual experience actively regulates ocular growth and refractive development in a wide variety of animal species.

4.2   Refractive status and visual environment

4.2.1   Prevalence of myopia: feral versus domestic/laboratory animals

It is generally thought that amongst wild species, particularly mammals, the most common refractive error is a low degree of hyperopia, and that myopia is quite rare (Duke-Elder, 1958; Curtin, 1985). However, much of the data that support this idea is anecdotal in nature and reflects measurements on a relatively small number of animals (e.g. Barrett, 1932). In addition, there are systematic errors associated with the techniques commonly employed to measure refractive errors in these animals (Glickstein and Millodot, 1970). Furthermore, it could reasonably be argued that other refractive errors might be more advantageous than low degrees of hyperopia (Walls, 1942), an idea advocated near the turn of the century by Johnson (1901) which is still widely held (cited by Hughes, 1977). In contrast, refractive state is believed to vary considerably more in domesticated species such as the laboratory rat (Mutti *et al.*, 1992) and the dog (Murphy *et al.*, 1992). Moreover, myopia is thought to be common, especially in non-human primates such as chimpanzees (Young, 1964; Young *et al.*, 1971) and in domesticated species like the rabbit that are frequently housed in small vivariums (Duke-Elder, 1958; Curtin, 1985).

Similarly, within a given species, the distribution of refractive errors can be quite different for animals that live predominately in visually open environments versus those raised under visually restricted laboratory conditions. For example, Rose and colleagues reported that the great majority (87%) of adult 'street' cats, i.e., wild cats which were believed to have never been restricted to a closed environment, were typically hyperopic (mean = 1.14 D, *n* = 12). In comparison, they found that 76% of adult cats that were raised in laboratory cages from infancy were typically myopic (mean = 0.8 D, *n* = 18) (Rose *et al.*, 1974; Belkin *et al.*, 1977). A similar trend has been observed in rhesus monkeys. In a large-scale study involving 1000 monkeys, Young (1964) found that newly captured rhesus monkeys were typically hyperopic (mean = 0.63 D, *n* = 299); and only 9.5% exhibited myopia. In contrast, for rhesus monkeys that had been born and raised in captivity or spent a substantial amount of their lives in a laboratory facility, the mean refractive error was significantly less hyperopic (mean = 0.06,

n = 701). Over 25% of the eyes of laboratory monkeys were myopic (Young and Leary, 1973). These results indicate that within a given species, caged animals are significantly more likely to be myopic than free-ranging animals.

The differences between feral and domestic/laboratory animals in the average static refractive error and, in particular, the prevalence of myopia have been considered by some investigators as evidence that near environments and/or the absence of distance vision promote the development of myopia (Barrett, 1932; Young and Leary, 1973; Rose *et al.*, 1974; Belkin *et al.*, 1977; Yinon, 1984). Based upon the assumption that domestic/laboratory animals are exposed to visual environments which in a time-averaged manner consist of shorter viewing distances, these results have been taken as evidence that something associated with the act of viewing near objects, most commonly assumed to be prolonged and excessive accommodation and/or convergence, leads to myopia.

Although these inter- and intra-species comparisons are largely in agreement with the idea that near viewing distances promote myopia, this line of evidence, which is somewhat analogous to comparing refractive error distributions for humans with different ethnic backgrounds or for humans from rural versus urban settings, is quite weak. Many factors could confound this analysis strategy. For example, a critical issue is the potential role of natural selection in eliminating myopia in feral animals. It is likely that evolutionary pressures for clear distance vision would be more acute in feral species and could reasonably provide a bias toward a low degree of hyperopia, especially over several generations. Genetic differences between domesticated and feral species could easily be paramount because even within a given animal species, it has been shown that the prevalence of myopia can vary substantially from one breed to the next (Murphy *et al.*, 1992), even in the absence of any obvious differences in visual ecology.

4.2.2   Peripheral refractive errors and viewing distance

In species with panoramic visual systems, there is a comparatively small decline in spatial resolution from the central part of the retina to the periphery. In order to take full advantage of this neural adaptation, it is necessary to maintain optimal optical focus over a wide expanse of visual space. The eyes of some species with panoramic vision exhibit systematic variations in refractive error across the visual field which appear to reflect an attempt to bring different viewing distances into focus simultaneously.

The possibility that peripheral variations in refractive error might serve as a 'static' accommodative mechanism to provide clear vision for near and far objects simultaneously was first recognized and confirmed in the eyes of stingrays (Walls, 1942; Sivak and Allen, 1975) and is best documented in the eyes of birds. It is well established that the pigeon eye exhibits systematic variations in refractive state across the visual field (Catania, 1964; Millodot and Blough, 1971; Nye, 1973). For example, the pigeon eye is typically emmetropic when refracted along the axis that normally corresponds to the frontal field, but shows increasing degrees of myopia as one moves from the pupillary axis into the lower visual field (Fitzke *et al.*, 1985). This refractive error gradient is not a measurement artifact because it is evident in both optical measurements like retinoscopy and in electrophysiologic assessments that indicate the eye's refractive status for the photoreceptor plane. Moreover, there is a clear vertical asymmetry in the pigeon eye. Measurements made above the pupillary axis show that the eye is emmetropic for the upper visual field.

Rather than a defect of vision, this lower-field myopia can be considered a beneficial adaptation for the pigeon. Consider the situation if the pigeon's eye was emmetropic across the entire visual field. Obviously when the pigeon was walking on the ground and foraging, it would be important for near objects to be in focus in order to feed efficiently. This could be accomplished by positive accommodation. However, in this case, the upper visual field, which would typically be receiving images from distant objects, would be relatively myopic and the animal would be less able to detect predators or alarm signals. In contrast, sector myopia in the lower visual field would allow the bird to keep near objects on the ground in focus while at the same time maintaining an optimal focus for the distant horizon and sky simply by keeping the eye in an unaccommodated state. In flight, the pigeon's head posture, normally beak down, ensures that emmetropic aspects of the eye view the frontal field.

Several observations support the idea that lower-field myopia is a functional adaptation to near viewing distances. In pigeons, the myopic gradient in the lower visual field matches the dioptric demands of the ground plane (Fitzke *et al.*, 1985).

For an unaccommodated, emmetropic eye positioned at a fixed distance above a flat plane, the dioptric demands for objects on the ground will vary with the sine of the angle of declination below the horizon. Fitzke *et al.* (1985) found that the lower-field myopia in the pigeon eye increased as the sine of the declination angle. Consequently, when a unaccommodated pigeon is standing on a flat plane and fixating a distant object on the horizon, the retinal image of the ground from the horizon to immediately beneath the animal would be in focus simultaneously.

The presence of the phenomenon of lower field myopia appears to vary with the visual ecology of the animal. Although lower-field myopia is common in ground-foraging birds (Hodos and Erichsen, 1990), it has not been found in raptors (Murphy *et al.*, 1995). For birds, like the hawk and kestrel which spend relatively little time on the ground and presumably require good distance vision in their lower field to identify and capture prey, lower-field myopia would offer little benefit.

If this anisotropy is a functional adaptation, then the degree of lower-field myopia should vary with an animal's height, or more specifically, as a function of the distance between the eye and ground. To a first approximation, inter-species comparisons of the degree of lower-field myopia are in agreement with this prediction (Figure 4.1A). Very small animals like the frog exhibit quite high degrees of myopia (Schaeffel *et al.*, 1994b), whereas large species such as the horse show little or no lower-field myopia (Sivak and Allen, 1975). Amongst ground-foraging birds, quails (height = 13 cm) show a much higher degree of lower-field myopia than cranes (height = 95 cm). Additionally, in the chick, the degree of myopia varies as a function of age in a manner that compensates for growth-related changes in height (Hodos and Erichsen, 1990). Thus, although the precision of the match between the degree of lower-field myopia and the dioptric demands posed by natural viewing conditions may vary between species and may be low in eyes with a large depth-of-field, all of the anisotropies observed for normally reared animals are in the appropriate direction and would significantly improve the range of clear panoramic vision.

However, perhaps the strongest evidence that lower-field myopia is a functional adaptation to chronic exposure to near viewing distances comes from studies which have demonstrated that it is possible to reverse the direction of this anisotropy

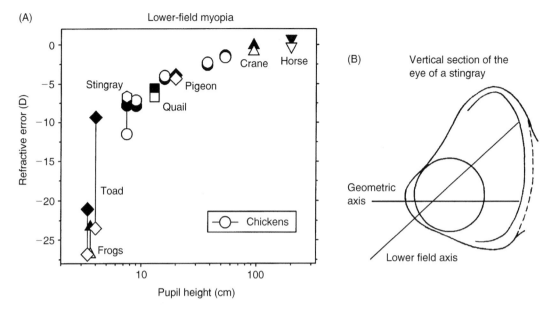

Figure 4.1 (A) Mean refractive state of the lower visual field for a variety of species plotted as a function of the vertical distance between the eye and ground. The refractive errors were measured for declination angles ranging between 30 and 70° below horizontal. The filled symbols for each species represent the measured degree of relative myopia, while the paired open symbols show the expected degree of relative myopia calculated using Fitzke *et al.*'s (1985) sine model. The data obtained for chickens at five different ages are illustrated by circles; the species for all other symbols are indicated. For some species, the absolute peripheral refractive errors, following correction for the 'small-eye' artifact of retinoscopy, are shown. In other cases, this artifact was minimized by expressing the degree of myopia as the difference between the refractive errors measured on the horizontal meridian versus the lower visual field. Data were taken from studies by Hodos and Erichsen (1990) (1-day, 6-week and adult chickens, quail, pigeons and cranes); Schaeffel *et al.* (1994b) (frogs, toads and 6-day and 28-day chicks); Sivak (1976) (stingrays); and Sivak and Allen (1975) (horse). (B) Schematic vertical section of the eye of a stingray demonstrating asymmetric vitreous chamber depth. (Redrawn from Walls, 1942.) *Note:* In this and all subsequent figures, negative and positive refractive errors indicate myopia and hyperopia, respectively

in young chicks by altering the animal's visual environment (Miles and Wallman, 1990). In contrast with normal birds, chicks reared in a low-ceiling environment become selectively more myopic in the upper visual field. This finding implies that visually mediated growth mechanisms may regulate local refractive development across the entire visual field and, thus, help to ensure a match between the eye's optimal focus and an animal's customary viewing conditions.

What is the structural basis for lower-field myopia? Anatomical studies have shown that in several species lower-field myopia is associated with asymmetries in the shape of the eye along the vertical meridian, with the dorsal portion of the retina being further away from the crystalline lens than either the inferior or central retina (Figure 4.1B) (Sivak, 1976). This effective increase in dorsal vitreous chamber depth would produce a rela-

tive shift in refractive state in the lower visual field towards myopia. Likewise, the upper-field myopia produced in chicks by the low-ceiling environment is associated with a relative increase in the dimensions of the inferior vitreous chamber (Miles and Wallman, 1990). Although the fact that lower-field myopia is also associated with astigmatism in some species (Schaeffel *et al.*, 1994b) suggests that systematic variations in optical power cannot be ruled out as a contributing factor, it appears that regional variations in axial length are a major factor. In this respect, it is possible that the alterations in the shape of the posterior globe associated with lower-field myopia are mediated by the same retinal mechanisms that are responsible for the local axial myopia produced by depriving a restricted portion of the retina of patterned visual inputs (Hodos and Kuenzel, 1984; Wallman *et al.*, 1987).

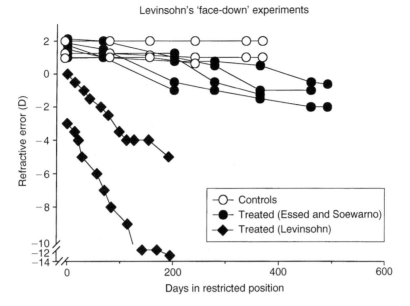

Figure 4.2 Effects of face posture on refractive error. Longitudinal refractive errors for monkeys that were secured in boxes which elevated their lower bodies and held their faces in the horizontal plane with their eyes looking in the downward direction (filled symbols). The open symbols represent data from control monkeys which were placed in boxes that held the monkeys in a normal, upright posture. The abscissa shows the length of the treatment period, with day 0 representing the start of the special rearing period. The stated goal of these experiments was to test the idea that maintaining the eyes in a downward direction promoted the development of myopia. (Data obtained from studies by Essed and Soewarno, 1928; Levinsohn 1919)

4.2.3 Prevalence of myopia–imposed near environments

Many of the factors that potentially confound comparisons between different species or populations of animals can be avoided by examining refractive changes in individual animals. A much stronger argument for the idea that near environments promote the development of myopia could be made if refractive changes in a given animal were clearly synchronized with a change in its visual environment. In this respect, there have been several attempts to alter the refractive status of monkeys via experimentally imposed alterations in the visual environment. Beginning in 1914, Levinsohn initiated a series of experiments that were intended to test the hypothesis that eye posture together with gravitational forces promote the development of myopia during prolonged nearwork (see Criswell and Goss, 1983). Levinsohn (1914) postulated that while reading, the plane of the face was frequently held in a horizontal position, and the eyes were typically oriented in a downward direction. According to his theory, in this situation, the downward pull of gravitational forces on the eye, which were thought to be resisted primarily by the optic

nerve at its insertion into the globe, would promote axial elongation and the concomitant development of myopia.

To test this hypothesis, Levinsohn and others placed young monkeys in boxes which held the animals' faces in the horizontal plane with the eyes pointing downward. The animals were typically secured in this restricted condition for 6 hours a day, 6 days a week for periods ranging between 4 weeks to well over a year. Although consistent results were not obtained in all studies (Marchesani, 1931), young monkeys subjected to this rearing strategy for extended periods exhibited myopic refractive error changes (Figure 4.2). In comparison, control monkeys that were held in similar boxes that were positioned in a normal upright orientation showed stable refractive errors.

For both theoretical and practical reasons, it is unlikely that Levinsohn's gravitational theory is correct. For example, the extraocular muscles would probably not allow a significant outward shift in eye position. Nevertheless, some aspect of this experimental manipulation resulted in significant myopic changes. Details of the visual scene that the experimental animals viewed while held in

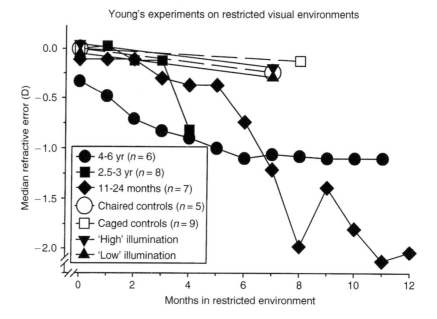

Figure 4.3 Effects of restricted, 'near', viewing conditions on the refractive status of monkeys. The median refractive error is plotted as a function of the duration of the observation period for different treatment groups. The filled symbols represent monkeys that were housed in the near environments. Control animals, which were housed in relatively unrestricted laboratory environments, are shown as open symbols. The critical features for each subject group are provided in the legend. Unless otherwise stated, the animals were 'adolescents'. Data obtained from Young (1961a, 1961b, 1962, 1963, 1965)

the head-down position were not provided, but photographs of monkeys in these rearing boxes indicate that the average viewing distance was probably relatively short (Levinsohn, 1919; Essed and Soewarno, 1928). However, attributing these myopic changes to restricted/near viewing conditions, while attractive, is clearly speculative.

The most direct test of the hypothesis that near environments promote the development of myopia was provided by a series of studies conducted by Young (1961a, 1961b, 1963). To simulate a near environment, monkeys (*Macaca nemestrina*) were placed in primate chairs which were covered with hoods made of a white diffusing material that restricted viewing distance to 20 inches or less. At 2- or 4-week intervals, the animals' refractive errors were measured and they were removed from the chairs for a 2-day period. For some monkeys, this rearing cycle was continued for periods up to 12 months.

Inspection of the refractive error data reported by Young suggests that many of the monkeys subjected to the restricted visual space became either more myopic or less hyperopic as a result of the experimental treatment (Figure 4.3). However, the

observed degree of myopia varied depending upon the animal's age at the onset of the restricted viewing conditions (Young, 1961b, 1963) and the level of illumination within the restricted environment (Young, 1962). For extended rearing periods and low photopic levels of illumination (4 foot candles), young monkeys between the ages of 11 and 24 months developed on average about 1.75 D of myopia. Based upon relative rates of axial development, 1 year of life for a macaque monkey is equivalent to about 3 years for a human infant (Kiely *et al.*, 1987). In comparison, monkeys that were 4–6 years of age only developed approximately 0.75 D of myopia over a comparable period in the restricted viewing conditions. These refractive changes appear to be permanent because the experimental animals failed to recover from the induced myopia when they were returned to a normal laboratory environment (Young, 1961a). However, it is curious that adolescent monkeys (presumably 4–6-year-olds) that were placed in restricted viewing conditions that were lighted by either very low illuminances (0.02 foot candles) or just slightly higher illuminances (26 foot candles) failed to develop myopia.

The precise aspect of Young's rearing strategy that caused some of the experimental animals to become myopic is not known. Young speculated that, while in the visually restricted environments, the monkeys converged and accommodated for the near viewing distances (Young, 1961b) and that prolonged high levels of accommodation somehow resulted in the myopic refractive changes. In support of this hypothesis, atropine-induced cycloplegia appeared to halt the progression of this myopia (Young, 1965). However, more recent experiments have indicated that topically applied atropine may prevent the development of myopia via direct pharmacological actions in the retina (Stone *et al.*, 1991). Thus, the paralysis of accommodation by atropine may not have been the key factor responsible for the interruption of myopia in Young's visually restricted monkeys. Consequently, the role of accommodation, or any other ocular process, in the development of restricted-environment myopia is still in question. In fact it could be argued that the myopia that Young observed was the result of form deprivation (Criswell and Goss, 1983; Wallman, 1993). While in the restricted environment, the monkeys could see their arms and components of the chair. However, the white translucent (diffusing) hoods that covered the monkeys were unpatterned and the investigator took care to ensure that external objects did not cast shadows on the hoods (Young, 1961b). As a result, it is possible that the hoods functioned much like a ganzfeld and that large aspects of the experimental monkeys' visual field were essentially deprived of form vision, a condition that readily promotes myopia in young monkeys (*see below*).

The lack of adequate experimental controls also makes Young's results difficult to interpret. In his series of studies, two control groups were employed to provide a reference for potential refractive error changes that may normally occur as a result of maintaining captive monkeys in a laboratory environment. One group, which was held in primate chairs that were not covered with visually restrictive hoods, showed relatively insignificant changes in refractive error that were equivalent to the small degree of myopia observed in the second control group of normal monkeys that were housed in traditional laboratory cages (*see* Figure 4.3) (Young, 1961a, 1962). These results indicate that normal adolescent monkeys exhibit relatively stable refractive errors in a normal laboratory environment, and that placing monkeys in chairs without further restricting their visual environment does not produce myopia. However, comparisons between either of these control groups and the experimental monkeys which were subjected to the restricted viewing conditions are confounded. All of the controls were exposed to significantly higher illumination levels (e.g. 40–50 foot candles) than the experimental monkeys that developed myopia (Young, 1962). Since even monkeys reared in hoods at high illumination levels (26 foot candles) failed to become myopic, the myopic changes found in the monkeys reared under hoods at low photopic levels of illumination must be interpreted cautiously. Overall, Young's findings are suggestive, but clearly not conclusive.

4.3   Form-deprivation myopia

Prior to 1977, the evidence that the visual environment influenced refractive development in laboratory animals was ambiguous, largely indirect, and primarily correlative in nature. However, during the course of their studies on the effects of visual experience on the developing nervous system, Hubel *et al.* (1976) made an important observation. Specifically, they noted that infant monkeys which had the lids of one eye surgically fused shortly after birth, a technique that was commonly employed to deprive an animal of patterned visual stimulation, developed high degrees of myopia. Wiesel and Raviola, recognizing the potential significance of these refractive changes, initiated a series of studies that demonstrated conclusively that the myopia associated with eyelid closure was produced by abnormal visual experience and that this phenomenon could serve as a useful animal model of human myopia (Wiesel and Raviola, 1977, 1979; Raviola and Wiesel, 1978, 1985).

4.3.2   The basic phenomenon

The effects of eyelid closure or form deprivation on the emmetropization process can best be appreciated by examining the refractive errors of monkeys where the lids of one eye were sutured closed early in life. As in human infants, both eyes of infant monkeys normally grow in a highly coordinated manner toward the ideal refractive state (Kiely *et al.*, 1987; Tigges *et al.*, 1990; Hung *et al.*, 1995). Consequently, the refractive error distribution for young adult monkeys exhibits the essential characteristics observed in young adult humans (Figure 4.4A). In particular, the distribution is leptokurtic, with the majority of monkeys showing either no refractive error or a low degree of hyperopia. The distribution of refractive errors for non-

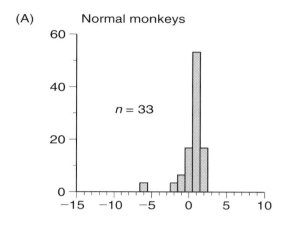

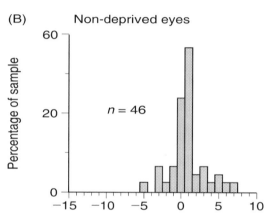

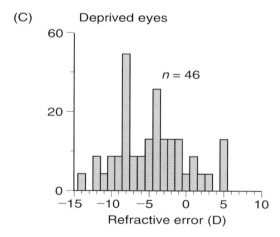

Figure 4.4 Frequency distributions of spherical-equivalent refractive errors for normal adult monkeys (A), the non-deprived (B) and deprived eyes (C) of monocularly lid-sutured monkeys. (Data obtained from Wiesel and Raviola, 1977; von Noorden and Crawford, 1978; Smith III *et al.*, 1987; Stone *et al.*, 1988; Raviola and Wiesel, 1990; Smith III *et al.*, 1994b)

deprived eyes of monocularly lid-sutured monkeys (Figure 4.4B) appears somewhat broader than the findings for normal monkeys, is highly peaked and centred at a low degree of hyperopia. In this case, the higher prevalence of moderate to high hyperopia in the non-deprived eyes can largely be attributed to the fact that some of the lid-sutured animals were under 3 months of age when the refractive data were obtained. However, it is also possible that the non-deprived eyes are not entirely normal. For example, there are some indications that unilateral manipulations can also produce subtle refractive error changes in the fellow eye (McBrien and Norton, 1992; Hung *et al.*, 1995). In contrast, the refractive error distribution for the form-deprived eyes of monkeys that had one eye sutured closed shortly after birth is clearly abnormal; it is quite broad and is dominated by large myopic refractive errors (Figure 4.4C).

A more precise indication of the effects of form deprivation can be obtained by comparing the refractive properties of the control and treated eyes in monocular lid-sutured monkeys. This is a powerful strategy because, assuming that the two eyes are independent (this is largely correct even though as noted above small interocular influences cannot be totally ruled out), interocular comparisons provide a very sensitive reference for assessing the direction and nature of any refractive error changes. Moreover, these within animal comparisons provide important controls for many of the variables that have often confounded investigations of the effects of visual experience on refractive development (e.g. natural selection pressures and potential genetic differences between subject populations). As shown in Figure 4.5, with few exceptions, deprived eyes are less hyperopic/more myopic than their fellow controls. It is important to note that an interocular asymmetry in image quality is not necessary to produce form-deprivation myopia. Binocular lid-sutured animals develop myopia in both eyes.

The induced myopic alterations appear to be axial in nature and can be attributed primarily to an increase in vitreous chamber depth; in monkeys, interocular differences in vitreous chamber depth correlate well with the degree of induced myopia (Figure 4.6) (Smith III *et al.*, 1987; Raviola and Wiesel, 1990). Although lid-sutured monkeys frequently exhibit astigmatism, there is no clear evidence that form deprivation alters corneal curvature, anterior chamber depth or lens thickness in higher primates (Raviola and Wiesel, 1985). However, in

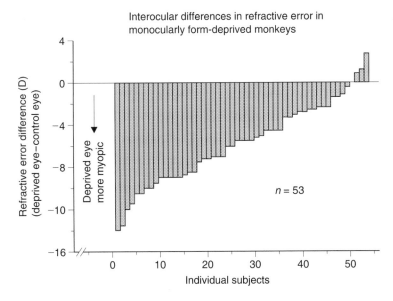

Figure 4.5 The type of refractive error produced by early form deprivation illustrated by the interocular differences in spherical-equivalent refractive error for individual monocularly form-deprived monkeys. Negative values indicate that the deprived eye was less hyperopic or more myopic than the fellow non-deprived eye. Subjects have been ordered by the degree of form-deprivation myopia. (Data obtained from Wiesel and Raviola, 1977; von Noorden and Crawford, 1978; Smith III *et al.*, 1987; Stone *et al.*, 1988; Raviola and Wiesel, 1990; Smith III *et al.*, 1994b)

addition to vitreous chamber elongation, anterior segment alterations have been observed in other form-deprived species (Yinon *et al.*, 1980; Wallman *et al.*, 1987). For example, in the tree shrew, a diurnal mammal closely related to primates, in addition to vitreous chamber elongation, lid suture results in a flatter cornea, a shallower anterior chamber, and a thinner crystalline lens (McBrien and Norton, 1992; *see also* Figure 4.9 below).

An important aspect of form-deprivation myopia is that, in addition to being a robust and consistent phenomenon in monkeys, it occurs in a wide range of animal species. Following the initial discovery in monkeys, form-deprivation myopia has been observed in cats (Gollender *et al.*, 1979; Kirby *et al.*, 1982; Yinon *et al.*, 1984), tree shrews (Sherman *et al.*, 1977; McKanna and Casagrande, 1978; Marsh-Tootle and Norton, 1989; McBrien and Norton, 1992), chickens (Wallman *et al.*, 1978; Yinon *et al.*, 1980; Hodos and Kuenzel, 1984; Hodos *et al.*, 1985), pigeons (Bagnoli *et al.*, 1985), barn owls (Knudsen, 1989), the American kestrel (Andison and Sivak, 1992), grey squirrels (McBrien *et al.*, 1993), and marmosets (Troilo and Judge, 1993). The degree of myopia and the speed at which the eye elongates vary from one species to the next and, in large part, reflect inter-species differences in eye size and relative maturational

rates. Species like the chicken, which have relatively small eyes and fast maturational rates, are capable of developing up to 20 D of myopia (Wallman *et al.*, 1978; Wallman and Adams, 1987), and changes in ocular growth rate can be demonstrated within a day of the onset of form deprivation (Weiss and Schaeffel, 1993). Most importantly, conditions which block or interfere with image formation in the human eye also disrupt emmetropization and typically result in axial myopia (Rob, 1977; O'Leary and Millodot, 1979; Hoyt *et al.*, 1981; Rabin *et al.*, 1981; Nathan *et al.*, 1985).

Since form-deprivation myopia occurs in such diverse species, it is likely that the visual system mechanisms that mediate these vision-dependent refractive changes are fundamental in an evolutionary sense and that these mechanisms are qualitatively similar in the eyes of a wide variety of animals. As a result, insight into the phenomenon of form-deprivation myopia and its underlying mechanisms gained in one species probably applies, at least in general terms, to other species and, in particular, to the human.

The degree of myopia produced by form deprivation depends on both internal and external factors. There is clear evidence that the susceptibility to form deprivation varies between individuals. In

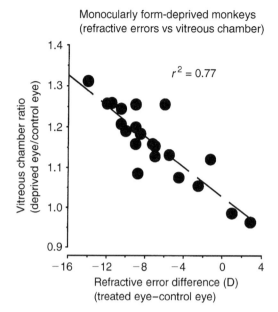

Monocularly form-deprived monkeys
(refractive errors vs vitreous chamber)

$r^2 = 0.77$

Figure 4.6 Comparison of interocular differences in spherical-equivalent refractive error and the ratio of vitreous chamber depths for individual monkeys that were monocularly form-deprived early in life. Vitreous chamber ratios greater than 1.0 indicate that the form-deprived eye had a longer vitreous chamber. Negative refractive error differences indicate that the form-deprived eye was relatively myopic. The axial nature of form-deprivation myopia is emphasized by the strong correlation between the interocular vitreous chamber ratios and the refractive error differences. (Data obtained from Stone *et al.*, 1988; Raviola and Wiesel, 1990; Ivone *et al.*, 1991)

binocularly deprived animals which are subjected to the same degree of form deprivation for similar periods of time, the degree of myopia varies substantially between animals, but it is highly correlated between the two eyes of a given animal. The variability between subjects is likely to reflect genetic differences in the sensitivity or efficiency of the mechanisms responsible for deprivation myopia (Schaeffel and Howland, 1991). Such differences could make certain individuals much more sensitive to environmental influences.

The period of form deprivation also has a significant impact on the degree of form-deprivation myopia (Smith III *et al.*, 1987, 1988; Raviola and Wiesel, 1990; McBrien and Norton, 1992; Troilo and Judge, 1993). Early form deprivation appears to disrupt the normal growth process resulting in rapid axial elongation. Within the normal growth period, this abnormal axial elongation continues as long as the eye is form-deprived. The effects of form deprivation on the rate of axial elongation decrease as the normal growth period comes to an end. Therefore, in general, the earlier the onset of deprivation and the longer the deprivation is maintained, the higher the degree of myopia (Figure 4.7). However, it should be noted that in a very young infant monkey even periods of deprivation as brief as two weeks can produce significant refractive anomalies.

Several additional factors can influence the degree of myopia observed at any given point in time. Firstly, in some species, form deprivation produces an initial transient hyperopic shift in refractive error that is then followed by the onset of deprivation myopia (McBrien and Norton, 1992; Troilo and Judge, 1993; Smith III and Hung, 1995). Although this initial hyperopic shift may be exaggerated by a mechanical flattening of the cornea produced by lid suture (McBrien and Norton, 1992), transient hyperopic shifts have also been observed in infant monkeys in which form deprivation was produced by diffuser spectacle lenses (Smith III and Hung, 1995). In this case, the transient hyperopia was associated with an initial relative reduction in axial growth in the deprived eye (Figure 4.8). Secondly, the eye's refractive status may continue to change after the end of the period of deprivation. In marmosets, parting the eyelids and restoring the potential for clear retinal images does not stop the abnormal vitreous chamber elongation and the formerly deprived eye can continue to become more myopic for a considerable period of time (Troilo and Judge, 1993). In other species, in particular the chicken (Wallman and Adams, 1987) and the macaque monkey, restoring normal visual experience while the animal is still within the normal growth period can lead to a substantial degree of recovery from myopia produced by a period of early form deprivation (*see* Figure 4.11). Given that numerous factors can influence the degree and type of refractive error produced by visual deprivation, it is not surprising that some clinical studies have reported that the refractive alterations associated with pathological conditions which optically mimic form deprivation are not as consistent as those obtained in controlled studies involving laboratory animals (von Noorden and Lewis, 1987).

It is thought that form deprivation does not produce myopia in adults, but rather that form deprivation only alters the eye's refractive state during a 'sensitive period' early in life. However, the effects

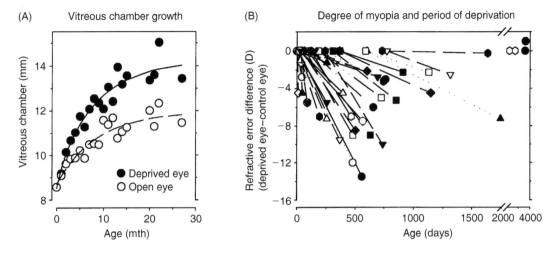

Figure 4.7 (A) Vitreous chamber depth plotted as a function of age for a monkey that had one eye sutured closed early in life. The deprived eye initially showed a relative acceleration in vitreous chamber growth which moderated as the overall rate of ocular growth declines with age. (Redrawn from Raviola and Wiesel, 1990.) (B) Interocular differences in spherical-equivalent refractive error plotted as a function of age for individual monocularly form-deprived monkeys. Only monkeys that developed a relative myopia in their treated eye are included. The first data point for each animal shows the age of onset for form deprivation. It was assumed that all monkeys were isometropic at the start of form deprivation. The second data point for each monkey indicates the age that deprivation was terminated and the degree of form-deprivation myopia. The slope of the line for a given animal indicates the rate at which form-deprivation myopia developed. In general, the earlier form deprivation is initiated, the faster myopia develops and, assuming deprivation is continued, the higher the degree of myopia. (Data obtained from Wiesel and Raviola, 1977; von Noorden and Crawford, 1978; Harwerth *et al.*, 1981; Smith III *et al.*, 1987; Stone *et al.*, 1988; Ivone *et al.*, 1991)

of form deprivation have only been studied in a few adult monkeys and it is possible that the duration of deprivation was simply too short to produce myopia. There are some suggestions that animals are still susceptible to the effects of abnormal visual experience after the age at which axial elongation normally stabilizes. For example, monkeys that had strabismus induced experimentally early in life frequently begin to develop abnormal refractive errors 2–3 years after the onset of anomalous binocular vision (Smith III *et al.*, 1994b; Kiorpes and Wallman, 1995). These observations raise the possibility that vision-dependent mechanisms are still capable of producing refractive error alterations relatively late in life. It will be important to resolve this issue because this information may have important implications for the phenomenon of late-onset myopia in the human population.

4.3.2   What causes deprivation myopia?

The phenomenon of deprivation myopia is a potentially invaluable tool for understanding the aetiology and pathogenesis for common forms of

myopia in humans. In establishing the relevance of deprivation myopia, it is critical to determine the exact cause of the abnormal ocular growth and the resulting refractive errors. This is particularly important, because many of the experimental protocols that are employed to produce form deprivation could possibly influence ocular growth through non-visual mechanisms. For example, surgical eyelid closure, the most common technique employed in monkeys to produce deprivation myopia, is also likely to alter the normal mechanical forces acting on the developing eye (McBrien and Norton, 1992) and to elevate local tissue temperature (Hodos *et al.*, 1987). Elevated temperature has been implicated as a contributing factor to the development of human myopia (Hirsch, 1957). Moreover, elevated ocular temperature in conjunction with increased intraocular pressure has been shown to produce myopia in laboratory animals (Maurice and Mushin, 1966; Tokoro, 1970; Mohan *et al.*, 1977).

Although form-deprivation techniques which involve direct physical contact with the globe can in some cases produce confounding ocular growth

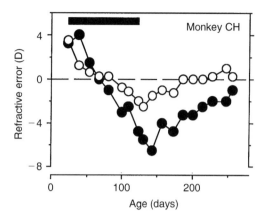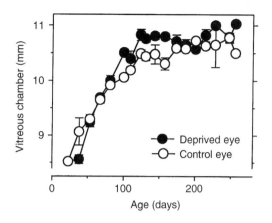

Figure 4.8 Refractive error (*left*) and vitreous chamber depth (*right*) plotted as a function of age for a monkey reared with a diffuser spectacle lens over one eye. The filled and open symbols represent the deprived and control eyes, respectively. The filled horizontal bar indicates the period of lens wear. This monkey showed an initial transient hyperopia that was associated with a relative reduction in vitreous chamber depth. Subsequently there was an acceleration in vitreous chamber growth rate and a concomitant myopic shift in refractive error. (Data from Smith III and Hung, 1995)

(McBrien and Norton, 1992; Hung and Smith III, 1996), the dramatic axial myopias associated with procedures like lid suture are not simply a consequence of secondary mechanical or thermal factors. Eyelid closure fails to produce myopia in monkeys that are reared in a totally dark environment (Raviola and Wiesel, 1978), which indicates that the mechanical aspects of lid suture alone are not sufficient to produce myopia. On the other hand, techniques which deprive the eye of form vision, but which avoid many of the mechanical aspects of eyelid closure, readily produce axial myopia (Wallman *et al.*, 1978; Wiesel and Raviola, 1979; Bartmann and Schaeffel, 1994; Smith III and Hung, 1995). Thus, it is the altered visual experience that promotes the development of myopia.

How much of an alteration in vision is necessary to produce deprivation myopia and what aspects of retinal stimulation are important for normal emmetropization? These are important questions. If deprivation myopia only occurs under extreme conditions that basically occlude the eye, then it is less likely that the mechanisms that are responsible for deprivation myopia are involved in normal ocular growth or in the genesis of common myopia. These extreme conditions would simply not be encountered during normal development.

Specific changes in the spectral composition of the retinal image are not necessary for the onset of deprivation myopia. Both eyelid suture, which strongly reduces retinal illumination in a

wavelength-dependent manner (Crawford and Marc, 1976), and optical diffusing lenses or corneal opacification, techniques which do not largely alter the spectral composition of light, produce deprivation myopia in monkeys (Wiesel and Raviola, 1979; Smith III and Hung, 1995). Reductions in retinal illumination also appear unnecessary. Rather than becoming myopic, monkeys that are reared in total darkness fail to undergo normal emmetropization and typically exhibit high degrees of hyperopia (Regal *et al.*, 1976; Guyton *et al.*, 1989). Furthermore, chickens reared with translucent diffusing lenses develop higher degrees of myopia than animals treated with opaque lenses which substantially reduce the degree of retinal illumination (Sivak *et al.*, 1989). Moreover, in the chicken, sectored diffuser lenses which disrupt image formation over half of the visual field, but which would not be expected to produce significant hemiretinal differences in retinal illumination, result in axial myopia only in the treated half of the retina (Wallman *et al.*, 1987).

As the name implies, it appears that a reduction in spatial detail triggers form-deprivation myopia. In agreement with this idea, the degree of deprivation myopia is correlated with the amount of image degradation. In the chicken, heavily frosted, translucent diffusing lenses produce high degrees of myopia whereas more lightly frosted lenses which allow higher image contrasts produce less myopia (Bartmann and Schaeffel, 1994). In the monkey,

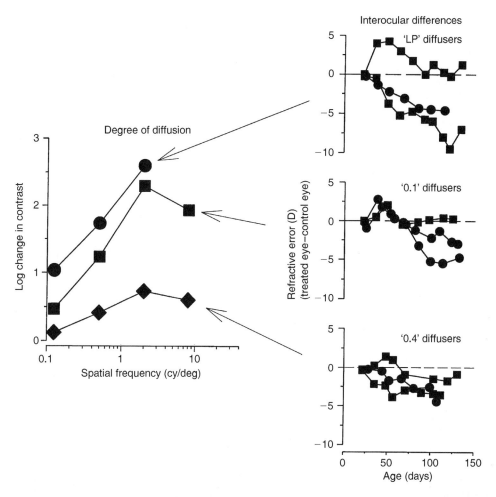

Figure 4.9 Reduction in behavioural contrast sensitivity plotted as a function of spatial frequency for a normal human observer obtained when viewing through the three different diffuser lenses (*left*). The circles, squares and diamonds represent data obtained with the three different diffuser lenses. The manufacturer designations (in the right column) provide an approximate indication of the visual acuity limit for an adult viewing through the diffuser lenses ('LP' = 'light perception'; '0.1' = 6/60; '0.4' = 6/15). (*Right*) Interocular refractive error differences plotted as a function of age for individual monkeys reared with one of three different diffuser lenses in front of one eye. Each function represents a single animal. Negative values indicate that the treated eye was more myopic/less hyperopic than the fellow control eye. The first point for each monkey represents the onset of lens wear. The arrows relate the strengths of the diffuser lenses for the three groups of monkeys. (Data from Smith III and Hung, 1995)

initial reports of the effect of diffuser contact lenses on eye growth suggested that moderate reductions in image contrast did not alter ocular growth (O'Leary *et al.*, 1992; Bradley *et al.*, 1996). However, it is likely that the results from these studies were confounded by non-visual aspects of contact lens wear. In infant monkeys, even soft, extended wear contact lenses can produce dramatic degrees of hyperopia which could surpass the expected axial myopia associated with form deprivation (Hung and Smith III, 1996).

As shown in Figure 4.9, diffuser spectacle lenses consistently produce myopia in infant monkeys, and the degree of myopia is correlated with the reduction in image contrast. Several aspects of these results are important. Firstly, the refractive error changes produced by the different diffuser lenses are qualitatively similar. And secondly, the contrast threshold for triggering the phenomenon of deprivation myopia is relatively low. Relatively modest levels of diffusion only reduced image contrast at high spatial frequencies by about 0.5 log units. Quantitatively similar reductions in image contrast can be produced by a relatively small degree of optical defocus. Yet, even these mild diffusers produced significant degrees of myopia.

The diffuser lens results indicate that deprivation myopia is a graded phenomenon, and that image degradation associated with relatively small amounts of chronic optical defocus could produce alterations in refractive error. In other words, the mechanisms that mediate deprivation myopia are probably sensitive enough to come into play during normal development. In this respect, it has been argued that the mechanisms that are responsible for deprivation myopia could participate in emmetropization (Wallman and Adams, 1987; Bartmann and Schaeffel, 1994; Hung *et al.*, 1995; Norton and Siegwart, 1995). An important implication of these results is that the potential for a clear, high-contrast retinal image is essential for normal emmetropization.

With respect to the potential role of deprivation mechanisms in normal ocular development, there are a number of interesting parallels between deprivation myopia in monkeys and the common forms of myopia in the human population. As in human myopes, the refractive errors of form-deprived monkeys can be attributed primarily to an increase in vitreous chamber depth, and on ophthalmoscopic examination, monkeys show anatomical features that resemble those seen in many myopic humans. For example, form-deprived monkeys exhibit myopic crescents at the optic disc (Raviola and Wiesel, 1985).

More importantly, the overall shape of monkey eyes with deprivation myopia is similar to that of human myopes. The average myopic human eye differs from emmetropic eyes in several ways. In addition to having longer vitreous chambers, myopes typically have thinner crystalline lenses, deeper anterior chambers and steeper corneas. In this regard, it has been hypothesized that myopic humans may become myopic because they inherit a different shaped eye than emmetropic individuals (Zadnik *et al.*, 1994). As shown in Figure 4.10, in comparison to controls and monkeys with experimental hyperopia, monkeys with myopia produced by diffuser lenses exhibit the hallmark characteristics of human myopia. These results show that vision-dependent mechanisms can alter the growth of the eye resulting in the characteristic distortions in ocular shape found in human myopes. Obviously, these results do not contradict the idea that individuals who develop myopia do so because they inherited an abnormally shaped eye. However,

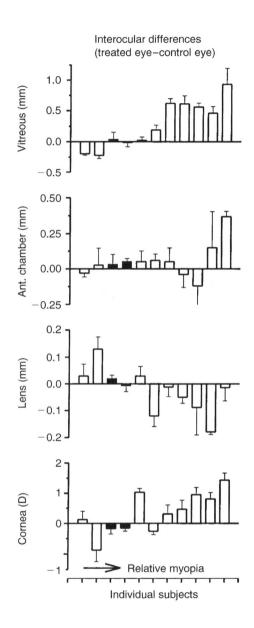

Figure 4.10 Interocular differences (right or treated eye–left or control eye) in ocular dimensions for individual control monkeys (*filled bars*) and monkeys reared with diffuser lenses over one eye (*open bars*). Positive values indicate that the measure for the treated eyes was greater than that for the fellow control eye. The subjects are arranged from left to right in order from the most hyperopic treated eye to the most myopic treated eye. Note that two of the deprived animals developed a relative hyperopia in their treated eyes. The monkey eyes with deprivation myopia are similar in shape to typical human eyes that have myopia. (Data from Smith III and Hung, 1995)

these results are significant because they demonstrate that in higher primates vision-dependent mechanisms are capable of transforming a normal eye into a stereotypical myopic eye.

4.4 Role of optical defocus in regulating emmetropization

Although the phenomenon of deprivation myopia clearly demonstrates that vision-dependent mechanisms can influence refractive development, its existence does not prove that visual feedback is involved in regulating early ocular growth or the process of emmetropization. However, as outlined below for the monkey, animals can recover from experimentally induced refractive errors. Moreover, changing the effective refractive status of the eye or the refractive balance between the two eyes with a spectacle lens will alter the normal emmetropization process, thereby causing the eye to grow in a manner that compensates for the imposed error. These experiments provide strong support for the idea that emmetropization involves a vision-dependent process that uses the error signals associated with optical defocus to regulate ocular growth. Additionally, as in the case of deprivation myopia, evidence for visual regulation of ocular growth has been found in a wide variety of species, including the chicken (Wallman and Adams, 1987; Schaeffel and Howland, 1988; Irving *et al.*, 1991, 1992; Schaeffel and Howland, 1991; Wildsoet and Wallman, 1995b), fish (Kröger and Fernald, 1994), tree shrew (Siegwart and Norton, 1993), marmoset (Troilo and Judge, 1993; Judge and Graham, 1995), guinea pig (McFadden and Wallman, 1995), and monkey (Hung *et al.*, 1995).

4.4.1 Recovery from experimental refractive errors

It was originally reported that form-deprivation myopia was permanent in infant monkeys (Raviola and Wiesel, 1985). However, as in the chick (Wallman and Adams, 1987; Troilo and Wallman, 1991), if unrestricted vision is restored at an early age, then the eyes of monkeys with experimentally-induced refractive errors are capable of a substantial degree of recovery (Figure 4.11). Upon removing the treatment lenses, infant monkeys with a hyperopic anisometropia produced by a contact lens rearing strategy show a rapid and systematic reduction in the hyperopia of the treated eye

which eliminates the induced anisometropia (Smith III *et al.*, 1994a). In a complimentary fashion, monkeys with myopic anisometropia produced by monocular form deprivation grow toward isometropia after the diffusing lenses are removed. In this case, the reduction in anisometropia is due principally to a reduction in the myopia of the deprived eye.

The exact cue that the eye uses to recover from experimental refractive errors is not known. It has been argued that recovery from abnormal refractive errors may be mediated, at least in part, by non-visual mechanisms that are sensitive to the overall shape of the eye (Troilo and Wallman, 1991). However, it is likely that vision-dependent mechanisms are involved since chickens with induced refractive errors fail to fully recover if they are put into dim light during the period of unrestricted vision (Gottlieb *et al.*, 1991).

The recovery from induced refractive errors comes about primarily as a result of changes in vitreous chamber elongation rates. Removing the diffuser lenses from a young monkey with form-deprivation myopia produces a dramatic reduction in the rate of axial growth. The abnormal axial elongation that produced the myopia virtually comes to a halt while the fellow eye continues to grow at a more normal rate (Figure 4.12). At the same time, the corneas, and possibly the crystalline lenses, become flatter in both eyes. The concomitant increase in the eye's focal length results in a systematic reduction of the myopia in the formerly deprived eye. Once the vitreous chamber depth of the fellow control eye catches up to that of the formerly deprived eye, the refractive errors in the two eyes are reasonably matched. Subsequently, the formerly deprived eye begins to grow again and both eyes adopt similar vitreous chamber growth rates. Recovery from hyperopia can also be attributed to alterations in axial growth rates. Upon restoring unrestricted vision, monkeys with hyperopic anisometropia exhibit a relative acceleration in axial growth in the treated eyes that eliminates interocular differences in refractive error (Smith III *et al.*, 1994a).

Due to the manner in which recovery from experimentally induced refractive errors is achieved, the ability of a given animal to recover will greatly depend upon the age at which unrestricted vision is restored. For example, it is unlikely that a monkey could recover fully from form-deprivation myopia if unrestricted vision was restored after the age at which the cornea had stopped flattening. Since it

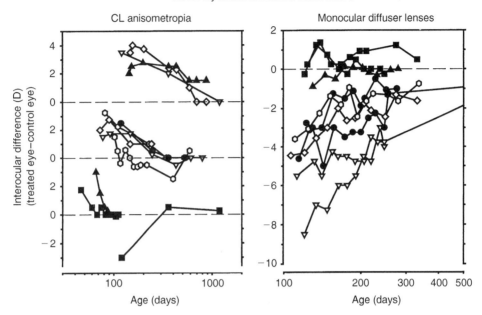

Figure 4.11 Interocular differences in spherical-equivalent refractive error plotted as a function of age for individual monkeys with anisometropia produced experimentally by rearing the animals with a high, negative-powered, contact lens on one eye (*left*) or with a diffuser spectacle lens in front of one eye (*right*). The first data point for each subject represents the degree and direction of anisometropia that existed at the end of the treatment period, i.e., at the start of the recovery period. Points plotted above the dashed zero lines indicate that the treated eye was more hyperopic or less myopic than the fellow control eye. To facilitate comparisons, some of the data in the left graph have been shifted vertically. All but one of the contact lens-reared monkeys exhibited hyperopic anisometropia whereas the majority of diffuser-reared monkeys showed myopic anisometropia. Both treatment groups exhibited evidence of recovery from the experimentally induced refractive errors; following removal of the stimulus for abnormal growth, almost every subject showed a systematic decrease in anisometropia. (From Smith III, 1997)

does not appear that vision-dependent mechanisms can result in an absolute reduction in axial length or in compensating corneal growth, simply stopping abnormal axial elongation would not compensate for the experimentally induced myopia unless the optical power of the eye could in some other way be decreased. Wallman (1993) has suggested that this age-dependent limitation in the ability of the primate eye to recover from myopia may explain why myopia that develops in teenage or adult humans is typically permanent. In contrast, normal infants that are myopic shortly after birth frequently show emmetropization (Gwiazda *et al.*, 1993a).

The ability of a monkey to recover from an induced refractive error may also be influenced by factors unrelated to the quality of the retinal image during post-treatment periods of unrestricted vision. Experimental manipulations that produce abnormal refractive errors can also

result in severe sensory deficits associated with amblyopia and strabismus (Smith III *et al.*, 1985; Harwerth *et al.*, 1981; Quick *et al.*, 1989). The presence of amblyopia or strabismus can preclude emmetropization and promote the development of anomalous refractive errors in both humans (Lepard, 1975; Abrahamsson, 1992) and monkeys (Smith III *et al.*, 1994b; Kiorpes and Wallman, 1995). Deviating and/or amblyopic eyes frequently fail to undergo emmetropization and instead can show increases in the magnitude of their refractive errors over long periods of time, particularly in the hyperopic direction. It is not known how these sensory deficits, which are thought to reflect primarily neural alterations in the visual cortex, influence ocular growth. However, it seems unlikely that monkeys that develop amblyopia and/or strabismus will fully recover from an experimentally induced refractive error.

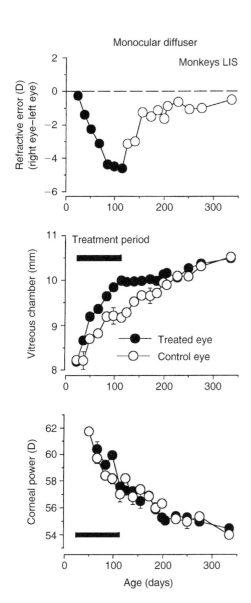

Monocular diffuser

Monkeys LIS

4.4.2 Compensation for optically induced anisometropia

The recovery phenomena described above demonstrate that the eyes of young monkeys can grow in a manner which eliminates an existing anisometropia, and are in agreement with the idea that ocular growth is regulated by optical defocus. A more rigorous test of the role of defocus in regulating emmetropization can be obtained by altering the effective refractive status of young animals using spectacle lenses, and determining whether their eyes grow in a manner that compensates for the optically induced error. For example, placing a negative lens in front of an emmetropic eye would optically simulate hyperopia. To compensate for the lens, i.e., to re-establish emmetropia, the eye would have to develop a degree of myopia equivalent to the power of the lens. On the other hand, a positive lens would produce an artificial myopia and would require the eye to become more hyperopic in order to re-establish the optimal refractive state.

Beginning with a series of studies by Frank Schaeffel and his colleagues (Schaeffel *et al.*, 1988; Schaeffel and Howland, 1991), it has been demonstrated that infants of several species, most notably the chicken, are capable of a high degree of differential interocular growth in response to viewing the world through anisometropic spectacle lenses. For example, young chicks are capable of fully compensating for lens powers between about −10 and +15 D (Irving *et al.*, 1992; Wildsoet and Wallman, 1995; Schmid and Wildsoet, 1996). However, early attempts to alter predictably refractive development in primates by experimentally imposing optical defocus did not consistently produce compensating ocular growth that would effectively eliminate an artificial refractive error (Smith III *et al.*, 1985; Crewther *et al.*, 1988; Chung, 1993; Smith III *et al.*, 1994a). It is likely that methodological issues, in particular the use of contact lenses which have been shown to produce refractive alterations in infant monkeys via non-visual mechanisms (Hung and Smith III, 1996), confounded many of these early studies. As shown below, young monkeys exhibit differential interocular growth in response to anisometropic spectacle lenses, though the magnitude of the interocular changes that can be produced is much smaller than that observed in sub-primate species like the chicken.

An impressive aspect of refractive development in young monkeys is that the two eyes of most

Figure 4.12 Longitudinal data from an infant monkey reared with a diffuser spectacle lens in front of one eye. (*Top*) Interocular differences in spherical-equivalent refractive error plotted as a function of age. Negative points indicate that the treated eye was less hyperopic or more myopic than the control eye. The filled symbols represent data obtained during the treatment period. (*Middle, bottom*) Vitreous chamber depth and corneal refractive power. The treated and control eyes are represented by the filled and open symbols, respectively. The horizontal bar shows the treatment period. (From Smith III, 1997)

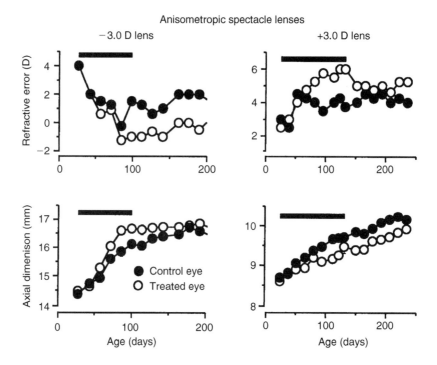

Figure 4.13 Spherical-equivalent refractive error (*top*) and either axial length (*bottom left*) or vitreous chamber depth (*bottom right*) plotted as a function of age of two monkeys reared −3 D (*left*) or +3.0 D lenses (*right*) in front of their treated eyes. The control eyes viewed through plano lenses. The filled horizontal bars indicate the treatment period when the animals wore the spectacle lenses. Both animals developed anisometropia that compensated for imbalance imposed by the treatment lenses. (From Smith III, 1997)

infants are well matched. Before 3–4 weeks of age, most normal infant monkeys exhibit moderate hyperopic errors between about 4 and 6 D. Over the next two months, there is a systematic and coordinated decrease in hyperopia in both eyes to levels typically between about 1.5 and 3 D of hyperopia. It appears that a low degree of hyperopia is the 'desired' refractive state for young monkeys. Throughout this early emmetropization, axial dimensions, corneal power and overall refractive status are nearly identical in the two eyes. However, low powered anisometropic spectacle lenses predictably disrupt the normal balance between the two eyes of infant monkeys.

Anisometropic spectacles optically simulate an interocular imbalance in the refractive state of young monkeys because infants are typically isometropic and because accommodation is yoked between the two eyes. The effective sign of the resulting optical defocus depends upon the subject's fixation pattern. Infant monkeys treated with negative lenses in front of one eye and a plano lens over their fellow eye typically

posture their accommodation for the control eye viewing through the plano lens. Consequently, the eye viewing through the negative lens experiences chronic hyperopic defocus (secondary focal point posterior to the retina) equal in magnitude to the power of the spectacle lens. It is interesting that anisometropic spectacles that consist of a positive lens and a plano lens also produce hyperopic defocus. Presumably because positive lenses compensate for the natural hyperopia in young monkeys and reduce accommodative demands for most objects, infant monkeys typically prefer to fixate with the eye viewing through the positive lens. As a result, the fellow eye viewing through the plano lens experiences chronic hyperopic defocus (Hung *et al.*, 1995).

As shown in Figure 4.13, during the course of wearing lenses that initially produce 3 D of anisometropia, the defocused eyes assume a faster axial growth rate than the 'in focus' eyes, and concomitantly infant monkeys develop over a period of months an anisometropia that is equal in magnitude to the power of the lens held in front of the

Interocular refractive error differences: anisometropic spectacles (treated eye–control eye)

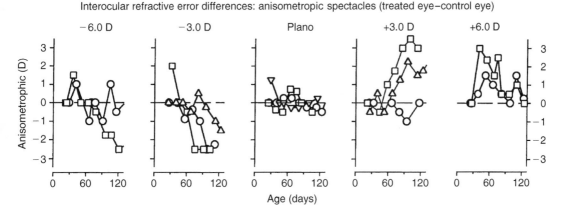

Figure 4.14 Interocular refractive error differences plotted as a function of age for individual monkeys reared with anisometropic spectacle lenses. Negative values indicate that the treated eye was more myopic or less hyperopic than the fellow control eye. The power of the anisometropic lenses is indicated above each graph. Control monkeys were reared with plano lenses in front of both eyes (*middle*). All data were obtained during the treatment period; the first point for each subject indicates the start of lens wear. (From Smith III, 1997)

treated eye. As a result, by the end of the treatment period, both eyes would be in focus simultaneously when the monkeys viewed through the anisometropic treatment lenses.

In essence, young monkeys appear to solve the imposed anisometropia by using a 'grow to clarity' strategy. The mechanisms that are responsible for the phenomenon of form-deprivation myopia could provide an effective means of balancing the refractive errors in the two eyes. By fixating with the effectively less hyperopic eye, the non-fixating eye experiences chronic hyperopic defocus. As illustrated in Figure 4.9 above, the resulting degree of defocus is capable of producing axial myopia. Thus, the initial unilateral defocus produced by anisometropic lenses would produce a relative acceleration in axial growth. However, once isometropia was re-established and clear vision was restored to both eyes, the stimulus for differential growth between the two eyes would be eliminated. Regardless of the nature of the mechanisms which mediate this differential growth, it is clear that the altered retinal imagery associated with optical defocus can produce differential interocular growth in infant monkeys. It seems reasonable to speculate that similar mechanisms may be responsible for the fact that low degrees of anisometropia are frequently transient in young human infants (Abrahamsson and Sjostrand, 1996) and that the overall magnitude of anisometropia in young infants decreases rapidly during early development (Almender *et al.*, 1990).

There is, however, a limit to the interocular refractive error changes that can predictably be produced with anisometropic lenses in infant monkeys. For example, monkeys reared with spectacle lenses that impose 6 D of anisometropia demonstrate interocular differences in ocular growth and refractive error that are larger than those found in control animals reared with zero-powered lenses over both eyes. And although these observed changes are in the appropriate direction, they are not large enough to completely compensate for the treatment lenses and are frequently transient in nature (Figure 4.14).

It is not known why infant monkeys exhibit inconsistent refractive error changes in response to the defocus associated with high degrees (6 D) of imposed anisometropia. However, in a somewhat analogous manner, young human infants with high anisometropias (e.g. over 3 D at 12 months of age) are more likely to retain their anisometropia as they get older and in some case the anisometropia may increase in magnitude (Abrahamsson and Sjostrand, 1996). Overall, these results are not consistent with the idea that defocus is the only visual cue that influences ocular growth, and that form-deprivation mechanisms alone are responsible for the differential axial growth found with lower degrees of anisometropia (e.g. 3 D). One possible explanation is that the higher degrees of anisometropia cause other visual system alterations (e.g. amblyopia) which somehow interfere with the effects of chronic defocus on ocular growth. This, however, is not a particularly satisfying explanation since monocular form deprivation, which produces profound sensory deficits, consistently results in exaggerated ocular growth and high degrees of myopic anisometropia. However, the high degrees of anisometropia that are produced by form deprivation rule out the possibility that the observed pattern of results is simply due to some physical limit on the magnitude of differential interocular growth in infant monkeys.

4.4.3   Compensation for bilateral spectacle lenses

In addition to altering the refractive balance between the two eyes, spectacle lenses can also produce predictable refractive changes in the fixating eyes of infant monkeys. An indication of compensating growth for 'in focus' eyes can be seen in the refractive histories of monkeys treated with positive-powered anisometropic lenses. For example, monkeys which fixate through low-powered positive lenses frequently exhibit either an absence of the normal reduction in hyperopia associated with emmetropization or a small increase in hyperopia in the fixating eye (Figure 4.13, *right*). However, in infant monkeys, the effects of optically imposed changes in the refractive status of fixating eyes can best be observed in animals reared with equal-powered, bilateral spectacle lenses. With binocular lenses, it is possible to impose myopia as well as hyperopia, and measures of the effective operating range of the emmetropization process will not be influenced by any potential interocular limitations in differential eye growth.

Infant monkeys show a remarkable degree of adaptability in response to binocular spectacle lenses. Following the introduction of negative lenses that impose moderate degrees of hyperopia (Figure 4.15 B,C), infant monkeys exhibit myopic shifts attaining refractive errors that are typically slightly less myopic than the nominal powers of the spectacle lenses. It is reasonable to argue that these animals have completely compensated for the treatment lenses because when viewing through the lenses, the animals effectively manifest a low degree of hyperopia, i.e., the near ideal refractive state for an infant monkey. Compelling evidence for compensation is also evident in monkeys fitted with moderate powered positive lenses. Positive lenses consistently prevent or greatly reduce the normal reduction in hyperopia that occurs in young monkeys so that the animals manifest a low degree of hyperopia with the treatment

lenses in place (Figure 4.15 D,E). It is apparent that in these animals there is little need for emmetropization because the spectacle lenses artificially produce the desired refractive state. This argument is bolstered by the observation that the positive lens-treated monkeys typically show clear signs of emmetropization during the recovery period following lens removal.

In infant primates, the emmetropization process appears to have a finite operating range. For imposed refractive errors ranging from 2 D of myopia to 8 D of hyperopia (open symbols, Figure 4.16), infant monkeys consistently exhibit evidence for compensating ocular growth. In other words, if an infant monkey (in this case 3–4 weeks of age) has a refractive error within this range, its eyes are capable of achieving the near ideal refractive state during emmetropization, i.e., a low degree of hyperopia. However, there are limits to the degree of compensating growth produced by spectacle lenses. For initial refractive errors outside this range, the emmetropization process either does not function or is simply unable to produce changes in ocular growth that are large enough to compensate for the initial error (Figure 4.15 A,F).

The effective emmetropization range for infant monkeys does not simply represent a limit in the degree to which the refractive error of an eye can change. It is possible to produce larger overall changes in refractive state as long as the imposed refractive errors fall within the effective operating range of the emmetropization process. As shown in Figure 4.17, by sequentially increasing the power of the treatment lenses in small increments in response to changes in the eye's refractive state, it is possible to produce larger refractive error changes and, in particular, significant increases in the absolute level of hyperopia in response to myopic defocus.

Like the anisometropia that develops in response to optically induced unilateral defocus, refractive compensation for changes in the fixating eye's effective refractive status come about primarily as a result of changes in the rate of axial elongation. For example, compare the rates of vitreous chamber elongation for the positive versus negative lens-treated monkeys illustrated in Figure 4.17. Positive lenses cause a relative reduction in vitreous chamber growth whereas negative lenses promote axial elongation.

4.4.4   Ocular mechanisms involved in lens compensation

With regard to the anisometropic changes described above, the idea that defocused retinal

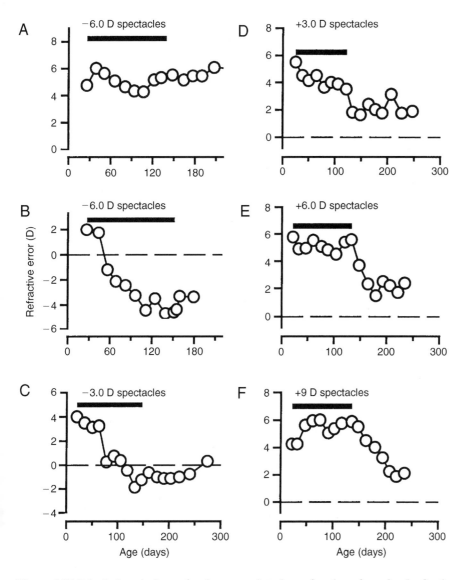

Figure 4.15 Spherical-equivalent refractive error plotted as a function of age for the fixating eyes of representative monkeys reared with equal-powered spectacle lenses over both eyes. The horizontal bars indicate the period of lens wear. The power of the lenses is shown for each monkey. (Data from Hung and Smith III, 1995; Hung *et al.*, 1996)

images accelerate axial growth and promote myopia whereas focused images slow down axial elongation can largely explain emmetropization in infant monkeys and the compensating changes produced in fixating eyes by spectacle lenses. Even though infant monkeys can accommodate to compensate for hyperopic focusing errors, it is likely that animals with significant degrees of hyperopia, whether natural errors or those imposed by negative lenses, do not always exert the full effort

required to maintain clear vision. Thus, in comparison with monkeys having a more ideal refractive state, these hyperopic monkeys would experience higher, time-averaged, degrees of defocus which would result in accelerated axial growth, presumably via form deprivation mechanisms. Subsequently, as these monkeys become less hyperopic, longer periods of clear vision would reduce axial growth rates. Accordingly, hyperopic monkeys that were corrected with positive lenses would experi-

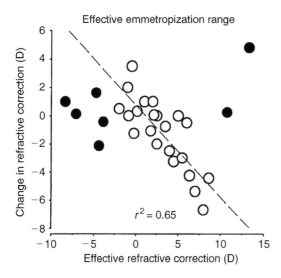

Effective emmetropization range

$r^2 = 0.65$

Figure 4.16 Change in the spherical-equivalent refractive error that occurred during the lens-rearing period for the fixating eyes of individual monkeys plotted as a function of the eyes' initial effective refractive error. Positive changes represent hyperopic shifts; negative values indicate that the monkey became less hyperopic or more myopic. The effective refractive error was defined as the natural refractive error correction minus the power of the spectacle lens placed in front of the eyes. Positive effective refractive errors represent eyes that showed a residual hyperopia when viewing through their spectacle lenses. The change in refractive error was correlated with the effective error for initial values between −2 and +8 D (open symbols). The filled symbols represent animals with initial errors that were apparently outside the effective operating range of the infant monkey's emmetropization process. (From Smith III, 1997)

ence greater periods of clear vision than uncorrected monkeys, show slower axial growth rates, and ultimately manifest more hyperopic refractive errors. Absolute hyperopic shifts in refractive error could come about if axial growth was dramatically reduced, but at the same time, the cornea continued to flatten.

However, form deprivation mechanisms alone cannot account for some findings in higher primates. In particular, high degrees of imposed hyperopia often fail to produce compensating growth in infant monkeys. For example, the monkey shown in Figure 4.15A was a 4.75 hyperope, and the −6.00 D treatment lenses imposed an initial effective hyperopic error of 10.75 D. However, despite the fact that young monkeys have a sufficiently large amplitude of accommodation to over-

come imposed errors of this magnitude, this monkey made no attempt to accommodate in order to obtain clear vision and, therefore, habitually experienced a high degree of hyperopic defocus. Interestingly, this animal showed no evidence of myopic growth; instead, it exhibited the same degree of hyperopia throughout the treatment period. Similarly, infant monkeys that habitually experience high degrees of defocus following the surgical removal of their crystalline lens also fail to show accelerated axial elongation (Wilson *et al.*, 1987). These results also suggest that factors other than the quality or clarity of the retinal image influence ocular growth.

Investigations in the chicken have provided substantial insight into how visual feedback could influence ocular development. Firstly, it appears that multiple vision-dependent mechanisms probably influence ocular development. In particular, several observations suggest that form-deprivation myopia and the myopia that develops in response to negative lenses are mediated via different mechanisms. Form-deprivation myopia is blocked by intravitreal injections of the neurotoxin, 6-hydroxydopamine (Schaeffel *et al.*, 1994a) and by continuous exposure to light (Bartmann *et al.*, 1994); however, the myopia produced by negative lenses is not. In addition, severing the optic nerve does not prevent form-deprivation myopia (Troilo *et al.*, 1987; Troilo and Wallman, 1991; Wildsoet and Pettigrew, 1988), but it reduces the myopia produced by negative lenses (Wildsoet and Wallman, 1995) and interferes with the recovery from form-deprivation myopia (Troilo *et al.*, 1997). Although different mechanisms seem to underlie deprivation- and lens-induced myopia in chicks, these mechanisms apparently share some common biochemical features because, for example, both phenomena are blocked by reserpine, an agent that lowers retinal levels of dopamine and serotonin (Schaeffel *et al.*, 1995).

Research in the chick also suggests that the developing eye is able to detect the sign of defocus and alter its growth in the appropriate direction to eliminate both myopic and hyperopic defocus. This idea grew out of the initial observations that positive lenses produced hyperopia whereas negative lenses produced myopia (Schaeffel *et al.*, 1988; Irving *et al.*, 1992). The best evidence for this hypothesis comes from recent experiments which have shown that chicks exhibit appropriate compensating growth for equivalent degrees of hyperopic and myopic defocus even when accommodation and all obvious behavioural cues to the

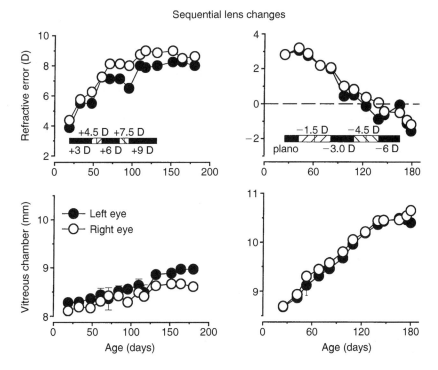

Figure 4.17 Refractive error (*top*) and vitreous chamber depth (*bottom*) plotted as a function of age for two representative monkeys that were treated with a series of increasing powered positive (*left*) or negative spectacle lenses (*right*). The period and the powers of the lenses are shown by the horizontal bars. Progressive increases in positive power produce a systematic increases in hyperopia, whereas progressive increases in negative power promoted myopia. In comparison to the negative lens-treated monkey, the hyperopic monkey also showed a much slower vitreous chamber growth rate. (From Smith III, 1997)

sign of the effective refractive error are excluded (Feldkaemper *et al.*, 1997). The fact that chicks compensate appropriately for myopic and hyperopic defocus in the presence of astigmatic blur also argues that the sign of defocus is important and that degraded images *per se* do not always produce axial myopia (McLean and Wallman, 1997).

Overall, it appears that, at least in the chick, the control of eye growth occurs on at least two levels, one of which is located entirely within the eye and is responsible for deprivation myopia and another which involves neural processes outside the eye and is involved in vision-dependent emmetropization. In addition, compensation for lens-induced hyperopic and myopic growth may be mediated by different processes because reserpine blocks compensation for negative lenses, but not for positive lenses (Schaeffel *et al.*, 1995). At the present time, it is unknown whether similar mechanisms are involved in regulating ocular growth in primates. Nevertheless, it is clear that no single mechanism can readily explain all of the vision-dependent

alterations in refractive error observed in monkeys. Regardless of the number and nature of these mechanisms, the overall weight of evidence clearly indicates that emmetropization in higher primates is regulated by optical defocus and that changes in the eye's effective focus produced by a spectacle lens can alter ocular growth and refractive development in infants.

4.5   Astigmatism and astigmatic compensation

The previous sections of this chapter have concentrated on spherical or spherical equivalent refractive errors, i.e., myopia and hyperopia. However, astigmatism is the most common refractive anomaly in the general population. Although relatively little is known about the genesis of astigmatism, research in laboratory animals has shed light on two major issues concerning astigmatism. Firstly, is uncorrected astigmatism a risk factor for the development of refractive error like myopia? Secondly, is there a vision-dependent 'sphericalization' process?

4.5.1   Astigmatism disrupts emmetropization

Although astigmatism could theoretically guide emmetropization (Wallman, 1993), in humans the presence of astigmatism early in life is frequently associated with spherical ametropia later in life, particularly myopia (Fulton *et al.*, 1982; Ehrlich *et al.*, 1995). It has logically been argued that this association comes about because the chronic image degradation produced by uncorrected astigmatism triggers the onset of form-deprivation myopia. Similarly, it is reasonable to hypothesize that uncorrected astigmatism, by disrupting normal emmetropization, could promote the development of anisometropia, another condition which is associated with the presence of early astigmatism (Ingram and Barr, 1979; Abrahamsson *et al.*, 1988). In studies of human refractive development, it is difficult to determine whether uncorrected astigmatism is a risk factor for the development of other refractive errors since additional factors may be responsible for both the astigmatism and the spherical refractive errors. However, by rearing infant monkeys with cylindrical lenses over one or both eyes it is possible to isolate the effects of astigmatic defocus on primate emmetropization.

At about 3 weeks of age, normal infant monkeys have relatively little corneal or refractive astigmatism (Smith III *et al.*, 1997). Consequently, viewing through cylindrical spectacle lenses which have a spherical equivalent power of zero (e.g. +1.50/−3.00×180) effectively simulates uncorrected astigmatism without altering the location of the circle of least confusion. In comparison with normal monkeys, cylinder-reared monkeys show atypical changes in ametropia and a much wider range of spherical-equivalent refractive errors (Figure 4.18). Many cylinder-reared monkeys showed little or no reduction in hyperopia with age or in some cases an increase in hyperopia. Others showed an overall reduction in hyperopia, but the course of emmetropization was interrupted by significant hyperopic shifts. Interestingly, few cylinder-reared monkeys exhibited a significant degree of myopia. The refractive balance between the two eyes was also frequently disrupted; in particular, many monkeys who wore cylindrical lenses over one eye showed a high prevalence of anisometropia. Another indication that astigmatism alters emmetropization was observed following lens removal;

many cylinder-reared monkeys showed significant changes in refractive error in one or both eyes, typically toward more normal, isometropic refractive errors.

In contrast with the idea that astigmatism disrupts emmetropization by initiating deprivation myopia, the high prevalence of hyperopia indicates that the refractive anomalies in cylinder-reared monkeys are not simply a consequence of an overall reduction in retinal image quality. Many cylinder-reared monkeys, like many young human infants (Dobson *et al.*, 1983), appear to adjust their accommodation for the least hyperopic meridian (Smith III *et al.*, 1997). Presumably because the vision-dependent mechanisms that regulate refractive development are insensitive to orientation cues, emmetropization is apparently directed toward the focal point for one of the meridians of the cylinder lens, with this typically (although not always) being the least hyperopic meridian. Consequently, many of the effects of astigmatism on refractive development could occur primarily because the eye does not grow in a manner that brings the circle of least confusion into focus, but instead emmetropization is directed toward one of the astigmatic line foci.

4.5.2   Sphericalization

In some respects, the changes in ocular astigmatism during early development are somewhat analogous to the reduction in spherical refractive errors associated with early emmetropization. Before one year of age, most human infants exhibit a significant degree of astigmatism. However, during normal maturation there is a systematic reduction in the magnitude of astigmatic error (Atkinson *et al.*, 1980; Ehrlich *et al.*, 1995). This pattern of refractive development raises the possibility that the eye can detect the presence of astigmatism and grow in a manner that eliminates this optical error.

Experiments to test the idea that there is a vision-dependent sphericalization process in young chicks have yielded contradictory results. Irving *et al.* (1991, 1992, 1995) found that young chicks reared with astigmatic errors imposed by cylindrical spectacle lenses developed refractive astigmatism which partially compensated for the induced astigmatic errors. The degree of compensation was greatest when the axis of the cylinder lenses was oriented obliquely. Even for oblique cylinders, the magnitude of refractive astigmatism that the animals developed during the treatment period (which

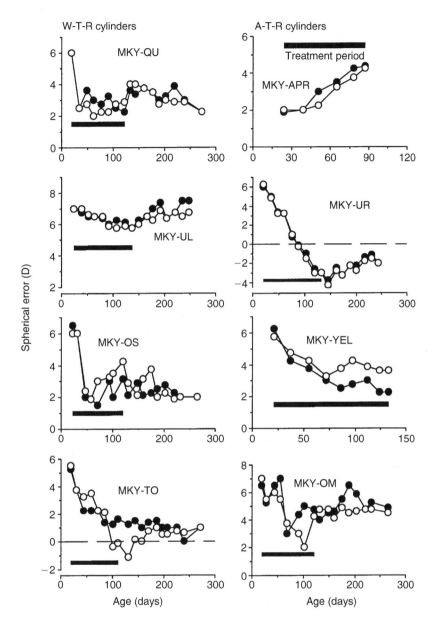

Figure 4.18 Spherical-equivalent refractive error plotted as a function of age for representative monkeys reared with either with- (W-T-R, *left*) or against-the-rule (A-T-R, *right*) cylinder lenses (+1.50/−3.00 × 90 or 180). The top four panels show data from animals reared with binocular lenses; the lower four panels represent data from monocularly treated monkeys. The filled horizontal bars indicate the lens-rearing period. (Redrawn from Smith III *et al.*, 1997)

was mostly corneal in nature) was only equivalent to approximately 60% of the total power of the cylinder lens. However, Laskowski and Howland (1996) and Schmid and Wildsoet (1997), using a similar rearing strategy, failed to find convincing evidence that young chicks developed refractive astigmatism which compensated for the astigmatic

defocus imposed by an external cylinder lens. Thus, the question of whether cylindrical lenses alter astigmatism in chicks is unresolved.

It should also be noted that infant monkeys reared with cylindrical lenses frequently develop significant degrees of refractive astigmatism (Smith III *et al.*, 1997). Longitudinal measures of corneal power indicate that the induced astigmatism is corneal in nature and is brought about by the decrease in refractive power that occurs if normal development is interrupted along one corneal meridian (Figure 4.19). The resulting astigmatism does not, however, optically compensate for the cylinder lenses. Regardless of whether the axis of the cylinder lens is positioned to simulate either with- or against-the-rule astigmatism, the axis of the induced astigmatism is typically oblique and when both eyes show astigmatism, the axes in the two eyes are mirror-symmetric and oblique in orientation (e.g. correcting minus cylinder lens axes of about 120–150° for the right eyes and 35–60° in left eyes). The mismatch between the orientation of the principal meridians of the eye and the axis of the cylindrical lens shifts the axis of the effective astigmatic error produced by viewing through the cylinder lenses. Consequently, even when the induced refractive astigmatism is similar in magnitude to the cylinder power of the treatment lenses, the monkeys still experience significant degrees of astigmatic defocus when viewing through the lenses.

The presence of astigmatism is not unique to monkeys reared with cylindrical lenses and, in this regard, the prevalence of astigmatism in monkeys with experimentally induced refractive errors produced by other rearing strategies provides insight into the genesis of the induced astigmatism (Huang *et al.*, 1997). Astigmatism occurs most frequently in animals who exhibit reduced vitreous chamber growth rates and hyperopic refractive errors (Figure 4.20). For example, in addition to the hyperopic cylinder-reared monkeys that showed high degrees of astigmatism, monkeys reared with bilateral positive lenses, especially those that demonstrated absolute increases in hyperopia (*see* Figure 4.17 for example), frequently developed high degrees of astigmatism. The astigmatic errors exhibited by animals reared with spherical lenses were also oblique, strongly correlated with changes in corneal shape, and followed a similar time course to those shown by cylinder-reared monkeys. In contrast, animals that exhibited an increase in axial elongation and/or developed myopia as a result of an experimental manipulation were rarely astigmatic. For example, diffuser-reared monkeys develop substantial degrees of axial myopia (*see* Figure 4.9), however, they exhibit very little corneal or refractive astigmatism. Similarly, the reduction in astigmatism observed in hyperopic monkeys following lens removal was typically associated with a concomitant reduction in hyperopia.

Thus, the results in infant monkeys show that vision-dependent processes are capable of altering the shape of the cornea and producing astigmatism. However, the resulting astigmatism does not appear to be an attempt to compensate for astigmatic defocus, and there is no convincing evidence for a vision-dependent sphericalization mechanism. To the contrary, the astigmatism observed in many monkeys with experimentally induced refractive errors appears to be a side-effect to a more general alteration in ocular growth, and is most common when axial growth is slowed. In this respect, the normal reduction in astigmatism observed in young human infants may be a consequence of the rapid axial elongation that occurs early in life.

4.6   Relation to human refractive error development

The weight of experimental evidence clearly indicates that fundamental aspects of ocular growth and refractive development in a wide range of animal species, including higher primates, are regulated by visual feedback associated with the eye's effective refractive status. This line of research raises intriguing questions about human refractive development, but, there are a number of issues that one should consider in attempting to extrapolate these results to the human condition. One of the foremost considerations is the degree to which results obtained in laboratory animals apply to human refractive development. In this respect, it is reassuring that many experimental manipulations yield qualitatively similar results in a wide variety of species. Despite obvious inter-species differences in ocular physiology (e.g. differences in the mechanism and pharmacology of accommodation; differences in the composition of the sclera), the eyes of different animals respond in fundamentally the same way to changes in the visual environment. Although there are clear quantitative differences in the magnitude and rapidity of vision-initiated changes in refractive development, there do not appear to be any fundamental differences between the most commonly studied species, the chicken, and the macaque monkey, the animal model which is most closely related to the human. Moreover, many normal aspects of refractive development in animals are analogous to aspects of

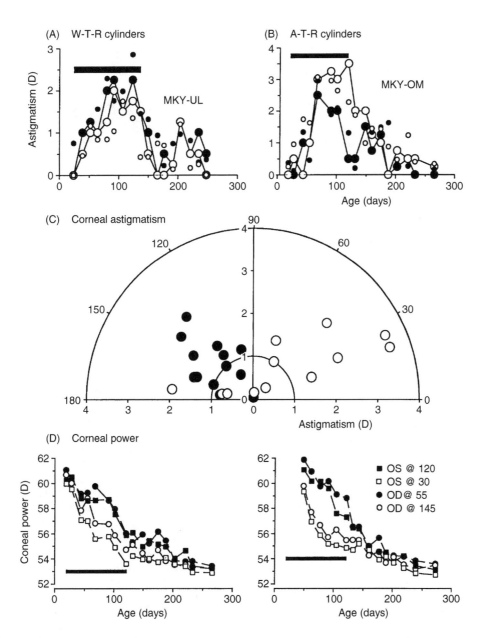

Figure 4.19 Magnitude of ocular (large circles) and corneal astigmatism (small circles) plotted as a function of age for both eyes (right = filled symbols; left = open symbols) of representative monkeys reared with cylinder lenses (+1.50/−3.00 × 90 or 180) oriented at axis 90° (W-T-R) or 180° (A-T-R) (A, B). The filled horizontal bar indicates the treatment period. (C) Polar plot of corneal astigmatism at the end of the treatment period for individual right (filled symbols) and left eyes (open symbols). The degree of astigmatism is represented by the distance from the origin; the direction of astigmatism is shown using minus-cylinder axis notation. (D) Corneal power for the principal meridians in the right (circles) and left (squares) eyes of two monkeys plotted as a function of age. The open and filled symbols represent the meridians corresponding to the minus-cylinder axis and the orthogonal power meridian, respectively. (Redrawn from Smith III *et al.*, 1997)

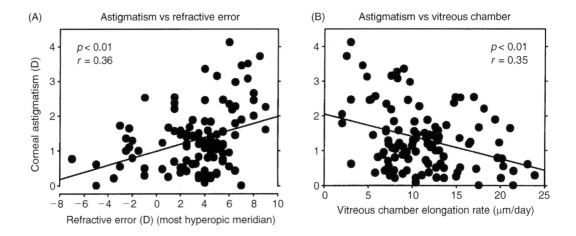

Figure 4.20 Corneal astigmatism at the end of the treatment period plotted as a function of refractive error (A) and vitreous chamber elongation rate (B) for individual eyes of monkeys with experimentally induced refractive errors. Corneal astigmatism was highest for hyperopic eyes and eyes that showed slow vitreous chamber growth rates. (Data from Huang *et al.*, 1997)

human refractive development (e.g. the phenomenon of emmetropization).

In view of the close similarities in ocular anatomy and the overall structure and function of their visual sensory and ocular-motor systems, it is generally considered that experimental results obtained in macaque monkeys can be extrapolated to humans with a very high degree of confidence. However, it is important to keep in mind that some inconsistencies have been observed between different species of macaque monkeys. Most notably, topically applied atropine and optic nerve section have been reported to block deprivation myopia in pigtail monkeys (*Macaca nemistrina*), but not in rhesus monkeys (*Macaca mulatta*; Raviola and Wiesel, 1985). Therefore, subtle genetic differences may cause the eyes to respond in a different manner to some environmental manipulations. Although this difference raises some concerns, in one sense this discrepancy is potentially important because it is also likely that the susceptibility to environmental factors varies between individual humans or humans from different ethnic backgrounds. In this respect, the differences between these two monkey species may provide additional parallels with human refractive development.

In extrapolating results from laboratory animals to humans it is important to take into account the different rates of ocular development. Based upon comparisons of the relative rates of axial elongation, infant monkeys mature about three times faster

than infant humans (Kiely *et al.*, 1987). Using this 3:1 ratio, the typical experimental observation period for infant monkeys corresponds to approximately the first 2–3 years in a human's life. Longitudinal refractive data indicates that the initial emmetropization in human infants is largely completed during this period (Gwiazda *et al.*, 1993a).

Reasonably, the results from monkeys suggest that human ocular growth during this period is regulated by visual feedback associated with the eye's effective refractive status. However, there have not been any systematic investigations of the effects of visual experience on older monkeys, in particular, animals with ages that are equivalent to those when adolescent humans most commonly develop refractive anomalies. Therefore, in the absence of other information, it is speculative to apply the available results from infant monkeys to explain refractive anomalies or guide management strategies for older humans. Recently, however, it has been demonstrated in the chicken (Papastergiou *et al.*, 1997) and tree shrew (Norton, personal communication) that form deprivation is capable of producing axial myopia in sexually mature animals, but in comparison with younger animals, the ocular responses are attenuated. Thus, it is possible that the same vision-dependent mechanisms that influence early ocular growth are also functioning later in life, but are simply not capable of producing refractive changes that are as dramatic as those observed in infants.

The refractive error experiments described above were conducted on essentially normal infant monkeys. The performance properties of the mechanisms that regulate ocular growth are known to vary between individuals (Schaeffel and Howland, 1991), and it is possible that the emmetropization mechanisms in infants with abnormal refractive errors are very different from those in the average child. If so, the principles derived from normal animals may not apply to refractive development in children with abnormal refractive errors. For example, high hyperopia in very young infants poses a risk for the development of amblyopia and strabismus which may be reduced by wearing correcting spectacles (Atkinson, 1993). However, lens-rearing experiments in monkeys suggest that hyperopic infants fully corrected with spectacles would not undergo emmetropization, but instead remain hyperopic. In agreement with this notion, there is some evidence that fully corrected, hyperopic infants are less likely to undergo emmetropization than uncorrected hyperopic infants (Ingram *et al.*, 1991). Thus, to avoid interfering with emmetropization, animal research would suggest that one should correct part, but not all of an infant's hyperopic error (*see* Atkinson, 1993). This management strategy is based on the assumption that highly hyperopic eyes have normal emmetropization mechanisms that respond to optical defocus in the same manner as those in the average child. However, it is very possible that vision-dependent, growth-regulating mechanisms are dysfunctional in these eyes–this may be why these eyes have abnormal refractive errors in the first place–and regardless of the eye's effective focus, the eye will always remain hyperopic. It will be important to gain a better understanding of potential individual differences in the response characteristics of the emmetropization process in order to design the optimal correction strategy for young infants–in this hypothetical case, a correction that would promote normal sensory and motor development as well as emmetropization.

The effects of interruptions in lens wear should also be considered when weighing the potential consequences of spectacle lenses on refractive development in very young human infants. In chicks, very brief daily periods of unrestricted vision are sufficient to prevent deprivation myopia (Napper *et al.*, 1995) and the myopia produced by wearing negative lenses (Schmid and Wildsoet, 1996). Additionally, the magnitude of hyperopia induced by positive lenses, although influenced to a smaller degree than induced myopic changes, decreases systematically in proportion to the length of daily periods of unrestricted vision (Schmid and Wildsoet, 1996). During the monkey experiments described above, lens wear was virtually continuous without any significant interruptions. With traditional correcting lenses, it is simply not possible to achieve similar compliance rates in human infants. At the present time, we do not know whether or not the inevitable interruptions in lens wear that occur in human infants will, in large part, negate any potential effects of correcting lenses on refractive development.

Although there are many unresolved issues related to the clinical application of experimental results from animals, these studies provide reason to question some time-honoured ideas and practices concerning the aetiology of refractive errors. In particular, the well-known association between near viewing environments and the prevalence of myopia, together with the recognized synchrony between myopia onset and the participation in near visual tasks, form the foundation for the 'use–abuse' theory of myopia (Weymouth and Hirsch, 1991). According to this classic theory, myopia is an adaptation to the near environment and something about the act of performing nearwork causes the eye to become myopic. It is often speculated that prolonged accommodation and/or convergence somehow promote axial elongation and myopia, possibly through mechanical forces exerted by the extraocular muscles or alterations in intraocular pressure. However, recent findings of accommodative dysfunction in human myopes and experimental findings in laboratory animals provide a different view of this association.

One of the most consistent and pervasive results from animal research is that degrading the quality of the retinal image typically results in axial myopia. At the same time, the preponderance of evidence suggests that accommodation may only influence ocular growth indirectly via its influence on retinal image quality (Raviola and Wiesel, 1985; Wallman, 1993). Assuming that these observations can legitimately be applied to humans, i.e., specifically that image degradation associated with optical defocus can promote axial myopia in humans, an alternative explanation for the association between nearwork and myopia is that the myopia develops as a consequence of low degrees of chronic optical defocus that come about in some individuals during nearwork. In support of this idea, children who develop myopia frequently exhibit higher than normal lags of accommodation in response to dioptric blur (Gwiazda *et al.*, 1993b,

1995). Since under-accommodating would degrade the quality of the retinal image, it is possible that the myopia seen in these individuals is a form of deprivation myopia. If this scenario is correct, then the treatment and management strategies that would evolve from this theoretical base would be different from those associated with the more traditional ideas of nearwork myopia. New insights into the potential aetiologies of common refractive anomalies and the resulting new treatment and management strategies for human refractive errors are the primary benefit of research on experimental refractive errors in laboratory animals.

References

Abrahamsson, M. (1992) Refraction changes in children developing convergent or divergent strabismus. *Br. J. Ophthalmol.* **76**, 723–727.

Abrahamsson, M. and Sjostrand, J. (1996) Natural history of infantile anisometropia. *Br. J. Ophthalmol.* **80**, 860–863.

Abrahamsson, M., Gabian, G. and Sjostrand, J. (1988) Changes in astigmatism between the ages of 1 and 4 years: a longitudinal study. *Br. J. Ophthalmol.* **72**, 145–149.

Almender, L. M., Peck, L. B. and Howland, H. C. (1990) Prevalence of anisometropia in volunteer laboratory and school screening populations. *Invest. Ophthalmol. Vis. Sci.* **31**, 2448–2455.

Andison, M. E. and Sivak, J. G. (1992) The refractive development of the eye of the American kestrel (*Falco sparverius*): a new avian model. *J. Comp. Physiol. [A]* **170**, 565–574.

Atkinson, J. (1993) Infant vision screening: prediction and prevention of strabismus and amblyopia from refractive screening in the Cambridge Photorefraction Program. In: *Early Visual Development, Normal and Abnormal* (K. Simons, ed.). Oxford University Press, pp. 335–348.

Atkinson, J., Braddick, O. J. and French, J. (1980) Infant astigmatism: its disappearance with age. *Vision Res.* **20**, 891–893.

Bagnoli, P., Porciatti, V. and Francesconi, W. (1985) Retinal and tectal responses to alternating gratings are unaffected by monocular deprivation in pigeons. *Brain Res.* **338**, 341–345.

Barrett, J. W. (1932) The causation of myopia. *Br. J. Ophthalmol.* **16**, 764–765.

Bartmann, M. and Schaeffel, F. (1994) A simple mechanism for emmetropization without cues from accommodation or colour. *Vision Res.* **34**, 873–876.

Bartmann, M., Schaeffel, F., Hagel, G. and Zrenner, E. (1994) Constant light affects retinal dopamine levels and blocks deprivation myopia but not lens-induced refractive errors in chickens. *Vis. Neurosci.* **11**, 199–208.

Belkin, M., Yinon, U., Rose, L. and Reisert, I. (1977) Effects of visual environment on refractive error of cats. *Doc. Ophthalmol.* **42**, 433–437.

Bradley, D. V., Fernandes, A., Tigges, M. and Boothe, R. G. (1996) Diffuser contact lenses retard axial elongation in infant rhesus monkeys. *Vision Res.* **36**, 509–514.

Catania, A. (1964) On the visual acuity of the pigeon. *J. Exp. Anal. Behav.* **7**, 361–366.

Chung, K. (1993) Critical review: effects of optical defocus on refractive development and ocular growth and relation to accommodation. *Optom. Vis. Sci.* **70**, 228–233.

Crawford, M. L. J. and Marc, R. E. (1976) Light transmission of the cat and monkey eyelids. *Vision Res.* **16**, 323–324.

Crewther, S. G., Nathan, J., Kiely, P. M., Brennan, N. A. and Crewther, D. P. (1988) The effect of defocusing contact lenses on refraction in cynomolgus monkeys. *Clin. Vis. Sci.* **3**, 221–228.

Criswell, M. H. and Goss, D. A. (1983) Myopia development in nonhuman primates–a literature review. *Am. J. Optom. Physiol. Opt.* **60**, 250–268.

Curtin, B. J. (1985) *The Myopias. Basic Science and Clinical Management.* Harper & Row.

Dobson, V., Howland, H. C., Moss, C. and Banks, M. S. (1983) Photorefraction of normal and astigmatic infants during viewing of patterned stimuli. *Vision Res.* **23**, 1043–1052.

Duke-Elder, W. S. (1958) *The Eye in Evolution*, Vol. 1. Henry Kimpton.

Ehrlich, D. L., Atkinson, J. and Braddick, O. (1995) Reduction of infant myopia: a longitudinal cycloplegic study. *Vision Res.* **35**, 1313–1324.

Essed, W. F. R. and Soewarno, M. (1928) Ueber experimentalmyopie bei Affen. *Klin. Monats. Augenheilk.* **80**, 56–62.

Feldkaemper, M., Diether, S., Schwahn, H. and Schaeffel, F. (1997) Are experimental myopia and hyperopia based on similar retinal processing. *Invest. Ophthalmol. Vis. Sci.* **38** (Suppl.), S542.

Fitzke, F. W., Hayes, B. P., Hodos, W. and Holden, A. L. (1985) Refractive sectors in the visual field of the pigeon eye. *J. Physiol. (Lond.)* **369**, 33–44.

Fulton, A. B., Hansen, R. M. and Petersen, R. A. (1982) The relation of myopia and astigmatism in developing eyes. *Ophthalmol.* **89**, 298–302.

Glickstein, M. and Millodot, M. (1970) Retinoscopy and eye size. *Science* **168**, 605–606.

Gollender, M., Thorn, F. and Erickson, P. (1979) Development of axial ocular dimensions following eye-lid suture in the cat. *Vision Res.* **19**, 221–223.

Goss, D. A. and Criswell, M. H. (1981) Myopia development in experimental animals. A literature review. *Am. J. Optom. Physiol. Opt.* **58**, 859–869.

Gottlieb, M. D., Marran, L., Xu, A., Nickla, D. L. and Wallman, J. (1991) The emmetropization process in chicks is compromised by dim light. *Invest. Ophthalmol. Vis. Sci.* **32** (Suppl.), 1203.

Guyton, D. L., Greene, P. R. and Scholz, R. T. (1989) Dark-rearing interference with emmetropization in the rhesus monkey. *Invest. Ophthalmol. Vis. Sci.* **30**, 761–764.

Gwiazda, J., Bauer, J., Thorn, F. and Held, R. (1995) Dynamic relationship between myopia and blur-driven accommodation in school-aged children. *Vision Res.* **35**, 1299–1304.

Gwiazda, J., Thorn, F., Bauer, J. and Held, R. (1993a) Emmetropization and the progression of manifest refraction in children followed from infancy to puberty. *Clin. Vis. Sci.* **8**, 337–344.

Gwiazda, J., Thorn, F., Bauer, J. and Held, R. (1993b) Myopic children show insufficient accommodative response to blur. *Invest. Ophthalmol. Vis. Sci.* **34**, 690–694.

Harwerth, R. S., Crawford, M. L. J., Smith III, E. L. and Boltz, R. L. (1981) Behavioral studies of stimulus deprivation amblyopia in monkey. *Vision Res.* **21**, 779–789.

Hirsch, M. (1957) The relationship between measles and myopia. *Am. J. Optom. Arch. Am. Acad. Optom.* **34**, 289.

Hodos, W. and Erichsen, J. (1990) Lower-field myopia in birds: an adaptation that keeps the ground in focus. *Vision Res.* **30**, 653–657.

Hodos, W. and Kuenzel, W. J. (1984) Retinal-image degradation produces ocular enlargement in chicks. *Invest. Ophthalmol. Vis. Sci.* **25**, 652–659.

Hodos, W., Fitzke, R. W., Hayes, B. P. and Holden, A. L. (1985) Experimental myopia in chicks: ocular refraction by electroretinography. *Invest. Ophthalmol. Vis. Sci.* **26**, 1423–1430.

Hodos, W., Revzin, A. M. and Keunzel, W. J. (1987) Thermal gradients in the chick eye: a contributing factor in experimental myopia. *Invest. Ophthalmol. Vis. Sci.* **28**, 1858–1866.

Hoyt, C. S., Stone, R. D., Fromer, C. and Billdon, F. A. (1981) Monocular axial myopia associated with neonatal eyelid closure in human infants. *Am. J. Ophthalmol.* **91**, 197–200.

Huang, J., Hung, L.-F. and Smith III, E. L. (1997) Astigmatism is associated with the development of axial hyperopia in young monkeys. *Invest. Ophthalmol. Vis. Sci.* **38** (Suppl.), S543.

Hubel, D. H., Wiesel, T. N. and LeVay, S. (1976) Functional architecture of area 17 in normal and monocularly deprived macaque monkeys. *Cold Spring Harb. Symp. Quant. Biol.* **40**, 581–589.

Hughes, A. (1977) The topography of vision in mammals. In: *The Visual System in Vertebrates* (F. Crescitelli, ed.), Vol. VII/5. Springer-Verlag, pp. 613–756.

Hung, L.-F. and Smith III, E. L. (1996) Extended-wear, soft, contact lenses produce hyperopia in young monkeys. *Optom. Vis. Sci.* **73**, 579–584.

Hung, L.-F., Crawford, M. L. J. and Smith III, E. L. (1995) Spectacle lenses alter eye growth and the refractive status of young monkeys. *Nature Med.* **1**, 761–765.

Ingram, R. M. and Barr, A. (1979) Changes in refraction between the ages of 1 and 3 1/2 years. *Br. J. Ophthalmol.* **63**, 339–342.

Ingram, R. M., Arnold, P. E., Dally, S. and Lucas, J. (1991) Emmetropization, squint, and reduced visual acuity after treatment. *Br. J. Ophthalmol.* **75**, 414–416.

Irving, E. L., Callender, M. G. and Sivak, J. G. (1991) Inducing myopia, hyperopia, and astigmatism in chicks. *Optom. Vis. Sci.* **68**, 364–368.

Irving, E. L., Sivak, J. G. and Callender, M. G. (1992) Refractive plasticity of the developing chick eye. *Ophthal. Physiol. Opt.* **12**, 448–456.

Irving, E. L., Callender, M. G. and Sivak, J. G. (1995) Inducing ametropias in hatchling chicks by defocus —aperture effects and cylindrical lenses. *Vis. Res.* **35**, 1165–1174.

Ivone, P. M., Tigges, M., Stone, R. A., Lambert, S. and Laties, A. M. (1991) Effects of apomorphine, a dopamine receptor agonist, on ocular refraction and axial elongation in a primate model of myopia. *Invest. Ophthalmol. Vis. Sci.* **32**, 1674–1677.

Judge, S. J. and Graham, B. (1995) Differential ocular growth of infant marmoset (*Callithrix jacchus jacchus*) induced by optical anisometropia combined with alternating occlusion. *J. Physiol. (Lond.)* **485**, 27p.

Kiely, P. M., Crewther, S. G., Nathan, J., Brennan, N. A., Efron, N. and Madigan, M. (1987) A comparison of ocular development of the cynomolgus monkey and man. *Clin. Vis. Sci.* **1**, 269–280.

Kiorpes, L. and Wallman, J. (1995) Does experimentally-induced amblyopia cause hyperopia in monkeys? *Vision Res.* **35**, 1289–1297.

Kirby, A. W., Sutton, L. and Weiss, H. (1982) Elongation of cat eyes following neonatal lid suture. *Invest. Ophthalmol. Vis. Sci.* **22**, 274–277.

Knudsen, E. I. (1989) Fused binocular vision is required for development of proper eye alignment in barn owls. *Vis. Neurosci.* **2**, 35–40.

Kröger, R. H. H. and Fernald, R. (1994) Regulation of eye growth in the African cichlid fish *Haplochromis burtoni*. *Vision Res.* **34**, 1807–1814.

Laskowski, F. H. and Howland, H. C. (1996) Effect of experimentally simulated astigmatism on eye growth and refractive development in chicks. *Invest. Ophthalmol. Vis. Sci.* **37** (Suppl.), 5687.

Lepard, C. W. (1975) Comparative changes in the error of refraction between fixing and amblyopic eyes during growth and development. *Am. J. Ophthalmol.* **80**, 485–490.

Levinsohn, F. G. (1914) Über den histologischen Befund Kurzsichtig gemachter Affenaugen und die Enstehung der Kurzsichtigkeit. *Albrect von Graefes Arch. Klin. Ophthalmol.* **88**, 452–472.

Levinsohn, F. G. (1919) Zur frage der kunstlich erzeugten kurzsichtigkeit bei affen. *Klin. Monats. Augenheilkd* **61**, 794–803.

Marchesani, O. (1931) Untersuchungen uber die myopie-genese. *Arch. Augenheilkd* **104**, 177–191.

Marsh-Tootle, W. and Norton, T. T. (1989) Refractive and structural measures of lid-sutured myopia in tree shrew. *Invest. Ophthalmol. Vis. Sci.* **30**, 2245–2257.

Maurice, D. M. and Mushin, A. S. (1966) Production of myopia in rabbits by raised body temperature and increased intraocular pressure. *Lancet* **474**, 1160–1162.

McBrien, N. A., Moghaddam, H. O., New, R. and Williams, L. R. (1993) Experimental myopia in a diurnal mammal (*Sciurus carolinensis*) with no accommodative ability. *J. Physiol. (Lond.)* **469**, 427–441.

McBrien, N. A. and Norton, T. T. (1992) The development of experimental myopia and ocular component dimensions in monocularly lid-sutured tree shrews (*Tupaia belangeri*). *Vision Res.* **32**, 843–852.

McFadden, S. and Wallman, J. (1995) Guinea pig eye growth compensates for spectacle lenses. *Invest. Ophthalmol. Vision Sci.* **36** (Suppl.), 758.

McKanna, J. A. and Casagrande, V. A. (1978) Reduced lens development in lid-suture myopia in tree shrews. *Exp. Eye Res.* **26**, 715–723.

McLean, R. and Wallman, J. (1997) Despite severe imposed astigmatic blur, chicks compensate for spectacle lenses. *Invest. Ophthalmol. Vis. Sci.* **38** (Suppl.), S542.

Miles, F. A. and Wallman, J. (1990) Local ocular compensation for imposed local refractive error. *Vision Res.* **30**, 339–349.

Millodot, M. and Blough, P. M. (1971) The refractive state of the pigeon eye. *Vision Res.* **11**, 1019–1022.

Mohan, M., Rao, V. A. and Dada, V. K. (1977) Experimental myopia in the rabbit. *Exp. Eye Res.* **25**, 33–38.

Murphy, C. J., Howland, M. and Howland, H. C. (1995) Raptors lack lower-field myopia. *Vision Res.* **35**, 1153–1155.

Murphy, C. J., Zadnik, K. and Mannis, M. J. (1992) Myopia and refractive error in dogs. *Invest. Ophthalmol. Vis. Sci.* **33**, 2459–2463.

Mutti, D. O., Zadnik, K., Johnson, C., Howland, H. and Murphy, C. J. (1992) Retinoscopic measurement of the refractive state of the rat. *Vision Res.* **32**, 583–586.

Napper, G. A., Brennan, N. A., Barrington, M., Squires, M., Vessey, G. A. and Vingrys, A. J. (1995) The duration of normal visual exposure necessary to prevent form deprivation myopia in chicks. *Vision Res.* **35**, 1337–1344.

Nathan, J., Kiely, P. M., Crewther, S. G. and Crewther, D. P. (1985) Disease-associated image degradation and spherical refractive errors in children. *Am. J. Optom. Physiol. Opt.* **62**, 680–688.

Norton, T. T. and Siegwart, J. T. (1995) Animal models of emmetropization: matching axial length to the focal plane. *J. Am. Optom. Assoc.* **66**, 405–414.

Nye, P. W. (1973) On the functional differences between frontal and lateral visual fields of the pigeon. *Vision Res.* **13**, 559–574.

O'Leary, D. J. and Millodot, M. (1979) Eyelid closure causes myopia in humans. *Experientia* **35**, 1478–1479.

O'Leary, D. J., Chung, K. M. and Othman, S. (1992) Contrast reduction without myopia induction in monkey. *Invest. Ophthalmol. Vis. Sci.* **33** (Suppl.), 712.

Papastergiou, G. I., Schmid, G. F., Laties, A. M., Pendrak, K., Lin, T. and Stone, R. A. (1997) Induction of axial elongation and myopic refractive shift in one year old chickens. *Invest. Ophthalmol. Vis. Sci.* **38** (Suppl.), S543.

Quick, M. W., Tigges, M., Gammon, J. A. and Boothe, R. G. (1989) Early abnormal visual experience induces strabismus in infant monkeys. *Invest. Ophthalmol. Vis. Sci.* **30**, 1012–1017.

Rabin, J., Van Sluyters, R. C. and Malach, R. (1981) Emmetropization: a vision-dependent phenomenon. *Invest. Ophthalmol. Vis. Sci.* **20**, 661–664.

Raviola, E. and Wiesel, T. N. (1978) Effect of dark-rearing on experimental myopia in monkeys. *Invest. Ophthalmol. Vis. Sci.* **17**, 485–488.

Raviola, E. and Wiesel, T. N. (1985) An animal model of myopia. *N. Engl. J. Med.* **312**, 1609–1615.

Raviola, E. and Wiesel, T. N. (1990) Neural control of eye growth and experimental myopia in primates. In: *Myopia and the Control of Eye Growth*. Ciba Foundation Symposium 155. Wiley, pp. 22–44.

Regal, D. M., Booth, R., Teller, D. Y. and Sackett, G. P. (1976) Visual acuity and visual responsiveness in dark-reared monkeys (*Macaca nemestrina*). *Vision Res.* **16**, 523–530.

Rob, R. M. (1977) Refractive errors associated with hemangiomas of the eyelids and orbit in infancy. *Am. J. Ophthalmol.* **83**, 52–58.

Rose, L., Yinon, U. and Belkin, M. (1974) Myopia induced in cats deprived of distance vision during development. *Vision Res.* **14**, 1029–1032.

Schaeffel, F. and Howland, H. (1991) Properties of the feedback loops controlling eye growth and refractive state in the chicken. *Vision Res.* **31**, 717–734.

Schaeffel, F. and Howland, H. C. (1988) Mathematical model of emmetropization in the chicken. *J. Opt. Soc. Am. [A]* **5**, 2080–2086.

Schaeffel, F., Bartmann, M., Hagel, G. and Zrenner, E. (1995) Studies on the role of the retinal dopamine/melatonin system in experimental refractive errors in chickens. *Vision Res.* **35**, 1247–1264.

Schaeffel, F., Glasser, A. and Howland, H. C. (1988) Accommodation, refractive error and eye growth in chickens. *Vision Res.* **28**, 639–657.

Schaeffel, F., Hagel, G., Bartmann, M., Kohler, K. and Zrenner, E. (1994a) 6-Hydroxydopamine does not affect lens-induced refractive errors but suppresses deprivation myopia. *Invest. Ophthalmol. Vis. Sci.* **34**, 143–149.

Schaeffel, F., Hagel, G. and Eikermann, J. (1994b) Lower-field myopia and astigmatism in amphibians and chickens. *J. Opt. Soc. Am. [A]* **11**, 487–495.

Schmid, K. L. and Wildsoet, C. F. (1996) Effects on the compensatory responses to positive and negative lenses of intermittent lens wear and ciliary nerve section in chicks. *Vision Res.* **36**, 1023–1036.

Schmid, K. L. and Wildsoet, C. F. (1997) Refractive astigmatism and its relation to emmetropization in the chick. *Vision Res.* (in press).

Sherman, S. M., Norton, T. T. and Casagrande, V. A. (1977) Myopia in the lid-sutured tree shrew (*Tupaia glis*). *Brain Res.* **124**, 154–157.

Siegwart, J. T. and Norton, T. T. (1993) Refractive and ocular changes in tree shrews raised with plus or minus lenses. *Invest. Ophthalmol. Vis. Sci.* **34** (Suppl.), 1208.

Sivak, J. G. (1976) The accommodative significance of the 'ramp' retina of the eye of the stingray. *Vision Res.* **16**, 945–950.

Sivak, J. G. and Allen, D. B. (1975) An evaluation of the 'ramp' retina of the horse eye. *Vision Res.* **15**, 1353–1356.

Sivak, J. G., Barrie, D. L. and Weerheim, J. A. (1989) Bilateral experimental myopia in chicks. *Optom. Vis. Sci.* **66**, 854–858.

Smith III, E. L. (1997) The role of optical defocus in primate emmetropization. *Optom. Vis. Sci.* (in press).

Smith III, E. L. and Hung, L.-F. (1995) Optical diffusion disrupts emmetropization and produces axial myopia in young monkeys. *Invest. Ophthalmol. Vis. Sci.* **36** (Suppl.), 758.

Smith III, E. L., Harwerth, R. S. and Crawford, M. L. J. (1985) Spatial contrast sensitivity deficits in monkeys produced by optically induced anisometropia. *Invest. Ophthalmol. Vis. Sci.* **26**, 330–342.

Smith III, E. L., Harwerth, R. S., Crawford, M. L. J. and von Noorden, G. K. (1987) Observations on the effects of form deprivation on the refractive status of the monkey. *Invest. Ophthalmol. Vis. Sci.* **28**, 1236–1245.

Smith III, E. L., Harwerth, R. S., Crawford, M. L. J. and von Noorden, G. K. (1988) The influence of the period of deprivation on experimental refractive errors. In: *Strabismus and Amblyopia* (G. Lennerstrand, G. K. von Noorden and E. Campos, eds), Vol. 49. Macmillan Press, pp. 197–206.

Smith III, E. L., Huang, J. and Hung, L.-F. (1997) Cylindrical spectacle lenses alter emmetropization and produce astigmatism in young monkeys. In: *Proceedings of the 6th International Congress on Myopia* (T. Tokoro, ed.) Springer (in press).

Smith III, E. L., Hung, L.-F. and Harwerth, R. S. (1994a) Effects of optically induced blur on the refractive status of young monkeys. *Vision Res.* **34**, 293–301.

Smith III, E. L., Hung, L.-F., Harwerth, R. S., Crawford, M. L. J. and von Noorden, G. K. (1994b) Experimentally induced strabismus can produce anisometropia in young monkeys. *Invest. Ophthalmol. Vis. Sci.* **35** (Suppl.), 1951.

Stone, R. A., Laties, A. M., Raviola, E. and Wiesel, T. N. (1988) Increase in retinal vasoactive intestinal polypeptide after eyelid fusion in primates. *Proc. Natl. Acad. Sci. USA* **85**, 257–260.

Stone, R. A., Lin, T. and Laties, A. M. (1991) Muscarinic antagonist effects on experimental chick myopia. *Exp. Eye Res.* **52**, 755–758.

Tigges, M., Tigges, J., Fernandes, A., Eggers, H. M. and Gammon, J. A. (1990) Postnatal axial eye elongation in normal and visually deprived rhesus monkeys. *Invest. Ophthalmol. Vis. Sci.* **31**, 1035–1046.

Tokoro, T. (1970) Experimental myopia in rabbits. *Invest. Ophthalmol.* **12**, 926–934.

Troilo, D. and Judge, S. J. (1993) Ocular development and visual deprivation myopia in the common marmoset (*Callithrix jacchus*). *Vision Res.* **33**, 1311–1324.

Troilo, D. and Wallman, J. (1991) The regulation of eye growth and refractive state: an experimental study of emmetropization. *Vision Res.* **31**, 1237–1250.

Troilo, C., Frances, E. and Yi, G. (1997) The temporal characteristics of eye growth control are affected by optic nerve section. *Invest. Ophthalmol. Vis. Sci.* **38** (Suppl.), S462.

Troilo, D., Gottlieb, M. D. and Wallman, J. (1987) Visual deprivation causes myopia in chicks with optic nerve section. *Curr. Eye Res.* **6**, 993–999.

von Noorden, G. K. and Crawford, M. L. J. (1978) Lid closure and refractive error in macaque monkeys. *Nature* **272**, 53–54.

von Noorden, G. K. and Lewis, R. A. (1987) Axial length in unilateral congenital cataracts and blepharoptosis. *Invest. Ophthalmol. Vis. Sci.* **28**, 750–752.

Wallman, J. (1993) Retinal control of eye growth and refraction. *Prog. Retinal Res.* **12**, 134–153.

Wallman, J. and Adams, J. I. (1987) Developmental aspects of experimental myopia in chicks: susceptibility, recovery and relation to emmetropization. *Vision Res.* **27**, 1139–1163.

Wallman, J., Gottlieb, M. D., Rajaram, V. and Fugate-Wentzek, L. (1987) Local retinal regions control local eye growth and myopia. *Science* **237**, 73–77.

Wallman, J., Turkel, J. and Trachtman, J. (1978) Extreme myopia produced by modest changes in early visual experience. *Science* **201**, 1249–1251.

Walls, G. L. (1942) *The Vertebrate Eye and Its Adaptive Radiation*. Cranbrook Institute of Science (Bloomfield Hills, Michigan).

Weiss, S. and Schaeffel, F. (1993) Diurnal growth rhythms in the chickens eye: relation to myopia development and retinal dopamine levels. *J. Comp. Physiol. [A]* **172**, 263–270.

Weymouth, F. W. and Hirsch, M. J. (1991) Theories, definitions, and classifications of refractive errors. In: *Refractive Anomalies. Research and Clinical Applications* (T. Grosvenor and M. Flom, eds). Butterworth-Heinemann, pp. 1–14.

Wiesel, T. N. and Raviola, E. (1977) Myopia and eye enlargement after neonatal lid fusion in monkeys. *Nature* **266**, 66–68.

Wiesel, T. N. and Raviola, E. (1979) Increase in axial length of the macaque monkey eye after corneal opacification. *Invest. Ophthalmol. Vis. Sci.* **18**, 1232–1236.

Wildsoet, C. and Pettigrew, J. D. (1988) Experimental myopia and anomalous eye growth patterns unaffected by optic nerve section in chickens: evidence for local control of eye growth. *Clin. Vision Sci.* **3**, 99–107.

Wildsoet, C. and Wallman, J. (1995) Choroidal and scleral mechanisms of compensation for spectacle lenses in chicks. *Vision Res.* **35**, 1175–1194.

Wilson, J. R., Fernandes, A., Chandler, C. V., Tigges, M., Boothe, R. G. and Gammon, J. A. (1987) Abnormal development of the axial length of aphakic monkey eyes. *Invest. Ophthalmol. Vis. Sci.* **28**, 2096–2099.

Yinon, U. (1984) Myopia induction in animals following alteration of the visual input during development: a review. *Curr. Eye Res.* **3**, 677–690.

Yinon, U., Koslowe, E. C. and Rassin, M. I. (1984) The optical effects of eyelid closure on the eyes of kittens reared in light and dark. *Curr. Eye Res.* **3**, 677–690.

Yinon, U., Rose, L. and Shapiro, A. (1980) Myopia in the eye of developing chicks following monocular and binocular lid closure. *Vision Res.* **20**, 137–141.

Young, F. A. (1961a) The development and retention of myopia by monkeys. *Am. J. Optom. Arch. Am. Acad. Optom.* **38**, 545–555.

Young, F. A. (1961b) The effect of restricted visual space on the primate eye. *Am. J. Ophthalmol.* **52**, 799–806.

Young, F. A. (1962) The effect of nearwork illumination level on monkey refraction. *Am. J. Optom. Arch. Am. Acad. Optom.* **39**, 60–67.

Young, F. A. (1963) The effect of restricted visual space on the refractive error of the young monkey eye. *Invest. Ophthalmol.* **2**, 571–577.

Young, F. A. (1964) The distribution of refractive errors in monkeys. *Exp. Eye Res.* **3**, 230–238.

Young, F. A. (1965) The effect of atropine on the development of myopia in monkeys. *Am. J. Optom. Arch. Am. Acad. Optom.* **42**, 439–449.

Young, F. A. and Leary, G. A. (1973) Visual-optical characteristics of caged and semifree-ranging monkeys. *Am. J. Physical Anthropol.* **38**, 377–382.

Young, F. A., Leary, G. A. and Garrer, D. N. (1971) Four years of annual studies of chimpanzee vision. *Am. J. Optom. Arch. Am. Acad. Optom.* **36**, 407–416.

Zadnik, K., Satariano, W. A., Mutti, D. O., Sholtz, R. I. and Adams, A. J. (1994) The effect of parental history of myopia on children's eye size. *J. Am. Med. Assoc.* **271**, 1323–1327.

Accommodation and myopia

Mark Rosenfield

5.1 Introduction

As discussed in the preceding chapters, the proposed association between the development of myopia and the performance of sustained near-vision tasks dates back to Kepler (1611, cited by Duke-Elder and Abrams, 1970). Numerous subsequent studies, including the classic works of Donders (1864) and Cohn (1886), have supported this proposal, although a mechanism linking the two has never been clearly elucidated. In attempting to produce a hypothesis which links the development of myopia with sustained near-visual activity, the action of accommodation would appear to be the obvious link as positive ocular accommodation produces an increase in the dioptric power of the eye via physiological changes in the crystalline lens. Since myopia occurs when the refractive power of the eye become excessive with respect to the axial length of the globe, this premise is appealing. However, the ocular refractive status refers to the locus within the eye conjugate with optical infinity during minimal accommodation (Rosenfield, 1997). Thus myopia can only be said to exist when the accommodative response is minimized (*see also* section 5.7 on pseudomyopia).

Nevertheless, the development of myopia, providing it remains uncorrected, will reduce the stimulus to blur-driven accommodation. Accordingly, one might conjecture that the onset of myopia represents an adaptive process to reduce the demand upon accommodation. However, it is unclear at the present time whether myopia develops as a result of an abnormal accommodative response, or alternatively that the accommodative stimulus is reduced as a consequence of myopic development.

The earliest suggestion of a link between accommodation and myopia appears to be that of Kepler (1611), who stated, 'but he who is from childhood occupied with study or fine work, speedily becomes accustomed to the vision of near objects, and with the advance of years this increases, so that remote objects are more and more imperfectly seen'. However, Kepler believed that accommodation was mediated via changes in the position of the retina, relative to the crystalline lens. Whilst numerous subsequent authors have also suggested that the development of myopia is related to the action of accommodation (e.g. Stansbury, 1948; Goldschmidt, 1968; Duke-Elder and Abrams, 1970; Curtin, 1970, 1985), to date no clear mechanism has been elucidated. A discussion of possible hypotheses whereby myopia could result from the action of the accommodative system appears in section 5.9.

5.2 School myopia

School myopia quite simply refers to myopia which first develops during the school years (Weymouth and Hirsch, 1991). Accordingly, this term describes the time of onset, but should not be taken to imply any specific aetiology. Nevertheless, many authors have assumed that school myopia results from the performance of nearwork, even when no justification for such an association exists.

Childhood myopia would be a better description, since this does not imply any specific aetiology.

The classic study of Cohn (1886) examined the prevalence of myopia in German schoolchildren and suggested that the onset of myopia was related to their poor working conditions, specifically the reduced illumination, contrast and close working distances under which nearwork was being performed. Interestingly, Cohn did not attribute the development of myopia solely to accommodation, but rather indicated that convergence and the downward posture of the head may also be significant factors. Many subsequent studies have also examined school (or childhood) myopia (e.g. Mäntyjärvi, 1983, 1987; Mäntyjärvi and Nousiainen, 1988; Kao *et al.*, 1988; Pärssinen, 1990, 1991, 1993; Javal, 1990), and whilst the action of accommodation has frequently been investigated in these studies, no consensus exists as to how variations in accommodation might lead to myopic development. This chapter will consider whether the inception of myopia might be related to variations in:

1 the amplitude of accommodation;
2 the within-task accommodative response;
3 the composition of the within-task accommodative response;
4 accommodative adaptation;

and each of these possibilities will be discussed in turn.

5.3   The amplitude of accommodation and myopic development

The amplitude of accommodation reflects the maximum accommodative response, and has been defined as the dioptric distance between the far-point (point conjugate with the retina when accommodation is fully relaxed) and the near-point (point conjugate with the retina when accommodation is fully exerted) of accommodation (Rosenfield, 1997). A number of studies have reported significant variations in this parameter with refractive error. For example, Fledelius (1981) observed mean amplitudes in groups of juvenile myopes, emmetropes and hyperopes of 13.8, 11.6 and 10.7 D, respectively. These differences were statistically significant. In addition, both Maddock *et al.* (1981) and McBrien and Millodot (1986a) subdivided their myopic population into either low

(<3 D) and high (>3 D) myopes, or early- (myopia onset at 13 years of age or earlier) and late- (myopia onset at 15 years of age or later) onset myopes. Since the late-onset myopes are also typically low myopes, both studies reported similar findings, with low myopes having higher amplitudes than high myopes. However, both myopic subgroups had higher amplitudes than either emmetropes or hyperopes. In contrast, Fisher *et al.* (1987) did not observe any significant variation in the nearpoint of accommodation with refractive error.

When considering the amplitude of accommodation in different refractive groups, care must be taken to consider the stimulus to ocular accommodation. For example, if the near point was located 10 cm in front of the spectacle plane of a fully corrected (by spectacle lenses) 5 D hyperope and 5 D myope (back vertex distance = 14 mm), then the ocular stimulus to accommodation would be 10.05 D and 7.72 D, respectively (Rosenfield, 1997). Conversely, if both of these subjects had ocular amplitudes of 10 D, then the near point of the hyperope and myope would be located 100.6 mm and 74.3 mm in front of their spectacle plane, respectively. Thus the myopic patient could appear to have a higher amplitude when, in fact, they are identical. It should be noted that the findings of McBrien and Millodot (1986a) are indeed ocular amplitudes, and while the Maddock *et al.* (1981) study did not specify whether the measurements were spectacle or ocular accommodation, the observation of higher amplitudes in low myopes when compared with high myopes cannot be explained with respect to ocular accommodation.

It is difficult to see how relatively small differences in the amplitude of accommodation in children and young adults could be related either to variations in the within-task accommodative response or the development of axial myopia. For example, McBrien and Millodot (1986a) reported mean amplitudes of accommodation in populations of emmetropes and late-onset myopes (mean age of both groups was 19.7 years) of 9.28 D and 10.77 D, respectively. When performing a typical near-vision task at a viewing distance of 33 cm (accommodative stimulus = 3 D), one would predict an accommodative response of approximately 2.6 D, reflecting the normal lag of accommodation (Morgan, 1944; Heath, 1956; Charman, 1982; Ciuffreda and Kenyon, 1983). Thus the emmetropic and late-onset myopic subjects would be exerting 28% and 24% of their total amplitude. It would seem unlikely that such small differences in the proportion of the total available accommodation could be a precursor to permanent changes in the refractive error of the eye. Furthermore, in younger children, the amplitude of accommodation would be higher, so that the proportion of the total available accommodation being used would be even smaller. Taking Duane's (1912) mean value of 13.8 D for the amplitude of accommodation in 8-year-olds, this would indicate that only 19% of the total accommodation is typically used. However, smaller children typically read at closer distances than adults (Chiu *et al.*, 1994), so that a greater accommodative response is probable. Nevertheless, it seems unlikely that the development of nearwork-induced myopia could result from relatively small variations in the total amplitude of accommodation.

5.4 Variations in the accommodative response and myopic development

As described earlier, the notion that myopia develops from variations in the accommodative response is appealing. Indeed, a number of studies cited below have demonstrated a reduced accommodative response in myopic individuals. However, when considering the effect of ametropia on the accommodative response, care must be taken to ensure that it is the ocular accommodative stimulus which is quantified, since this will vary with refractive error (Bennett and Rabbetts, 1989; Rosenfield, 1997). For example, consider an emmetropic individual viewing a near target located 333 mm in front of the principal point of their eye. Here, the accommodative stimulus will be 1/0.333 or 3.00 D. If the same object is viewed by a myopic subject who is fully corrected by a −5.00 D spectacle lens at a back vertex distance of 14 mm, then the ocular accommodative stimulus is only 2.63 D. Additionally, if this same patient were to be corrected by an appropriately powered contact lens (in this case −4.67 D), then the ocular accommodative stimulus becomes equal to that of the emmetrope, i.e., 3.00 D. Accordingly, one might anticipate a lower accommodative response in a myopic patient corrected with spectacles, when compared with an emmetrope, due to the reduced accommodative stimulus. (For a more detailed explanation and procedure for calculating ocular accommodation, *see* Rosenfield, 1997).

Nevertheless, several studies have observed reduced accommodative responses in myopic individuals, when compared with emmetropes. For

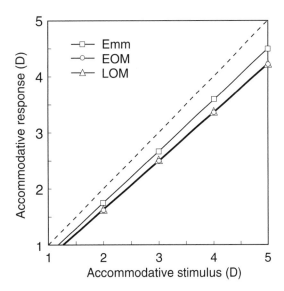

Figure 5.1 Mean accommodative stimulus–response functions for populations (each comprising *n* = 10) of emmetropes (Emm), early-onset myopes (EOM), i.e., myopia onset at 13 years of age or earlier, and late-onset myopes (LOM), i.e., myopia onset at 15 years of age or later. Responses for the EOM and LOM group were almost identical. (Redrawn based upon the mean equations presented by McBrien and Millodot, 1986b. However, confidence limits for these functions were not provided)

example, Ramsdale (1979) used a laser optometer to compare the accommodative responses for stimuli ranging from −2 to +7 D, and reported that the myopic group exhibited lower responses at all stimulus levels. However, a subsequent paper by Ramsdale (1985) reported no significant difference between the accommodative responses of myopic and emmetropic subjects. McBrien and Millodot (1986b) used a Canon R-1 infra-red optometer to assess the effect of refractive error on accommodation, and also reported lower responses in myopes. These results are illustrated in Figure 5.1. It should be noted that in McBrien and Millodot's study, all ametropic subjects were corrected with soft contact lenses, and therefore both the stimuli and responses reflect ocular accommodation. However, the magnitude of the differences was relatively small, only 0.15 D for the 5 D stimulus, and this difference is less than the degree of repeatability of the Canon R-1 infra-red optometer used by McBrien and Millodot (Rosenfield and Chiu, 1995). Studies by Rosenfield and Gilmartin (1988a), Tokoro (1988), Bullimore *et al.* (1992) and Gwiazda *et al.* (1993a) have also reported

Table 5.1 Mean differences in within-task accommodative response to a 3 D accommodative stimulus in populations of myopes and emmetropes

Study	Mean difference (D)
Bullimore *et al.* (1992)	0 D (active condition)[a]
Gwiazda *et al.* (1993a)	0 D (positive lens series)[b]
Bullimore *et al.* (1992)	0.08 D (passive condition)[a]
McBrien and Millodot (1986b)	0.16 D (late-onset myopes)[c]
McBrien and Millodot (1986b)	≈ 0.16 D (early-onset myopes)[c]
Gwiazda *et al.* (1993a)	≈ 0.20 D (decreasing distance series)[b]
Rosenfield and Gilmartin (1988a)	0.22 D
Ramsdale (1979)	≈ 0.50 D
Gwiazda *et al.* (1995)	≈ 0.60 D[d]
Gwiazda *et al.* (1993a)	≈ 0.90 D (negative lens series)[b]

Results are shown in ascending order of differences. In every case the mean accommodative response for the myopic group was less than that observed for the emmetropic subjects.
[a] Accommodation was assessed with subjects both passively reading numbers (passive condition) and adding the numbers (active condition).
[b] Accommodation was stimulated by varying target distance (decreasing distance series), by introducing minus lenses while viewing a target at 4 m (negative lens series) and by introducing positive lenses while viewing a target at 0.25 m (positive lens series).
[c] Late-onset myopia: myopia onset at 15 years of age or later. Early-onset myopia: myopia onset at 13 years of age or earlier.
[d] Only the slope of the accommodative stimulus–response function was provided. The response to a 3 D stimulus was calculated assuming a *y*-intercept of +0.25 D.

lower accommodative responses in myopic individuals (Table 5.1).

The observations cited above do indeed support the proposal of a reduced accommodative response in at least a proportion of myopic individuals. Again, it is unclear whether these variations in response are a precursor to, or occur after the refractive error development. Furthermore, it is questionable whether the magnitude of the observed differences is sufficiently large to be sig-

nificant when considering the aetiology of the ametropia. This is discussed further in section 5.9.

5.5   Variations in the composition of the accommodative response

As noted above, differences in the magnitude of the total accommodative response between myopes and emmetropes have been reported. In addition, variations in the composition of the aggregate accommodative response may also exist. Taking Heath's (1956) classification of accommodation, which is analogous to the classification of vergence proposed by Maddox (1893), four accommodative subcomponents exist, namely tonic, proximally induced, convergent (including disparity) and blur-driven accommodation.

5.5.1   Variations in tonic accommodation

In the absence of an adequate visual stimulus, accommodation adopts an intermediate position of approximately 0.5–1.0 D. Since this position was believed to reflect the level of tonic innervation to the ciliary muscle, this has been termed tonic accommodation (Rosenfield *et al.*, 1993). However, the response (typically measured by placing the subject in total darkness), probably represents an aggregate response resulting from multiple stimuli (Rosenfield *et al.*, 1993).

In considering the relationship between myopia and tonic accommodation, Ramazzini in 1713 (cited by Owens, 1991) reported that prolonged nearwork would produce changes in 'tonus of the membranes and fibres of the eye'. More recently, Van Alphen (1961) considered the ciliary muscle and choroid to act as a single functional unit which could behave as a continuous sheet of smooth muscle surrounding the eye. He speculated that the resistance to stretch was directly related to the contractive state or tone of the ciliary muscle. Van Alphen suggested that the intraocular pressure of the globe is counterbalanced by a combination of the tension in the choroid and the degree of scleral elasticity. Since the tension of the choroid is dependent upon the tonus of the ciliary muscle; the ability to resist intraocular forces will be a function of ciliary tonus. The presence of high ciliary muscle tone would produce increased resistance to intraocular pressure and thereby lower the resulting tension on the sclera. In contrast, for subjects having lower ciliary muscle tone, higher intraocular pressure would be more likely to result in scleral stretching. Thus Van Alphen's model of emmetropization would predict that hyperopic subjects would exhibit higher levels of tonic accommodation whilst those myopes whose increased axial length resulted from an inability to resist intraocular forces would have lower tonic accommodation values (*see* Chapter 6).

While many workers have attempted to demonstrate a relationship between the level of tonic accommodation and refractive error, examination of the data failed to reveal any consistent pattern. Suzumura (1979), Gawron (1981) and Simonelli (1983) indicated that myopic subjects had higher dioptric tonic accommodation values, while Ramsdale (1985) and Maddock *et al.* (1981) reported lower levels of tonic accommodation in myopes. Furthermore, Carreras (1951), Smith (1983), Gilmartin *et al.* (1984) and Whitefoot and Charman (1992) did not demonstrate any significant correlation between tonic accommodation and refractive error. To resolve this issue, other studies have divided their myopic subjects into subgroups in order to identify whether categories of tonic accommodation levels exist within these subgroups. Several investigators (McBrien and Millodot, 1986b; Rosenfield and Gilmartin, 1988a, 1988b; Bullimore *et al.*, 1988; Rosenfield and Gilmartin, 1989; Gilmartin and Bullimore, 1991; Bullimore *et al.*, 1992) have subdivided myopic subjects into late-onset myopes (LOMs), i.e., myopic onset at 15 years of age or later, and early-onset myopes (EOMs), i.e., myopic onset prior to 15 years of age. The rationale behind this differentiation was that stabilization of the refractive error normally takes place around 15 years of age (Brown, 1938, 1942; Slataper, 1950; Goss and Winkler, 1983), and therefore the myopia developing at or beyond 15 years–and following the cessation of bodily growth (Goldschmidt, 1968)–is more likely to be environmental in origin. However, more recent studies have demonstrated the development of axial myopia in subjects older than 15 years of age (McBrien and Millodot, 1987a; Bullimore *et al.*, 1992; Goss and Jackson, 1993; Grosvenor, 1994; Fledelius, 1995; Lin *et al.*, 1996). Furthermore, one might question whether it is reasonable to assign different aetiologies on the basis of age of onset. For example, a number of systemic conditions which first manifest themselves in mid or late-adulthood such as Huntington's and Parkinson's disease have a clear hereditary basis (Aminoff, 1996).

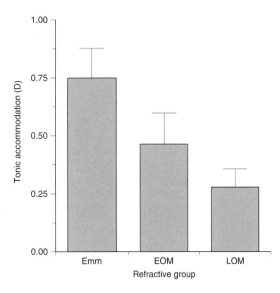

Figure 5.2 Mean dioptric levels of tonic accommodation in populations (each comprising $n = 17$) of emmetropes (Emm), early-onset myopes (EOM), i.e., myopia onset prior to 15 years of age, and late-onset myopes (LOM), i.e., myopia onset after 15 years of age. Error bars indicate 1 SEM. (From Rosenfield and Gilmartin, 1987a)

Even when adopting the myopic subdivisions described above, results comparing tonic accommodation and refractive error have been equivocal. Several studies (McBrien and Millodot, 1987b; Bullimore *et al.*, 1988; Rosenfield and Gilmartin, 1987a, 1987b) have observed lower dioptric values of tonic accommodation in LOMs. An example of these differences in tonic accommodation values is illustrated in Figure 5.2. However, other investigations have failed to reproduce this observation of significantly lower tonic accommodation in LOMs (Rosenfield and Gilmartin, 1989, 1990). Furthermore, Fisher *et al.* (1987) divided their myopic population on the basis of degree of refractive error rather than age of myopia onset, and did not demonstrate any significant variation in tonic accommodation between populations of high myopes (i.e., >4.00 D of myopia), low myopes (ranging from 0.75 to 4.00 D), emmetropes and hyperopes. However, when their results were combined with those of others ($n = 136$), there was a suggestion that high myopes and high hyperopes may have exhibited an increase in baseline tonic accommodation. On the basis of all the findings described above, one must infer that the evidence for variations in baseline tonic accommodation between refractive groups is inconclusive.

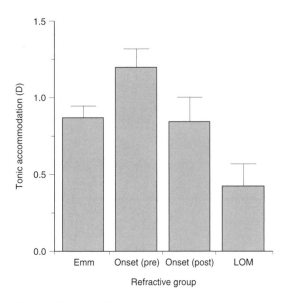

Figure 5.3 Mean dioptric values of tonic accommodation in populations of emmetropes (Emm; *n* = 25), late-onset myopes (LOM), i.e., myopia onset at 15 years of age or later (*n* = 7) and an onset group (*n* = 6) who switched from emmetropia to myopia during the course of the 2–3-year study. Onset (pre) and onset (post) indicates the findings at the time these subjects were emmetropic and myopic, respectively. (Redrawn from Jiang, 1995)

In addition, Jiang (1995) measured values of tonic accommodation in subjects who were initially emmetropic and became myopic, when compared with individuals who either remained emmetropic or were already myopic (late-onset myopes) upon entering the study. Interestingly, Jiang observed that in the 'became myopic' group, the initial mean tonic accommodation value (obtained while the subjects were still emmetropic) was significantly higher than that found for a group who remained emmetropic. The late-onset myopes (i.e., those individuals who had been myopic for a significant period of time) exhibited the lowest tonic accommodation levels. This is illustrated in Figure 5.3. These results strongly suggest that any decline in baseline tonic accommodation occurs after the manifestation of refractive changes. This conclusion is also supported by the findings of Adams and McBrien (1993), who reported that changes in tonic accommodation occur concurrently with refractive development. In a two-year longitudinal study, Adams and McBrien observed no significant difference between the initial values of tonic accommodation in subjects who remained emmetropic versus those individuals who were initially emmetropic but became myopic. However, this latter group (i.e., the 'became myopic' group) exhibited lower levels of tonic accommodation following myopic development. Accordingly, it was concluded that changes in tonic accommodation occur concurrently with refractive development and cannot be used as a predictor of potential myopia.

5.5.2 Variations in proximally induced accommodation

Proximally induced accommodation (PIA) may be defined as accommodation resulting from knowledge of apparent nearness of an object of regard (Rosenfield and Gilmartin, 1990). A number of recent investigations have demonstrated that awareness of target proximity can produce a significant increase in the open-loop accommodative response (Rosenfield and Gilmartin, 1990; Wick and Currie, 1991; Rosenfield *et al.*, 1991; Rosenfield and Ciuffreda, 1991). Rosenfield and Gilmartin compared PIA in populations of emmetropes and late-onset myopes (myopia onset at 15 years of age or later) by examining the open-loop accommodative response to targets placed at viewing distances of 5 m (0.2 D) and 0.33 m (3 D). The accommodation and vergence loops were opened by subjects viewing targets monocularly through 0.5 mm pinholes. The results are illustrated in Figure 5.4, and it may be observed that the late-onset myopic group exhibited significantly lower levels of PIA throughout the 60 second measurement period.

While there is no clear explanation as to the origin of the lower PIA response in late-onset myopes, three possibilities appear to exist. Firstly, the myopic subjects perceive the target to be further away than the emmetropes. This seems unlikely, although may be worthy of further testing. In high myopes (e.g. greater than 8.00 D), it is conceivable that the retinal image size minification produced by correction with concave spectacle lenses might be responsible for differences in apparent distance perception. However, the late-onset myopes tested by Rosenfield and Gilmartin (1990) required a mean refractive correction of only −2.00 D (range −1.00 to −3.25 D), and for the purposes of the experiment more soft contact lenses. Accordingly, it seems unlikely that these differences were due to variations in apparent perceived distance.

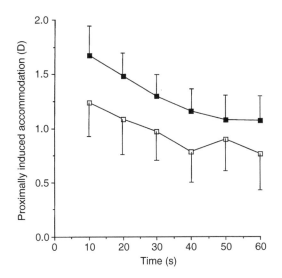

Figure 5.4 Mean values of proximally induced accommodation (PIA) for 10 emmetropes (closed squares) and 10 late-onset myopes (open squares) during the course of a 60 s fixation period. PIA was calculated as the difference in open-loop accommodative responses when viewing targets located at distances of 5 m and 0.33 m. Error bars indicate ±1 SEM. (From Rosenfield and Gilmartin, 1990)

A second possible explanation for the reduced PIA response might be related to reduced proximal gain in late-onset myopes. Thus both emmetropes and myopes would perceive the target to be at the same apparent distance, but a lower gain factor would result in a reduced PIA response. If this is indeed the case, then it would be of interest to examine whether the proximally induced vergence gain is also lower in myopes. These lower gain factors could be responsible for the reduced aggregate accommodative response which has been reported in myopes (Ramsdale, 1979; McBrien and Millodot, 1986b; Rosenfield and Gilmartin, 1988a; Tokoro, 1988; Bullimore *et al.*, 1992; Gwiazda *et al.*, 1993a).

Thirdly, PIA may be an aggregate response being composed of both proximal accommodation (PA) and proximal vergence (PV) stimulating convergent accommodation. Thus:

$$PIA = PA + PV (CA/C)$$

where CA/C represents the convergent accommodation to convergence ratio (Fry, 1940; Kent 1958; Morgan, 1968; Kersten and Legge, 1983). If the CA/C ratio were to be lower in late-onset myopes, then this would produce a reduced PIA response.

However, Rosenfield and Gilmartin (1988c) demonstrated no significant difference between the CA/C ratios of emmetropes, early- and late-onset myopes. Accordingly, the most likely explanation for lower PIA in late-onset myopes would appear to be reduced proximal gain.

5.5.3 Variations in convergent (or disparity-induced) accommodation

Under closed-loop conditions, with negative feedback mechanisms allowed to operate, the output of the vergence system will initiate an accommodative response. This is termed convergent accommodation (Fry, 1940; Kent 1958; Morgan, 1968; Kersten and Legge, 1983). Rosenfield and Gilmartin (1988c) assessed the CA/C ratio in populations of late-onset myopes, early-onset myopes and emmetropes, and observed no significant difference in the values of this ratio between refractive groups. In all cases the magnitude of CA/C was approximately 0.4 D/6Δ. Subsequent investigations by Jones (1990a) and Jiang (1995) have confirmed this finding of equivalent CA/C ratios in both emmetropes and myopes.

Additionally, two further studies by Rosenfield and Gilmartin (1987b, 1988a) examined disparity-induced accommodation in groups of myopes and emmetropes. Disparity-induced accommodation was defined as changes in the closed-loop accommodative response following the introduction of a disparity stimulus. This is in contrast to the measurement of convergent accommodation, where the accommodation loop is opened (for example by having the subject view through a small diameter pinhole, Ward and Charman, 1987).

Rosenfield and Gilmartin (1988b) measured the closed-loop accommodative response to a target located at a viewing distance of 33 cm in populations of emmetropes and late-onset myopes. Retinal disparity was induced by the introduction of base-out prisms, and the accommodative response measured over a 10 minute fixation period. The results are illustrated in Figure 5.5. It may be observed that with zero supplementary disparity stimulus, the accommodative response of the late-onset myopic group was significantly lower than that of the emmetropes. However, following the introduction of a 6Δ base-out prism, the accommodative responses became equivalent. These results might be explained in two ways. Firstly, the introduction of a disparity stimulus induced a greater amount of convergent accommodation in the myopes. However, the finding of equivalent

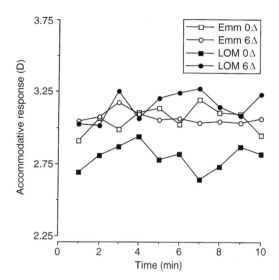

Figure 5.5 Mean accommodative responses for 10 emmetropes and 10 late-onset myopes (LOMs) during the course of a 10 min near-vision task performed at a viewing distance of 0.33 m. The task was performed both with a 6Δ base-out prism before the right eye, and without a supplementary disparity stimulus (0Δ). Error bars have been omitted for clarity but SEMs for the emmetropes and LOMs were approximately ±0.10 D and ±0.17 D, respectively. (From Rosenfield and Gilmartin, 1988a)

CA/C ratios in myopes and emmetropes would not support this theory (Rosenfield and Gilmartin, 1988c; Jones, 1990a; Jiang, 1995). Alternatively, following the introduction of base-out prism under closed-loop conditions, one would predict that the increased convergent accommodation would be accompanied by a decrease in blur-driven accommodation in order to keep the overall accommodative response relatively constant (Rosenfield, 1997). Thus the increase in disparity-induced accommodation in the late-onset myopes may result from a failure to relax blur-driven accommodation following the introduction of the disparity stimulus. This relative insensitivity to the presence of retinal blur, which may alter the interaction of the various accommodative subcomponents, may be an important factor in the aetiology of myopia and will be discussed in section 5.9.

5.5.4   Variations in blur-driven accommodation

While the aggregate accommodative response has been widely investigated in myopic individuals,

there have been relatively few investigations examining changes in accommodation produced solely by the effects of retinal defocus (i.e., blur-driven accommodation). In order to ensure that the other accommodative stimuli are controlled, such measurements should be recorded under monocular conditions with a fixed target, thereby ensuring that the stimuli to convergent and proximally induced accommodation remain constant. One of the few studies that examined changes in the accommodative response to monocular stimuli presented via a Badal optometer, which would maintain a constant retinal image size (Bennett and Rabbetts, 1989) was that of Rosenfield and Gilmartin (1987b). This study reported that blur-induced accommodation was significantly lower in early-onset myopes (i.e., myopia onset prior to 15 years of age). However, the initial levels of accommodation recorded for late-onset myopes and emmetropes were equivalent.

Gwiazda *et al.* (1993a) also claimed that myopic children exhibited reduced accommodative gain to blur-stimuli. Concave lenses were used to vary the accommodative stimulus, and mean slopes of the accommodative stimulus-response function of 0.61 and 0.20 D/D were reported for the emmetropic and myopic populations, respectively. However, such poor responses (for both groups) would be at almost pathological levels, and it seems unlikely that the children ever saw the target clearly. Recent reports by Chen and O'Leary (1997) and Rosenfield *et al.* (1997) have demonstrated that both children (between 3 and 14 years of age) and young adults typically demonstrate a stimulus–response gradient of approximately 0.90 D/D when the accommodative stimulus is varied by altering the physical location of the target. Additionally, it is well established in the clinical setting that when minus lenses are used to stimulate accommodation, particularly in young children, considerable encouragement must be given for them to accommodate appropriately. Gwiazda *et al.* (1993a) reported a mean accommodative response in their myopic group of only 0.70 D for a 3.5 D accommodative stimulus. It is apparent that this represents a grossly abnormal accommodative response.

An investigation by Abbott *et al.* (1998) adopted a very similar protocol to that of Gwiazda *et al.* (1993a) to investigate the accommodative stimulus–response function in populations of young adult (18–31 years of age) emmetropes and myopes. Abbott *et al.* reported a significantly reduced accommodative response in progressing myopes when changes in accommodation were stimulated using minus lenses (while concurrently viewing a distant target). However, when either variations in target distance, or the introduction of plus lenses (while concurrently viewing a near target) were used to stimulate changes in accommodation, then no significant difference in accommodative response was observed between the refractive groups. When using the minus lens procedure to stimulate changes in accommodation, the mean gradient of the stimulus–response function for progressing and stable myopes was 0.70 and 0.84 D/D, respectively. This difference was statistically significant. It is also of interest to note that these gradient values were considerably higher than those reported by Gwiazda *et al.* (1993a).

Jones (1990a) and Ramsdale (1979) also examined the gradient of the monocular accommodative stimulus–response function, and all reported lower slopes in myopic populations. However, these studies did not indicate whether a Badal optical stimulus was used. Thus it is possible that variations in retinal image size as the target viewing distance was changed could have induced changes in proximally induced accommodation resulting from a shift in the apparent distance of the stimulus. However, a recent study by Hung *et al.* (1995a) suggested that the relative contribution of proximally induced accommodation to the closed-loop accommodative response was extremely small (typically not exceeding 4% of the overall response). Accordingly, it may reasonably be concluded that the lower stimulus–response gradients observed in these studies do indeed reflect reduced blur-induced accommodation in myopes.

These differences in blur-induced accommodation may reflect variations in the ability of myopic individuals to detect the presence of retinal defocus. Jones (1990b) observed similar pupillary diameters in myopic and emmetropic populations, thereby discounting the possibility that variations in pupil size could produce differences in blur sensitivity. However, Abraham-Cohen *et al.* (1997) directly compared the ability of myopic and emmetropic individuals to detect the presence of blur. Subjects (12 myopes, 12 emmetropes) were cyclopleged, and viewed a near bipartite target through an appropriate near addition lens via a 2 mm artificial pupil. One half of the target remained fixed while the other half was alternatively moved forward or backward until subjects first reported a difference in clarity between the two halves of the target. The mean blur threshold for the emmetropic and myopic groups was ±0.11 D and ±0.18 D, respectively. Thus the emmetropic group detected the presence of blur significantly earlier than the myopes.

A recent report by Jiang (1997) presented a modified control model of accommodation which included an accommodative sensory gain input. This operator was added to reflect those changes in stimulus conditions (e.g. luminance, spatial frequency and contrast) which alter the gradient of the accommodative stimulus–response function. Also, an effective threshold (ET) was defined as the accommodative deadspace divided by the accommodative sensory gain. Analysing data from 13 emmetropic subjects and 10 late-onset myopes (i.e., myopia onset at 15 years of age or later), Jiang reported that the mean value of ET was significantly higher in the myopic group when compared with the emmetropes. This finding again suggests decreased sensitivity to the presence of retinal defocus in myopes.

However, it is critical to determine whether these changes in sensitivity to retinal defocus occur before or after the development of myopia. Gwiazda *et al.* (1995) noted that a group of children who were emmetropic at the time of testing but subsequently became myopic exhibited slopes and ranges of accommodation that were similar to the other emmetropes. This result strongly suggests that changes in blur-induced accommodation occur after the onset of myopia and therefore cannot be regarded as a precursor to refractive error development.

5.6 Accommodative adaptation

Whilst the level of tonic accommodation has been shown to be relatively stable over both short- and long-term periods (Miller, 1978; Mershon and Amerson, 1980; Heron *et al.*, 1981; Owens and Higgins, 1983; Krumholz *et al.*, 1986), other investigations have demonstrated that the magnitude of tonic accommodation appears to change transiently following a period of sustained fixation (Ebenholtz, 1983; Schor, 1986; Fisher *et al.*, 1987; Gilmartin and Bullimore, 1987; Owens and Wolf-Kelly, 1987; Rosenfield and Gilmartin, 1988b; Rosenfield *et al.*, 1994). The expressions 'accommodative adaptation' and 'accommodative hysteresis' have been adopted to describe this

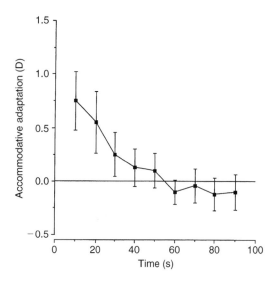

Figure 5.6 Mean accommodative adaptation (measured with respect to the pre-task tonic accommodation level) against time for the 90 s period immediately following completion of a 3 min near-vision task carried out at a viewing distance of 33 cm (3 D) in 10 emmetropic subjects. Error bars indicate ±1 SEM. (From Rosenfield and Gilmartin, 1988b)

apparent post-task shift in tonic accommodation relative to the pre-task level (Ebenholtz, 1983; Schor, 1986; Rosenfield *et al.*, 1992a).

It is important to note that during accommodative adaptation, the actual tonic output does not change. Immediately following the removal of a sustained accommodative stimulus, the output of the fast blur-driven accommodative response (FBAR) will dissipate rapidly, whereas the slow blur-driven accommodative response (SBAR) will exhibit a slower rate of decay. Therefore, the apparent post-task increase in tonic accommodation actually reflects the prolonged rate of decay of SBAR (Rosenfield and Gilmartin, 1988b). This is illustrated in Figure 5.6. There is no evidence that any change in baseline tonic innervation actually takes place (Hung 1992; Rosenfield *et al.*, 1994). While the pre-task measurement may indeed reflect baseline tonic accommodation (provided all other exogenous accommodation stimuli have been eliminated, and the output of SBAR has decayed fully), the accommodative output measured immediately following task completion will be a composite response including both tonic accommodation and the sustained output of SBAR. It is the maintained output of SBAR that is responsible for the apparent shift in the open-loop response, while the actual level of tonic accommodation

probably remains constant. It should be noted that measurement of the true level of tonic accommodation immediately following completion of a sustained near-vision task is virtually impossible, as it will always be masked by the SBAR.

The term 'accommodative adaptation' is analogous to the vergence or prism adaptation which may be observed when an increased vergence demand is maintained over a sustained period of time (Henson and North, 1980; Schor, 1986; Sethi, 1986). For a review of factors which may influence accommodative adaptation, *see* Rosenfield *et al.* (1993, 1994).

Over the past two decades, many workers have debated the possible association between tonic accommodation, accommodative adaptation and refractive error development. Unfortunately, some investigations have failed to differentiate between accommodative adaptation and actual refractive changes. By definition, *myopia exists when the far point lies at a finite distance in front of the eye while the accommodative response is at its minimum value.* Thus, this definition refers to the ability of the optical components of the eye to produce a focused image of an infinitely distant object of regard on the retina. Therefore, myopia refers exclusively to a proximal shift in the far point, and its presence cannot be defined or implicated in terms of the magnitude of either the near point of accommodation, tonic accommodation or accommodative adaptation.

Ebenholtz (1983) suggested that the slow decay of 'post-task tonic accommodation' following a period of near fixation may play a role in the aetiology of axial myopia. Although more recent evidence using infra-red optometers (Schor, 1986; Gilmartin and Bullimore, 1987; Rosenfield and Gilmartin, 1988b) would not support Ebenholtz's data which indicated that the adaptation induced following sustained near-fixation would require over 10 hours to decay, a link may still exist between the adaptive response and environmentally induced myopia.

Several studies have examined accommodative adaptation in different refractive groups (Fisher *et al.*, 1987; McBrien and Millodot, 1987b; Rosenfield and Gilmartin, 1988b, 1989; Gilmartin and Bullimore, 1991; Morse and Smith, 1993). Both Gilmartin and Bullimore (1991) and Rosenfield and Gilmartin (1988b) demonstrated that following a period of sustained near vision, populations of emmetropes and LOMs exhibited different regression patterns of accommodative adaptation. This is

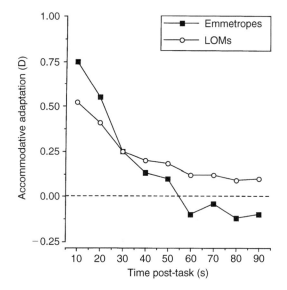

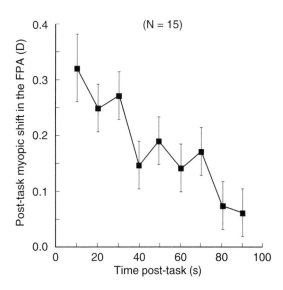

Figure 5.7 Mean accommodative adaptation (measured with respect to pre-task TA) during the 90 s period immediately following completion of a 3 min near-vision task performed at a viewing distance of 33 cm (3 D) in 10 emmetropic subjects and 10 late-onset myopes (LOMs). Error bars have been omitted for clarity but SEMs were of the order of ±0.17 D. (From Rosenfield and Gilmartin, 1988b)

Figure 5.8 Mean post-task myopic shift in the so-called 'far point of accommodation' (FPA) (also called closed-loop adaptation or 'transient myopia') measured with respect to the pre-task level, during the 90 s period immediately following completion of a 10 min near-vision task performed at a viewing distance of 20 cm (5 D) in 15 visually normal subjects. Error bars indicate ±1 SEM. (Data from Blustein *et al.*, 1993; figure reproduced from Rosenfield, 1994)

illustrated in Figure 5.7. It may be observed that immediately following the near-vision task, emmetropes initially show a larger shift, and furthermore exhibited a steeper regression gradient when compared with LOMs. McBrien and Millodot (1988) also reported differences in accommodative adaptation between LOMs, EOMs, emmetropes and hypermetropes. They observed that LOMs showed increased adaptation 1 minute following task completion when compared with the other refractive groups. Interestingly, they did not observe any adaptation following a 15 minute task located at 5 D in either the emmetropic or EOM refractive groups. This finding may be related to the adopted time-course of the measurements. McBrien and Millodot assessed accommodative adaptation by examining post-task tonic accommodation 1, 7 and 15 minutes following task completion. Data from several studies (Gilmartin and Bullimore, 1987; Rosenfield and Gilmartin, 1988b, 1989; Gilmartin and Bullimore, 1991) has indicated that a substantial proportion of the regression of accommodative adaptation is completed within 1 minute following task completion. This may explain the apparent absence of recorded adaptation in these subjects.

5.6.1 Adaptation under closed-loop conditions

In addition to examining accommodative adaptation under open-loop conditions, typically achieved by making the pre- and post-task measurements in total darkness, other studies have examined adaptation under closed-loop viewing conditions (e.g. Ehrlich, 1997; Rosenfield *et al.*, 1992b; Ciuffreda and Ordonez, 1995; Ong and Ciuffreda, 1997). Here, pre- and post-task measurements of accommodation were assessed while subjects viewed a distant target, typically a visual acuity chart. Thus normal blur-feedback mechanisms were allowed to operate. Under these conditions, a transient increase in the post-task response was observed immediately following completion of the near-vision task. This is illustrated in Figure 5.8. These measurements have erroneously been referred to as pre- and post-task measures of the far point of accommodation (FPA). While the pre-task value does indeed represent the FPA, the post-task reading will be the combined response of the FPA plus the residual output of the SBAR. Since the FPA is defined as the point conjugate with the retina in the unaccommodated eye (Emsley, 1953), it will be apparent that this post-task measurement cannot accurately be referred to as the FPA.

Additionally, a number of investigators have described this closed-loop accommodative adaptation as 'transient myopia' (e.g. Rosenfield and Ciuffreda, 1994; Ong and Ciuffreda, 1995). This term is unfortunate, since myopia (or any refractive error) can only be quantified when the accommodative response is minified. Clearly this is not the case here, due to the sustained output of SBAR. The accommodative adaptation observed under closed-loop conditions is smaller than that recorded in the open-loop situation (e.g. in total darkness) due to the effect of blur-feedback. In darkness, positive adaptation of approximately 1.0 D (Rosenfield and Gilmartin, 1988b; Bullimore and Gilmartin, 1989) is typically observed immediately following a sustained near-vision task. Under closed-loop viewing, the magnitude of the adaptive shift is typically of the order of +0.2–0.3 D in asymptomatic individuals (Rosenfield *et al.*, 1992b; Ciuffreda and Ordonez, 1995). Thus the magnitude of closed-loop adaptation lies either close to or within the limits of repeatability of an infra-red optometer (Rosenfield and Chiu, 1995). The reduction in adaptation under closed-loop conditions is produced by the effect of blur-driven accommodation. The magnitude of adaptation produced under open-loop viewing (around 1.0 D) would produce a defocused view of the distant target were it not compensated for by the action of blur-driven accommodation. Thus the degree of adaptation observed under closed-loop conditions does not reflect the total adaptation. However, one might argue that this represents the shift observed under naturalistic conditions, since nearwork is habitually performed under closed-loop viewing, with blur-feedback present.

5.6.2 Accommodative adaptation, SBAR and the aggregate accommodative response

In considering how accommodative adaptation might be related to the development of nearwork-induced myopia, it is necessary to examine the contribution of SBAR to the aggregate accommodative response. Schor *et al.* (1986) reported that accommodative adaptation resulting from the increased output of SBAR decreased the lag of accommodation, although they only presented data for a single subject. However, this finding would be consistent with vergence adaptation, where the output of slow fusional vergence reduces the magnitude of fixation disparity (i.e., the vergence error)

in asymptomatic individuals (Ogle *et al.*, 1967). Rosenfield and Gilmartin (1998) examined both the within-task accommodative response and accommodative adaptation (assessed under open-loop conditions) induced by a sustained 10 minute near-vision task at a viewing distance of 33 cm. Subjects were divided into two subgroups on the basis of their adaptative response. Firstly, an adaptive group (*n* = 11), where the magnitude of adaptation exceeded +0.30 D, and secondly, a non-adaptive group (*n* = 7) where the degree of adaptation for each individual was less than +0.30 D. The mean lags of accommodation for the two groups during the course of the 10 min task are shown in Figure 5.9. The reduction in the lag of accommodation during the course of the near task in the adaptor group was significant, whereas no significant change in lag was observed in the non-adaptor group. These findings confirm that SBAR does indeed serve to increase the accuracy of the accommodative response.

What remains unclear, however, is whether accommodative adaptation (assessed under either open-loop or closed-loop conditions) is actually related to the development of permanent myopia. One possibility is that reduced or absent accommodative adaptation might lead to increased retinal defocus, which might ultimately stimulate vitreous elongation. This notion will be discussed further in sections 5.9.1 and 10.3. Longitudinal studies are required to demonstrate whether differences in either the magnitude or rate of decay of accommodative adaptation are actually associated with myopia development, occur after the refractive changes have taken place, or are totally unrelated to refractive error development.

5.7 Accommodative spasm and pseudomyopia

Suchoff and Petito (1986) defined accommodative spasm as a condition in which a greater accommodative response than is considered normal is observed for a given accommodative stimulus. However, since a lead of accommodation (i.e., accommodative response exceeding the magnitude of the dioptric stimulus) is a normal finding when viewing distant objects of regard, and occasionally when viewing near objects (Heath, 1956; Charman 1982; Rosenfield, 1997), accommodative spasm should be restricted to those conditions where the accommodative response exceeds the stimulus by an amount greater than the depth-of-focus of the

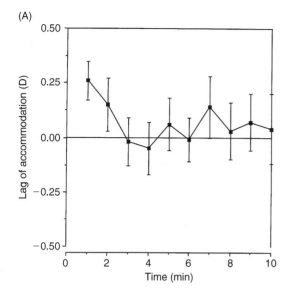

(A)

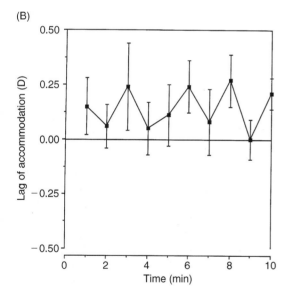

(B)

Figure 5.9 Mean lag of accommodation during the course of a continuous 10 min near-vision task for 11 subjects exhibiting accommodative adaptation (A) and 7 non-adaptors (B). Positive and negative values indicate a lag and lead of accommodation, respectively. The adaptors demonstrated a significant reduction in the lag of accommodation during the course of the task, whereas no significant change in lag was observed in the non-adaptive subjects. (Error bars indicate ±1 SEM)

eye (typically of the order of ±0.30 D) (Campbell, 1957; Charman and Whitefoot, 1977).

Duke-Elder and Abrams (1970) indicated that this condition was first described adequately by

Von Graefe in 1856, and was named by Leipreich in 1861 (Mishra *et al.*, 1995). It is generally produced by increased parasympathetic innervation to the ciliary muscle. Symptoms may include asthenopia, headaches, ocular fatigue, blurred vision, diplopia (from excessive accommodative convergence), and a requirement to perform nearwork at abnormally close distances (Borish, 1970; Duke-Elder and Abrams, 1970; Stenson and Raskind, 1970; Cooper, 1987; Griffin, 1988; Rutstein *et al.*, 1988). Its origin may be organic or functional, although the organic type is relatively rare (Duke-Elder and Abrams, 1970).

Functional accommodative spasm most frequently occurs immediately following periods of prolonged nearwork. Other factors such as poor illumination, glare, stress and general debility have also been associated with this condition. While it has been described as resembling the fatigue-cramps of other muscles (Duke-Elder and Abrams, 1970), it must be noted that accommodation is produced by contraction of the ciliary smooth muscle which has different physiological properties from striated muscle. Indeed, Guyton (1986) indicated that under normal functioning conditions, fatigue at the neural–smooth muscular junction probably occurs only at the most exhausting levels of muscular activity. This is consistent with the difficulty in producing accommodative fatigue (Rosenfield, 1997).

Pseudomyopia (also called spurious myopia) is an apparent myopic shift resulting from a failure to relax accommodation fully. If a cycloplegic drug is administered, then the myopic shift will disappear. Clearly this is not true myopia, since the latter is quantified by the location of the far point while the accommodative response is minimized (Rosenfield, 1997). Pseudomyopia is typically transient in nature, although on occasions, may become permanent (Curtin, 1985). It is demonstrated by a significant difference in refractive error under cycloplegic and non-cycloplegic conditions (Prangen, 1922; Alexander, 1940; Sollom, 1966). It should be suspected if a significantly greater amount (more than 1 D) of plus power (i.e., more hyperopia or less myopia) is found on retinoscopy when compared with the subjective refractive findings, if the patient appears to have an abnormally low amplitude of accommodation for their age, or increases in eso posture are observed (Irvine, 1947), particularly towards the end of a working day. Curtin (1985) noted that pseudomyopia may be produced by oedema of the ciliary body, swelling or increased refractive index of the crystalline lens, anterior displacement of the crystalline lens, changes in the refractive index of the aqueous or vitreous or increases in axial length.

What is of particular interest is whether periods of accommodative spasm or transient pseudomyopia could be a precursor to permanent myopia which remains present even when a cycloplegic agent is administered (i.e., in the absence of accommodation). Sato (1957, 1981) suggested that myopia was produced by increased crystalline lens power resulting from changes in the tonus of the ciliary muscle. These variations in muscle tonus were produced by sustained periods of accommodation. Unfortunately, Sato dismissed axial elongation as a cause of nearwork-induced myopia, whereas recent studies have demonstrated that almost all young-adult-onset myopia is indeed axial in origin (Adams, 1987; McBrien and Millodot, 1987a; Bullimore *et al.*, 1992; Goss and Jackson, 1993; Grosvenor, 1994; Fledelius, 1995; McBrien and Adams, 1997).

Later, Young (1981) proposed that the development of myopia was a two-stage process, with the first phase being an 'induced tonic change' in the ciliary muscle which keeps the lens in a continuously accommodated posture (i.e., pseudomyopia). This sustained accommodative response would lead to the second stage of myopia development, namely increased axial length of the globe. Young suggested that the increased intraocular pressure produced by sustained accommodation might be responsible for the increase in axial length. This notion will be discussed further in sections 5.8 and 5.9.

Biometric data from Zadnik *et al.* (1994, 1995) would not support the proposal that myopia results from excessive ciliary muscle tone. Mutti *et al.* (1996) pointed out that if high ciliary tonus was a precursor to permanent myopia, then myopes would be predicted to exhibit a thicker and more steeply curved crystalline lens. In contrast, myopic children tended to have thinner lenses (Zadnik *et al.*, 1995), and additionally, children with two myopic parents (who were considered to be more likely to develop myopia) had flatter crystalline lens radii, when compared with children with one or no myopic parents (Zadnik *et al.*, 1994).

5.8 Accommodation, intraocular pressure and myopia

Since the vast majority of young-adult-onset myopia is produced by an increase in the axial length of the globe (McBrien and Millodot, 1987a; Bullimore *et al.*, 1992; Goss and Jackson, 1993; Grosvenor, 1994; McBrien and Adams, 1997), one must establish a mechanism which is capable of producing this axial elongation. One proposal is that the force exerted by the intraocular pressure (IOP) on the coats of the eye might be responsible for this dimensional shift. In an excellent review of this topic, Pruett (1988) noted that there were two possible mechanisms which might link IOP and myopia development. Firstly, the sclera of a myopic individual may be more prone to stretch (or creep) in response to the stresses imposed by IOP, and furthermore, may have poor memory or hysteresis so that it gradually becomes deformed permanently. Secondly, myopic eyes may have higher IOP. The latter notion is supported by the findings of Tomlinson and Phillips (1970), Abdalla and Hamdi (1970), Barraquer (1974; cited by Stuart-Black Kelly, 1981) and Edwards and Brown (1993), who all observed higher levels of IOP in myopic individuals. Indeed, Tomlinson and Phillips (1970) reported a statistically significant, but weak ($r^2 = 0.14$) correlation between IOP and the axial length of the globe in 75 subjects of between 18 and 27 years of age. However, one must again question whether the changes in IOP occur prior to, or following myopia development. For example, an increase in axial length might alter the functional structure of the trabecular meshwork, resulting in decreased aqueous outflow and a rise in IOP. Alternatively, increased aqueous production may produce distension of the globe (Bill, 1965; Tomlinson and Phillips, 1970). Indeed, a recent longitudinal study by Edwards and Brown (1996) demonstrated an increase in IOP after the development of myopia. However, they had a relatively small sample size (only 13 children developed myopia) and indeed stated that the findings need to be confirmed in a larger population. Nevertheless, if myopia does indeed result from accommodation, then one possible mechanism might be that periods of sustained accommodation lead to variations in IOP. Over extended periods of time, these small but sustained IOP shifts might ultimately induce an increase in the axial length of the globe.

In a review of this topic, Stansbury (1948) cited a number of workers including Ware (1813) and von Arlt (1856) who stated that myopia was produced by raised intraocular tension during accommodation. However, several investigations using Goldmann applanation tonometry (Armaly and Rubin, 1961; Mauger *et al.*, 1984) concluded that accommodation produced a significant reduction in IOP. Armaly and Rubin (1961) observed a mean reduction in IOP of 4.5 mmHg in young patients (20–25 years of age) while viewing a 4 D accommodative stimulus. In a subsequent paper, Armaly and Jepson (1962) concluded that increased accommodation produced a simultaneous increase in both aqueous outflow facility and in the rate of aqueous inflow, and the overall change in IOP was dependent upon the relative magnitude of these two shifts. This is consistent with earlier anatomical observations of changes in the valve action of the angle (Burian and Allen, 1955) and trabecular pore size (Flocks and Zweng, 1957) with increased accommodation (Allen and Burian, 1965).

In contrast to these findings using applanation tonometry, direct measurements of vitreous chamber pressure have demonstrated increased pressure with accommodation. For example, Young (1975) implanted a radiosonde pressure transducer into the vitreous chamber in two monkeys (*Macaca nemestrina*), and observed an increase in vitreous pressure with decreasing fixation distance. The increase in vitreous pressure was approximately 6 mmHg when viewing a target at a fixation distance of 30 cm. Furthermore, the increase in vitreous chamber pressure was maintained as long as the accommodation response was sustained, but decreased when accommodation relaxed. However, it is unclear whether implantation of the pressure transducer–described as having the diameter of an 'aspirin tablet' (Young, 1975)–would itself have any effect on the vitreous chamber pressure.

An explanation for the apparent discrepancy between the IOP and vitreous chamber pressure findings with increased accommodation has been proposed by Young and Leary (1991). They indicated that corneal applanation measured the pressure of the anterior chamber, whereas the implanted transducer assessed the vitreous chamber pressure. Young and Leary noted that for opposing pressure shifts to occur, a membrane would have to separate these two chambers of the eye. While they hypothesized that the hyaloid membrane might separate the anterior and posterior chambers, they also noted that if a water-soluble dye was injected into the vitreous chamber of a monkey, it became visible in the anterior chamber 15 minutes later (Suzuki, 1973; Young and Leary, 1991). Thus the precise form and characteristics of any separating membrane between the anterior and vitreous chambers which would be capable of producing a pressure differential remains uncertain.

In addition, it is important to consider that any changes in IOP which might occur during sustained periods of nearwork may not be related to the accommodative response. Variations in IOP may also be produced by convergence (Greene, 1980, 1991; Moses *et al.*, 1982), pressure from the eye lids during blinking and lid squeezing (Coleman and Trokel, 1969) and downward head posture (Tokoro *et al.*, 1989). Indeed, the IOP changes produced by these non-accommodative functions can be markedly greater than the typical pressure changes produced by accommodation. For example, Coleman and Trokel (1969) reported increases in IOP of 5–10 mmHg during both voluntary blinking and levo-version, and increases of over 80 mmHg during lid squeezing.

It will be apparent that at the present time there is very limited data to support the proposal that increased axial length of the globe is mediated via increased intraocular (or vitreal) pressure produced by the action of accommodation. The pressure changes are relatively small, and presumably would have to be maintained for extremely prolonged periods of time, in order to affect the sclera, i.e., the most rigid tunic of the eye (Graebel and Van Alphen, 1977; Bell, 1978; Phillips and McBrien, 1995). Furthermore, Greene (1980) noted that increased vitreous pressure generated by the choroid would result in a decline in the pressure within the suprachoroidal space (Van Alphen, 1961), so that these forces would not be transmitted to the sclera. Finally, until the effects of accommodation on the forces within the globe are clarified, it is impossible to substantiate any claims for an association between accommodation, IOP and myopia.

5.9 Possible mechanisms linking accommodation with myopia development

If the development of myopia is indeed associated with the actions of the accommodative system, then it is critical that the mechanism linking the two be definitively outlined. To date, one must conclude that no clear model has yet been established. Nevertheless, many workers have speculated as to how the actions of accommodation might lead to myopia development, and these will be considered in this section.

It is important to note that the vast majority of myopia which develops during childhood and young adulthood is axial in nature, being produced by an increase in vitreous chamber depth (Wibaut, 1926; Tron, 1940; Sorsby *et al.*, 1961; Sorsby and Leary, 1970; Larsen, 1971a, 1971b; Adams, 1987; McBrien and Millodot, 1987a; Bullimore *et al.*, 1992; Goss and Jackson, 1993; Grosvenor, 1994; Zadnik *et al.*, 1994; Fledelius, 1995; McBrien and Adams, 1997). This finding would appear to rule out the proposal that myopia results from the crystalline lens being permanently deformed, i.e., a failure to relax accommodation fully. However, some workers, as outlined in section 5.7, have suggested that myopia development may be a two-stage process, with sustained accommodation being the precursor to vitreous chamber elongation. Again it must be emphasized that myopia (or any refractive error) can only be said to exist under conditions of minimal accommodation. If the instillation of a cycloplegic agent eliminates the refractive shift (as will occur in pseudomyopia), then no change in the refractive error of the eye can be said to have taken place.

Three possible mechanisms have been proposed to link accommodation with myopia development, namely:

1   variations in intraocular pressure;
2   retinal defocus;
3   retinal stretching.

Possible associations between intraocular pressure, accommodation and myopia were discussed in section 5.8.

5.9.1   Accommodation, retinal defocus and myopia

A number of studies have proposed that the stimulus for axial elongation is the presence of a defocused retinal image. The eye is presumed to adjust the location of the retina in order to reduce the diameter of the retinal blur circle. The rationale for this theory is derived from animal studies which have demonstrated that degraded retinal images produce substantial myopia in a variety of different species (*see* Chapters 3 and 4). For example, Schaeffel *et al.* (1988) and Irving *et al.* (1991, 1992) demonstrated that if plus and minus lenses are placed before the eyes of newly hatched chicks, to induce myopia and hyperopia, respectively, then the subsequent growth of the eye compensates for the induced refractive error. Thus, an eye which viewed through a plus lens (to induce myopia) developed a relatively shorter axial length (i.e.,

became hyperopic) in order to compensate for the induced refractive error. Similarly, eyes which wore minus lenses exhibited increased vitreous chamber depth (i.e., axial myopia). Furthermore, these compensatory growth and refractive changes were unaffected by lesions of the Edinger-Westphal nucleus to eliminate accommodation (Schaeffel *et al.*, 1990; Troilo, 1990; Troilo and Wallman, 1991). In contrast, Ni and Smith (1989) observed in kittens that introduction of both plus and minus lenses produced axial myopia. Furthermore, while Hung *et al.* (1995b) reported that plus and minus lenses produced axial elongation and myopia in the predicted direction in infant rhesus monkeys, a subsequent paper by Hung and Smith (1996) observed that both plus and minus contact lenses produced hyperopia in the same species.

It will be apparent that this effect appears to be species-dependent, but at least in some animals, the location of the retina is successfully adjusted to minimize the degree of retinal defocus. Interestingly, Wallman *et al.* (1992) and Wildsoet and Wallman (1995) have proposed that these refractive changes observed in chicks may be induced at least in the initial stages by changes in choroidal thickness, although subsequent growth of the sclera makes the refractive changes more permanent and allows the choroid to return to its original thickness (Wildsoet, 1997). However, Zadnik and Mutti (1995) pointed out that changes in choroidal thickness do not appear to be a significant long-term factor in human refractive error development. An investigation of human myopic eyes using magnetic resonance imaging (MRI) revealed a mean difference in choroidal thickness between groups of hyperopes and myopes of only 0.4 mm (equivalent to approximately 1.3 D), whereas the mean difference in refractive error was 10.25 D (Cheng *et al.*, 1992).

If retinal defocus is a precursor to axial elongation, then it is unclear when the critical image degradation occurs. Two possibilities appear to exist: either during the course of a sustained near-vision task, or immediately following task completion. As was noted in section 5.4, several studies have observed reduced within-task accommodative responses in myopic individuals, when compared with emmetropes (Ramsdale, 1979; McBrien and Millodot, 1986b; Rosenfield and Gilmartin, 1988a; Tokoro, 1988; Bullimore *et al.*, 1992; Gwiazda *et al.*, 1993a). One might suggest that these reduced responses could be responsible for retinal defocus. The mean difference in accommodative response between emmetropes and myopes for a typical reading distance of 0.33 m (accommodative stimulus = 3 D) recorded in a number of studies is shown in Table 5.1. It may be observed that the mean difference varied from 0 to 0.90 D. These results would suggest that extended intervals of retinal defocus may occur during periods of reading in certain individuals.

As will be discussed later in Chapter 10, section 10.3, these differences in within-task accommodative response may also be associated with variations in the magnitude of accommodative adaptation induced during the course of a sustained near-vision task. As indicated previously (section 5.6.2), a role of accommodative adaptation is to increase the accuracy of the aggregate accommodative response (Schor *et al.*, 1986; Rosenfield and Gilmartin, 1998) (see Figure 5.9). Accordingly, those individuals lacking appropriate adaptive responses are likely to demonstrate an increased lag of accommodation to a near stimulus. Furthermore, as discussed in section 10.3, reduced adaptation will also be associated with diminished sympathetic innervation to the ciliary muscle, asthenopia, esophoria at near and an increased AC/A ratio. All of these five factors have previously been associated with the development of myopia in young adults (Curtin, 1985; Gilmartin and Bullimore, 1987; Rosenfield and Gilmartin, 1987a; Goss and Grosvenor, 1990; Gwiazda *et al.*, 1993a).

Alternatively, the accommodative adaptation observed immediately following a sustained near task might also produce transient periods of retinal defocus. As was indicated in section 5.6.1, if a subject views a distant target (under closed-loop conditions) immediately following a continuous period of near-work, then a transient increase in accommodation of approximately 0.2 D is frequently observed (Ehrlich, 1987; Rosenfield *et al.*, 1992b), although shifts exceeding 1.00 D have also been reported (Ong and Ciuffreda, 1995, 1997). This adaptation reflects the relatively prolonged rate of decay of the SBAR. Accordingly, during this initial post-task period, subjects may experience blur when viewing distant objects. This is a relatively common symptom in young-adult subjects. In an informal survey of optometry students (Rosenfield and Chiu, unpublished data), 83 subjects were questioned as to whether they ever experienced blurred distance vision following periods of reading. Forty-five per cent of the respondents reported that this occurred occasionally (i.e., approximately 25% of the time), while 26% of the

individuals indicated that this occurred often (i.e., at least 50% of the time).

It is uncertain which of these two potential periods of defocus is more likely to contribute to the development of permanent axial myopia. If the sign of the defocus is critical, then this would support the proposal that an increased lag of accommodation during the course of the near-task would be responsible. With a reduced accommodative response, the target will be focused behind the retina, a situation which would be improved by an increase in axial length. In contrast, when viewing a distant object immediately following sustained near fixation (with accommodative adaptation), the image of the distant object will be formed in front of the retina–a situation which would not be helped by an increase in the axial length of the globe. Thus if the sign of the optical defocus is critical, then this would support the proposal that the defocus present during the course of the sustained task is most relevant. Furthermore, the increased within-task lag of accommodation observed in myopes may be sustained throughout the period of nearwork (Rosenfield and Gilmartin, 1988a), whereas the transient adaptive shifts observed following nearwork typically dissipate within 50 s of task completion (Gilmartin and Bullimore, 1987; Rosenfield *et al.*, 1992b; Gilmartin and Winfield, 1995).

In addition, the magnitude of the within-task lag of accommodation in myopes is significantly greater than that observed in emmetropes (Ramsdale, 1979; McBrien and Millodot, 1986b; Rosenfield and Gilmartin, 1988a; Tokoro, 1988; Bullimore *et al.*, 1992; Gwiazda *et al.*, 1993a). However, studies comparing accommodative adaptation in populations of emmetropes and myopes have recorded mixed results. For example, Rosenfield and Gilmartin (1988b) observed that immediately following a near-vision task, emmetropes show both a greater degree of adaptation (assessed under open-loop conditions) and a more rapid rate of decay when compared with late-onset myopes. This finding would suggest that emmetropes have a greater degree of retinal defocus than myopes, although it dissipates more rapidly. In contrast, when assessing post-task adaptation under closed-loop conditions, Ciuffreda and Wallis (1997) observed significantly greater adaptation in myopic subjects, when compared with both emmetropes and hyperopes. It is unclear whether the magnitude or duration of the retinal defocus is more relevant. Furthermore, Morse and Smith (1993) concluded that accommodative adaptation was associated with the pre-task level of tonic accommodation rather than the baseline refractive error.

In an examination of accommodation and convergence parameters in emmetropic subjects before they became myopic, both Goss (1991) and Portello *et al.* (1997) observed a significantly greater lag of accommodation, as assessed by the binocular cross-cylinder test (Rosenfield, 1997), in the 'became myopic' group, when compared with those individuals who remained emmetropic. These findings support the proposal that it is the defocus occurring during the course of a near-vision task, rather than that present immediately following task completion, that is more likely to be related to myopia development.

In considering how retinal defocus might be a precursor to axial elongation, Goss (1988) hypothesized that the defocused retinal image might lead to increased production of growth-inducing substances, or growth factors, which would stimulate an increase in the axial length of the globe. In a detailed review, Goss and Wickham (1995) suggested that young adult-onset myopia may reflect variations in scleral fibrocyte sensitivity to a growth-inducing chemical mediator such as human growth hormone (HGH). In addition to the release of these systemic growth factors, local chemical mediators, such as glutamate (Redburn, 1989) may also be responsible for inducing scleral growth (Goss and Wickham, 1995).

While this hypothesis is fascinating, caution must be exercised when applying it to human child- and young adult-onset myopia. Firstly, much of the biochemical evidence has been obtained in chicks, who have quite different scleral histology and biochemistry when compared with mammals. The mammalian sclera consists of type I collagen fibres and a proteoglycan matrix, whereas the avian sclera contains both dense white connective tissue and a hyaline cartilage layer (Goss and Wickham, 1995). Additionally, Zadnik and Mutti (1995) noted that axial elongation following experimentally induced myopia occurred through increased mitosis and protein synthesis in the chick (Christensen and Wallman, 1991) but via scleral reorganization in the mammalian tree shrew (Norton *et al.*, 1992).

Secondly, the only evidence that retinal image defocus produces myopia in humans comes from cases of severe image degradation. For example, Rabin *et al.* (1981) reported that disruption of pattern vision in young humans by conditions such as persistent pupillary membrane, vitreous debris or traumatic cataract were accompanied by substantial amounts of myopia. Myopia in humans has also been associated with lid haemangioma (Robb, 1977), ptosis (O'Leary and Millodot, 1979), and neonatal lid closure (Hoyt *et al.*, 1981). It seems quite unrealistic to equate the degree of image degradation produced by these severe conditions with the loss of retinal image contrast produced, for example, by an increase in lag of accommodation of approximately 0.50 D. Furthermore, Nathan *et al.* (1985) reported that ocular pathology which primarily impaired foveal vision in children (e.g. albinism and maculopathies) was frequently associated with hyperopia.

Thirdly, almost all of the experimental animal studies have been performed on neonates. However, in considering the effects of nearwork and specifically accommodation on myopia development, studies should be performed on older animals. To date, such experiments have not been conducted (Zadnik and Mutti, 1995).

The retinal defocus theory would suggest that if myopia is to be avoided, then the presence of a sharply focused retinal image is critical. This would imply that subjects must wear a precise refractive correction at all times. However, this statement should be taken with extreme caution when considering the refractive correction of children under 6 years of age. Gwiazda *et al.* (1993b) demonstrated a broad range of refractive errors in children under 6 months of age (see Section 10.2.2), which developed into the more typical leptokurtotic refractive distribution (Stenstrom, 1948) by 6 years of age, with a high prevalence of emmetropia. These changes may reflect a period of 'emmetropization' (Staub, 1900, cited by Medina, 1987a) whereby a regulating mechanism produces coordinated growth of the ocular components. The effect of wearing a refractive correction on this process of emmetropization is unclear (Hung *et al.*, 1995b; Wildsoet, 1997), although Medina (1987b) suggested that refractive correction could 'defeat the emmetropization process'. This is supported by the findings of both Dobson *et al.* (1986) and Ingram *et al.* (1991), who reported that infants wearing a full-time hyperopic correction tended to remain hyperopic, in contrast with those individuals whose hyperopia remained uncorrected.

Nevertheless, the notion that a full refractive correction must be prescribed in older children and young adults (to avoid even small amounts of retinal defocus) runs contrary to the proposal that myopia should be less than fully corrected in order to preclude further refractive development (*see*

Goss, 1982, 1994 for a review). Indeed, if the sign of the retinal defocus is critical, then hyperopic blur resulting from the retinal image being focused behind the retina must be avoided. This may be particularly critical at near, where bifocals may be prescribed to reduce, but not necessarily eliminate the lag of accommodation. Further work is required to determine whether precise refractive correction at all viewing distances does indeed inhibit myopic development and/or progression.

5.9.2 Accommodation, retinal stretching and myopia

An alternative proposal is that the action of accommodation exerts stresses directly upon the sclera, resulting in retinal stretching (Bell, 1978). Moses (1981) noted that the ora serrata moves forward by approximately 0.05 mm with each dioptre of accommodation in young observers. Enoch (1975) calculated that a 0.5 mm retinal advance (resulting from 10 D of accommodation) would produce a 30 mm^2 (or 2.4%) increase in the surface area of the retina. This model assumes that the retina is stretched about a non-compressible vitreous. What remains unclear, however, is whether this forward movement of the choroid and retina actually results in any change in the sclera, particularly at the posterior pole, where the axial elongation that leads to permanent myopia primarily occurs (Greene, 1991). Furthermore, the effects of accommodation need to be considered at naturalistic response levels (i.e., around 3 D) rather than at stimulus demands that approach the amplitude of accommodation.

5.10 Conclusions

As noted earlier, the proposal that nearwork-induced myopia is mediated via the actions of accommodation appears to be reasonable. The increased refractive power of the eye produced by accommodation, were it to be maintained permanently, is likely to result in myopia. However, the majority of permanent myopia is produced by an increase in vitreous chamber depth (Sorsby *et al.*, 1961; Sorsby and Leary, 1970; Larsen, 1971a, 1971b). To date, no mechanism has clearly been elucidated which demonstrates how variations in accommodation could lead to increased axial length of the globe.

One difficulty is that the development of myopia itself alters the accommodative demand. If an association does indeed exist between accommodation and refractive error development, then this must be demonstrated prior to myopia onset. For example, the ocular accommodative stimulus for a fully corrected myopic individual is lower than for an emmetrope viewing the same stimulus (Rosenfield, 1997). Accordingly, one would predict lower accommodative responses in myopes. However, it does appear that the increased lag of accommodation observed in myopes actually exceeds that which would be predicted by calculating the ocular accommodative stimulus (McBrien and Millodot, 1986b; Rosenfield and Gilmartin, 1988a; Bullimore *et al.*, 1992). Nevertheless, it is unclear whether this larger accommodative error, which might result from decreased accommodative adaptation, is actually related to the aetiology of the ametropia. Another possibility is that myopic subjects simply fail to detect the retinal defocus, and so their accommodative response is less accurate. If this were true, then one might also predict greater variation in the within-task accommodative response to a fixed, sustained stimulus. It would be of interest to compare the blur-driven accommodative responses to small amounts of retinal defocus in emmetropes, myopes who wear a full-time refractive correction, and myopes who either wear a part-time correction, or a full-time partial correction. Alternatively, some myopes may be 'lazy accommodators', i.e., they detect retinal defocus, but fail to accommodate the required amount to provide an optimal image of the object of regard –perhaps due to enhanced 'blur interpretation', i.e., an improved ability to resolve defocused retinal images. Again it must be emphasized that even if differences in accommodative responsivity do exist prior to myopia onset, this does not provide firm evidence that accommodation is an aetiological factor in refractive error development.

It should also be noted that attempts to retard myopia development or progression by accommodative control have been disappointing. Myopia control using cycloplegic agents, bifocals, biofeedback or undercorrection will be discussed in detail in Chapter 9. These findings generally do not support the proposal that myopia develops via an accommodative mechanism. However, a key reason why attempts to control myopic progression have been relatively unsuccessful may relate to the absence of subject pre-selection. A particular treatment regime may work successfully in a subgroup of myopes, but if applied indiscriminately to every myopic individual, may, when the results are averaged across all patients, show no significant effect. One could argue that if accommodative control is successful in slowing myopic progression in at least a subset of patients, then this might provide evidence that accommodation does plays a role in these individuals. Thus it is essential to identify these 'accommodative myopes' before commencing therapy. The clinical parameters described by Goss (1991), most notably the presence of esophoria at near (Goss and Jackson, 1996) may be valuable here. This proposal is supported by the findings of Oakley and Young (1975), Neetens and Evans (1985) and Goss (1994), who all reported that bifocal therapy for myopia control was more successful in those patients exhibiting esophoria at near. It should be noted that approximately 25% of the population between 10 and 20 years of age exhibit esophoria at near (Hirsch *et al.*, 1948).

If one is to demonstrate that myopia development is related to the actions of accommodation, then a model clearly linking the two must be demonstrated. Simply because two events occur simultaneously does not confirm an association. While the effects of accommodation on retinal defocus, variations in intraocular pressure and retinal stretching have all been hypothesized to produce myopia, longitudinal data must be provided to verify whether any of these or other factors are indeed precursors to myopia development. Until this data is available, then any association between myopia development and the actions of ocular accommodation must be considered unproven.

References

Abbott, M. L., Schmid, K. L. and Strang, N. C. (1998) Differences in the accommodation stimulus response curves of adult myopes and emmetropes. *Ophthal. Physiol. Opt.* **18**, 13–20.

Abdalla, M. I. and Hamdi, M. (1970) Applanation ocular tension in myopia and emmetropia. *Br. J. Ophthalmol.* **54**, 122–125.

Abraham-Cohen, J. A., Rosenfield, M. and Jang, C. (1997) Blur sensitivity in myopes. *Optom. Vis. Sci.* **74** (Suppl.), 177.

Adams, A. J. (1987) Axial length elongation, not corneal curvature, as a basis of adult onset myopia. *Am. J. Optom. Physiol. Opt.* **64**, 150–151.

Adams, D. W. and McBrien, N. A. (1993) A longitudinal study of the relationship between tonic accommodation (dark focus) and refractive error in adulthood. *Invest. Ophthalmol. Vis. Sci.* (Suppl.) **34**, 1308.

Alexander, G. F. (1940) Spasm of accommodation. *Trans. Ophthalmol. Soc. UK* **60**, 207–212.

Allen, L. and Burian, H. M. (1965) The valve action of the trabecular meshwork. *Am. J. Ophthalmol.* **59**, 382–389.

Aminoff, M. J. (1996) Nervous system. In: *Current Medical Diagnosis and Treatment*, 35th edn (L. M. Tierney, S. J. McPhee and M. A. Papadakis, eds). Appleton & Lange, pp. 858–914.

Armaly, M. F. and Jepson, N. C. (1962) Accommodation and the dynamics of the steady-state intraocular pressure. *Invest. Ophthalmol.* **1**, 480–483.

Armaly, M. F. and Rubin, M. L. (1961) Accommodation and applanation tonometry. *Arch. Ophthalmol.* **65**, 415–423.

Bell, G. R. (1978) A review of the sclera and its role in myopia. *J. Am. Optom. Assoc.* **49**, 1399–1403.

Bennett, A. G. and Rabbetts, R. B. (1989) *Clinical Visual Optics*, 2nd edn. Butterworth-Heinemann.

Bill, A. (1965) The aqueous humor drainage mechanism in the cynomolgus monkey (*Macaca irus*) with evidence for unconventional routes. *Invest. Ophthalmol.* **4**, 911–919.

Blustein, G. H., Rosenfield, M. and Ciuffreda, K. J. (1993) Does dark accommodation really change following sustained near fixation? *Optom. Vis. Sci.* (Suppl.) **70**, 16.

Borish, I. M. (1970) *Clinical Refraction*, 3rd edn. Professional Press, pp. 93–94.

Brown, E. V. L. (1938) Net average yearly change in refraction of atropinized eyes from birth to beyond middle life. *Acta Ophthalmol.* **19**, 719–734.

Brown, E. V. L. (1942) Use–abuse theory of changes in refraction versus biologic theory. *Arch. Ophthalmol.* **28**, 845–850.

Bullimore, M. A. and Gilmartin, B. (1989) The measurement of adaptation of tonic accommodation under two open-loop conditions. *Ophthal. Physiol. Opt.* **9**, 72–75.

Bullimore, M. A., Boyd, T., Mather, H. E. and Gilmartin, B. (1988) Near retinoscopy and refractive error. *Clin. Exp. Optom.* **71**, 114–118.

Bullimore, M. A., Gilmartin, B. and Royston, J. M. (1992) Steady-state accommodation and ocular biometry in late-onset myopia. *Doc. Ophthalmol.* **80**, 143–155.

Burian, H. M. and Allen, L. (1955) Mechanical changes during accommodation observed by gonioscopy. *Arch. Ophthalmol.* **54**, 66–72.

Campbell, F. W. (1957) The depth of field of the human eye. *Optica Acta* **4**, 157–164.

Carreras, M. (1951) La miopia nocturna e influencia sobre la misma de la amplitud de acomodacion. *Archos. Soc. Oftal. Hisp.-Am.* **11**, 1443–1489.

Charman, W. N. (1982) The accommodative resting point and refractive error. *Ophthal. Opt.* **21**, 469–473.

Charman, W. N. and Whitefoot, H. (1977) Pupil diameter and the depth-of-field of the human eye as measured by laser speckle. *Optica Acta* **24**, 1211–1216.

Chen, A. H. and O'Leary, D. J. (1997) The accommodative response curve in children. *Invest. Ophthalmol. Vis. Sci.* **38**, S982.

Cheng, H. M., Singh, O. S., Kwong, K. K. *et al.* (1992) Shape of the myopic eye as seen with high-resolution magnetic resonance imaging. *Optom. Vis. Sci.* **69**, 698–701.

Chiu, N. N., Rosenfield, M. and Solan, H. (1994) Habitual reading and writing distances in children. *Optom. Vis. Sci.* (Suppl.) **71**, 126.

Christensen, A. M. and Wallman, J. (1991) Evidence that increased scleral growth underlies visual deprivation myopia in chicks. *Invest. Ophthalmol. Vis. Sci.* **32**, 2143–2150.

Ciuffreda, K. J. and Kenyon, R. V. (1983) Accommodative vergence and accommodation in normals, amblyopes and strabismics. In: *Vergence Eye Movements: Basic and Clinical Aspects* (C. M. Schor and K. J. Ciuffreda, eds). Butterworths, pp. 101–173.

Ciuffreda, K. J. and Ordonez, X. (1995) Abnormal transient myopia in symptomatic individuals after sustained nearwork. *Optom. Vis. Sci.* **72**, 506–510.

Ciuffreda, K. J. and Wallis, D. (1997) Accommodative after effects and refractive state. *Invest. Ophthalmol. Vis. Sci.* **38**, S543.

Cohn, H. (1886) *The Hygiene of the Eye in Schools* (English translation by W. P. Turnbull). Simpkin, Marshall & Co.

Coleman, D. J. and Trokel, S. (1969) Direct-recorded intraocular pressure variations in a human subject. *Arch Ophthalmol.* **82**, 637–640.

Cooper, J. (1987) Accommodative dysfunction. In: *Diagnosis and Management in Vision Care* (J. F. Amos, ed.). Butterworths, pp. 431–459.

Curtin, B. J. (1970) Myopia: a review of its etiology, pathogenesis and treatment. *Surv. Ophthalmol.* **15**, 1–17.

Curtin, B. J. (1985) *The Myopias. Basic Science and Clinical Management.* Harper & Row.

Dobson, V., Sebris, S. L. and Carlson, M. R. (1986) Do glasses prevent emmetropization in strabismic infants? *Invest. Ophthalmol. Vis. Sci.* (Suppl.) **27**, 2.

Donders, F. C. (1864) *On the Anomalies of Accommodation and Refraction of the Eye* (translated by W. D. Moore). The New Sydenham Society.

Duane, A. (1912) Normal values of the accommodation at all ages. *J. Am. Med. Assoc.* **59**, 1010–1013.

Duke-Elder, S. and Abrams, D. (1970) *System of Ophthalmology*, Vol. V: *Ophthalmic Optics and Refraction*. C. V. Mosby.

Ebenholtz, S. M. (1983) Accommodative hysteresis: a precursor for induced myopia? *Invest. Ophthalmol. Vis. Sci.* **24**, 513–515.

Edwards, M. H. and Brown, B. (1993) Intraocular pressure in a selected sample of myopic and nonmyopic Chinese children. *Optom. Vis. Sci.* **70**, 15–17.

Edwards, M. H. and Brown, B. (1996) IOP in myopic children: the relationship between increases in IOP and the development of myopia. *Ophthal. Physiol. Opt.* **16**, 243–246.

Ehrlich, D. L. (1987) Near vision stress: vergence adaptation and accommodative fatigue. *Ophthal. Physiol. Opt.* **7**, 353–357.

Emsley, H. H. (1953) *Visual Optics*, vol. I, 5th edn. Butterworths.

Enoch, J. M. (1975) Marked accommodation, retinal stretch, monocular space perception and retinal receptor orientation. *Am. J. Optom. Physiol. Opt.* **52**, 376–392.

Fisher, S. K., Ciuffreda, K. J. and Levine, S. (1987) Tonic accommodation, accommodative hysteresis, and refractive error. *Am. J. Optom. Physiol. Opt.* **64**, 799–809.

Fledelius, H. C. (1981) Accommodation and juvenile myopia. *Doc. Ophthalmol. Proc. Series* No. 28 (H. C. Fledelius, P. H. Alsbirk and E. Goldschmidt, eds). Dr W. Junk, pp. 103–108.

Fledelius, H. C. (1995) Adult onset myopia–oculometric features. *Acta Ophthalmol. Scand.* **73**, 397–401.

Flocks, M. and Zweng, H. C. (1957) Studies on the mode of action of pilocarpine on aqueous outflow. *Am. J. Ophthalmol.* **44**, 380–388.

Fry, G. A. (1940) Skiametric measurement of convergent accommodation. *Optom. Weekly* **31**, 353–356.

Gawron, V. J. (1981) Differences among myopes, emmetropes, and hyperopes. *Am. J. Optom. Physiol. Opt.* **58**, 753–760.

Gilmartin, B. and Bullimore, M. A. (1987) Sustained near-vision augments inhibitory sympathetic innervation of the ciliary muscle. *Clin. Vis. Sci.* **1**, 197–208.

Gilmartin, B. and Bullimore, M. A. (1991) Adaptation of tonic accommodation to sustained visual tasks in emmetropia and late-onset myopia. *Optom. Vis. Sci.* **68**, 22–26.

Gilmartin, B. and Winfield, N. R. (1995) The effect of topical β-adrenoceptor antagonists on accommodation in emmetropia and myopia. *Vis. Res.* **35**, 1305–1312.

Gilmartin, B., Hogan, R. E. and Thompson, S. M. (1984) The effect of timolol maleate on tonic accommodation, tonic vergence, and pupil diameter. *Invest. Ophthalmol. Vis. Sci.* **25**, 763–770.

Goldschmidt, E. (1968) On the etiology of myopia. An epidemiological study. *Acta Ophthalmol.* (Suppl.) **98**, 1–172.

Goss, D. A. (1982) Attempts to reduce the rate of increase of myopia in young people–a critical literature review. *Am. J. Optom. Physiol. Opt.* **59**, 828–841.

Goss, D. A. (1988) Retinal image-mediated ocular growth as a possible etiological factor in juvenile-onset myopia. Vision Science Syposium, A Tribute to Gordon G. Heath. Indiana University, pp. 165–183.

Goss, D. A. (1991) Clinical accommodation and heterophoria findings preceding juvenile onset of myopia. *Optom. Vis. Sci.* **68**, 110–116.

Goss, D. A. (1994) Effect of spectacle correction on the progression of myopia in children–a literature review. *J. Am. Optom. Assoc.* **65**, 117–128.

Goss, D. A. and Grosvenor, T. (1990) Rates of childhood myopia progression with bifocals as a function of nearpoint phoria: consistency of three studies. *Optom. Vis. Sci.*, **67**, 637–640.

Goss, D. A. and Jackson, T. W. (1993) Cross-sectional study of changes in the ocular components in school children. *Applied Optics* **32**, 4169–4173.

Goss, D. A. and Jackson, T. W. (1996) Clinical findings before the onset of myopia in youth: 3. Heterophoria. *Optom. Vis. Sci.* **73**, 269–278.

Goss, D. A. and Wickham, M. G. (1995) Retinal-image mediated ocular growth as a mechanism for juvenile onset myopia and for emmetropization. *Doc. Ophthalmol.* **90**, 341–375.

Goss, D. A. and Winkler, R. L. (1983) Progression of myopia in youth: age of cessation. *Am. J. Optom. Physiol. Opt.* **60**, 651–658.

Graebel, W. P. and Van Alphen, G. W. H. M. (1977) The elasticity of sclera and choroid of the human eye, and its implications on scleral rigidity and accommodation. *J. Biomed. Eng.* **99**, 203–208.

Greene, P. R. (1980) Mechanical considerations in myopia: relative effects of accommodation, convergence, intraocular pressure, and the extraocular muscles. *Am. J. Optom. Physiol. Opt.* **57**, 902–914.

Greene, P. R. (1991) Mechanical considerations in myopia. In: *Refractive Anomalies. Research and Clinical Applications* (T. Grosvenor and M. C. Flom, eds). Butterworth–Heinemann, pp. 287–309.

Griffin, J. R. (1988) *Binocular Anomalies. Procedures for Vision Therapy*, 2nd edn. Professional Press, pp. 381–382.

Grosvenor, T. (1994) Refractive component changes in adult-onset myopia: evidence from five studies. *Clin. Exp. Optom.* **77**, 196–205.

Guyton, A. C. (1986) *Textbook of Medical Physiology*, 7th edn. W. B. Saunders, pp. 138.

Gwiazda, J., Bauer, J., Thorn, F. and Held, R. (1995) A dynamic relationship between myopia and blur-driven accommodation in school-aged children. *Vision Res.* **35**, 1299–1304.

Gwiazda, J., Thorn, F., Bauer, J. and Held, R. (1993a) Myopic children show insufficient accommodative response to blur. *Invest. Ophthalmol. Vis. Sci.* **34**, 690–694.

Gwiazda, J., Thorn, F., Bauer, J. and Held, R. (1993b) Emmetropization and the progression of manifest refraction in children followed from infancy to puberty. *Clin. Vis. Sci.* **8**, 337–344.

Heath, G. G. (1956) Components of accommodation. *Am. J. Optom. Arch. Am. Acad. Optom.* **33**, 569–579.

Henson, D. B. and North, R. V. (1980) Adaptation to prism-induced heterophoria. *Am. J. Optom. Physiol. Opt.* **57**, 129–137.

Heron, G., Smith, A. C. and Winn, B. (1981) The influence of method on the stability of the dark focus position of accommodation. *Ophthal. Physiol. Opt.* **1**, 79–80.

Hirsch, M. J., Alpern, M. and Schultz, H. L. (1948) The variation of phoria with age. *Am. J. Optom. Arch. Am. Acad. Optom.* **25**, 535–541.

Hoyt, C. S., Stone, R. D., Fromer C. and Billson, F. A. (1981) Monocular axial myopia associated with neonatal eyelid closure in human infants. *Am. J. Ophthalmol.* **91**, 197–200.

Hung, G. K. (1992) Adaptation model of accommodation and vergence. *Ophthal. Physiol. Opt.* **12**, 319–326.

Hung, L. F. and Smith, E. L. (1996) Extended-wear, soft, contact lenses produce hyperopia in young monkeys. *Optom. Vis. Sci.* **73**, 579–584.

Hung, G. K., Ciuffreda, K. J. and Rosenfield, M. (1995a) Proximal contribution to a linear static model of accommodation and vergence. *Ophthal. Physiol. Opt.* **16**, 31–41.

Hung, L. F., Crawford, M. L. J. and Smith, E. L. (1995b) Spectacle lenses alter eye growth and the refractive status of young monkeys. *Nature Med.* **1**, 761–765.

Ingram, R. M., Arnold, P. E., Dally, S. and Lucas, J. (1991) Emmetropisation, squint, and reduced visual acuity after treatment. *Br. J. Ophthalmol.* **75**, 414–416.

Irvine, G. (1947) A survey of esophoria and ciliary spasm. *Br. J. Ophthalmol.* **31**, 289–304.

Irving, E. L., Callender, M. G. and Sivak, J. G. (1991) Inducing myopia, hyperopia, and astigmatism in chicks. *Optom. Vis. Sci.* **68**, 364–368.

Irving, E. L., Sivak, J. G. and Callender, M. G. (1992) Refractive plasticity of the developing chick eye. *Ophthal. Physiol. Opt.* **12**, 448–456.

Javal, E. (1990) Essay on the physiology of reading (translated by K. J. Ciuffreda and N. Bassil). *Ophthal. Physiol. Opt.* **10**, 381–384.

Jiang, B. C. (1995) Parameters of accommodative and vergence systems and the development of late-onset myopia. *Invest. Ophthalmol. Vis. Sci.* **36**, 1737–1742.

Jiang, B. C. (1997) Integration of a sensory component into the accommodation model reveals differences between emmetropia and late-onset myopia. *Invest. Ophthalmol. Vis. Sci.* **38**, 1511–1516.

Jones, R. (1990a) Accommodative and convergence control system parameters are abnormal in myopia. *Invest. Ophthalmol. Vis. Sci.* (Suppl.) **31**, 81.

Jones, R. (1990b) Do women and myopes have larger pupils? *Invest. Ophthalmol. Vis. Sci.* **31**, 1413–1415.

Kao, S. C., Lu, H. Y. and Liu, J. H. (1988) Atropine effect on school myopia. A preliminary report. *Acta Ophthalmol.* (Suppl.) **185**, 132–133.

Kent, P. R. (1958) Convergence accommodation. *Am. J. Optom. Arch. Am. Acad. Optom.* **35**, 393–406.

Kersten, D. and Legge, G. E. (1983) Convergence accommodation. *J. Opt. Soc. Am.* **73**, 332–338.

Krumholz, D. M., Fox, R. S. and Ciuffreda, K. J. (1986) Short-term changes in tonic accommodation. *Invest. Ophthalmol. Vis. Sci.* **27**, 552–557.

Larsen, J. S. (1971a) The sagittal growth of the eye. Pt II. Ultrasonic measurement of the axial diameter of the lens and the anterior segment from birth to puberty. *Acta Ophthalmol.* **49**, 427–440.

Larsen, J. S. (1971b) The sagittal growth of the eye. Pt III. Ultrasonic measurement of the posterior segment from birth to puberty. *Acta Ophthalmol.* **49**, 441–453.

Lin, L. L.-K., Shih, Y.-F., Lee, Y.-C. *et al.* (1996) Changes in ocular refraction and its components among medical students. A 5-year longitudinal study. *Optom. Vis. Sci.* **73**, 495–498.

Maddock, R. J., Millodot, M., Leat, S. and Johnson, C. A. (1981) Accommodation responses and refractive error. *Invest. Ophthalmol. Vis. Sci.* **20**, 387–391.

Maddox, E. E. (1893) *The Clinical Use of Prisms and the Decentering of Lenses.* John Wright & Sons, pp. 83–106.

Mäntyjärvi, M. (1983) Incidence of myopia in a population of Finnish school children. *Acta Ophthalmol.* **61**, 417–423.

Mäntyjärvi, M. (1987) Accommodation in hyperopic and myopic schoolchildren. *J. Ped. Ophthalmol. Strab.* **24**, 37–41.

Mäntyjärvi, M. and Nousianen, I. (1988) Refraction and accommodation in diabetic school children. *Acta Ophthalmol.* **66**, 267–271.

Mauger, R. R., Likens, C. P. and Applebaum, M. (1984) Effects of accommodation and repeated applanation tonometry on intraocular pressure. *Am. J. Optom. Physiol. Opt.* **61**, 28–30.

McBrien, N. A. and Adams, D. W. (1997) A longitudinal investigation of adult-onset and adult-progression of myopia in an occupational group. *Invest. Ophthalmol. Vis. Sci.* **38**, 321–333.

McBrien, N. A. and Millodot, M. (1986a) Amplitude of accommodation and refractive error. *Invest. Ophthalmol. Vis. Sci.* **27**, 1187–1190.

McBrien, N. A. and Millodot, M. (1986b) The effect of refractive error on the accommodative response gradient. *Ophthal. Physiol. Opt.* **6**, 145–149.

McBrien, N. A. and Millodot, M. (1987a) A biometric investigation of late onset myopic eyes. *Acta Ophthalmol.* **65**, 461–468.

McBrien, N. A. and Millodot, M. (1987b) The relationship between tonic accommodation and refractive error. *Invest. Ophthalmol. Vis. Sci.* **28**, 997–1004.

McBrien, N. A. and Millodot, M. (1988) Differences in adaptation of tonic accommodation with refractive state. *Invest. Ophthalmol. Vis. Sci.* **29**, 460–469.

Medina, A. (1987a) A model for emmetropization. The effect of corrective lenses. *Acta Ophthalmol.* **65**, 565–571.

Medina, A. (1987b) A model for emmetropization. Predicting the progression of ametropia. *Ophthalmologica* **194**, 133–139.

Mershon, D. H. and Amerson, T. L. (1980) Stability of measures of the dark focus of accommodation. *Invest. Ophthalmol. Vis. Sci.* **19**, 217–221.

Miller, R. J. (1978) Temporal stability of the dark focus of accommodation. *Am. J. Optom. Physiol. Opt.* **55**, 447–450.

Mishra, A. K., Batra, A. and Bhatia, R. P. (1995) Pseudo-myopia: a case report. *Ann. Ophthalmol.* **27**, 348–349.

Morgan, M. W. (1944) Accommodation and its relationship to convergence. *Am. J. Optom. Arch. Am. Acad. Optom.* **21**, 83–95.

Morgan, M. W. (1968) Accommodation and vergence. *Am. J. Optom. Arch. Am. Acad. Optom.* **45**, 417–454.

Morse, S. E. and Smith, E. L. (1993) Long-term adaptational aftereffects of accommodation are associated with distal dark focus and not with late onset myopia. *Invest. Ophthalmol. Vis. Sci.* (Suppl.) **34**, 1308.

Moses, R. A. (1981) Accommodation. In: *Adler's Physiology of the Eye. Clinical Application* (R. A. Moses, ed.). C. V. Mosby, pp. 304–325.

Moses, R. A., Lurie, P. and Wette, R. (1982) Horizontal gaze position effect on intraocular pressure. *Invest. Ophthalmol. Vis. Sci.* **22**, 551–553.

Mutti, D. O., Adams, A. J. and Zadnik, K. (1996) Author's reply. *Invest. Ophthalmol. Vis. Sci.* **37**, 2534.

Nathan, J., Kiely, P. M., Crewther, S. G. and Crewther, D. P. (1985) Disease-associated visual image degradation and spherical refractive errors in children. *Am. J. Optom. Physiol. Opt.* **62**, 680–688.

Neetens, A. and Evans, P. (1985) The use of bifocals as an alternative in the management of low grade myopia. *Bull. Soc. Belge Ophthalmol.* **214**, 79–85.

Ni, J. and Smith, E. L. (1989) Effect of chronic optical defocus on the kitten's refractive status. *Vis. Res.* **29**, 929–938.

Norton, T. T., Rada, J. A. and Hassell, J. R. (1992) Extracellular matrix changes in the sclera of tree shrews with induced myopia. *Invest. Ophthalmol. Vis. Sci.* (Suppl.) **33**, 1054.

Oakley, K. H. and Young, F. A. (1975) Bifocal control of myopia. *Am. J. Optom. Physiol. Opt.* **52**, 758–764.

Ogle, K. N., Martens, T. G. and Dyer, J. A. (1967) *Oculomotor Imbalance in Binocular Vision and Fixation Disparity.* Lea & Febiger.

O'Leary, D. J. and Millodot, M. (1979) Eyelid closure causes myopia in humans. *Experientia* **35**, 1478–1479.

Ong, E. and Ciuffreda, K. J. (1995) Nearwork-induced transient myopia. A critical review. *Doc. Ophthalmol.* **91**, 57–85.

Ong, E. and Ciuffreda, K. J. (1997) Accommodation, nearwork and myopia. *Optometric Extension Program.*

Owens, D. A. (1991) Near work, accommodative tonus, and myopia. In: *Refractive Anomalies. Research and Clinical Applications* (T. Grosvenor and M. C. r ioin, eds). Butterworth-Heinemann, pp. 318–344.

Owens, R. L. and Higgins, K. E. (1983) Long-term stability of the dark focus of accommodation. *Am. J. Optom. Physiol. Opt.* **60**, 32–38.

Owens, D. A. and Wolf-Kelly, K. (1987) Near work, visual fatigue, and variations in oculomotor tonus. *Invest. Ophthalmol. Vis. Sci.* **28**, 743–749.

Pärssinen, O. (1990) Anisometropia and changes in anisometropia in school myopia. *Optom. Vis. Sci.* **67**, 256–259.

Pärssinen, O. (1991) Astigmatism and school myopia. *Acta Ophthalmol.* **69**, 786–790.

Pärssinen, T. O. (1993) Corneal refraction and topography in school myopia. *C.L.A.O. J.* **19**, 69–72.

Phillips, J. R. and McBrien, N. A. (1995) Form deprivation myopia: elastic properties of sclera. *Ophthal. Physiol. Opt.* **15**, 357–362.

Portello, J. K., Rosenfield, M. and O'Dwyer, M. (1997) Clinical characteristics of pre-myopic individuals. *Optom. Vis. Sci.* **74** (Suppl.), 176.

Prangen, A. D. (1922) Spasm of the accommodation. In: *Transactions of the Section on Ophthalmology.* AMA Press, pp. 282–292.

Pruett, R. C. (1988) Progressive myopia and intraocular pressure: what is the linkage? *Acta Ophthalmol.* **185** (Suppl.), 117–127.

Rabin, J., Van Sluyters, R. C. and Malach R. (1981) Emmetropization: a vision-dependent phenomenon. *Invest. Ophthalmol. Vis. Sci.* **20**, 561–564.

Ramsdale, C. (1979) Monocular and binocular accommodation. *Ophthal. Opt.* **19**, 606–622.

Ramsdale, C. (1985) The effect of ametropia on the accommodative response. *Acta Ophthalmol.* **63**, 167–174.

Redburn, D. A. (1989) Co-transmitter roles of melatonin and glutamate in the outer plexiform layer of mammalian retina. In: *Extracellular and Intracellular Messengers in the Vertebrate Retina* (D. A. Redburn and H. Pasantes-Morales, eds). Alan R. Liss, pp. 191–205.

Robb, R. M. (1977) Refractive errors associated with hemangiomas of the eyelids and orbit in infancy. *Am. J. Ophthalmol.* **83**, 52–58.

Rosenfield, M. (1994) Accommodation and myopia: Are they really related? *J. Behav. Optom.* **5**, 3–11, 25.

Rosenfield, M. (1997) Accommodation. In: *The Ocular Examination. Measurement and Findings* (K. Zadnik, ed.). W. B. Saunders, pp. 87–121.

Rosenfield, M. and Chiu, N. N. (1995) Repeatability of subjective and objective refraction. *Optom. Vis. Sci.* **72**, 577–579.

Rosenfield, M. and Ciuffreda, K. J. (1991) Effect of surround propinquity on the open-loop accommodative response. *Invest. Ophthalmol. Vis. Sci.* **32**, 142–147.

Rosenfield, M. and Ciuffreda, K. J. (1994) Cognitive demand and transient nearwork-induced myopia. *Optom. Vis. Sci.* **71**, 381–385.

Rosenfield, M. and Gilmartin, B. (1987a) Effect of a near-vision task on the response AC/A of a myopic population. *Ophthal. Physiol. Opt.* **7**, 225–233.

Rosenfield, M. and Gilmartin, B. (1987b) Synkinesis of accommodation and vergence in late-onset myopia. *Am. J. Optom. Physiol. Opt.* **64**, 929–937.

Rosenfield, M. and Gilmartin, B. (1988a) Disparity-induced accommodation in late-onset myopia. *Ophthal. Physiol. Opt.* **8**, 353–355.

Rosenfield, M. and Gilmartin, B. (1988b) Accommodative adaptation induced by sustained disparity-vergence. *Am. J. Optom. Physiol. Opt.* **65**, 118–126.

Rosenfield, M. and Gilmartin, B. (1988c) Assessment of the CA/C ratio in a myopic population. *Am. J. Optom. Physiol. Opt.* **65**, 168–173.

Rosenfield, M. and Gilmartin, B. (1989) Temporal aspects of accommodative adaptation. *Optom. Vis. Sci.* **66**, 229–234.

Rosenfield, M. and Gilmartin, B. (1990) Effect of target proximity on the open-loop accommodative response. *Optom. Vis. Sci.* **67**, 74–79.

Rosenfield, M. and Gilmartin, B. (1998) Accommodative adaptation during sustained near-vision reduces accommodative error. *Invest. Ophthalmol. Vis. Sci.* **39**, S639.

Rosenfield, M., Ciuffreda, K. J. and Gilmartin, B. (1992a) Factors influencing accommodative adaptation. *Optom. Vis. Sci.* **69**, 270–275.

Rosenfield, M., Ciuffreda, K. J. and Hung, G. K. (1991) The linearity of proximally-induced accommodation and vergence. *Invest. Ophthalmol. Vis. Sci.* **32**, 2985–2991.

Rosenfield, M., Ciuffreda, K. J. and Novogrodsky, L. (1992) Contribution of accommodation and disparity-vergence to transient nearwork-induced myopic shifts. *Ophthal. Physiol. Opt.* **12**, 433–436.

Rosenfield, M., Ciuffreda, K. J., Hung, G. K. and Gilmartin, B. (1993) Tonic accommodation: a review. I. Basic aspects. *Ophthal. Physiol. Opt.* **13**, 266–284.

Rosenfield, M., Ciuffreda, K. J., Hung, G. K. and Gilmartin, B. (1994) Tonic accommodation: a review. II. Accommodative adaptation and clinical aspects. *Ophthal. Physiol. Opt.* **14**, 265–277.

Rosenfield, M., Rappon, J. M., James, M. F. and Portello, J. K. (1997) Repeatability of the accommodation stimulus response curve. *Optom. Vis. Sci.* **74** (Suppl.), 181.

Rutstein, R. P., Daum, K. M. and Amos, J. F. (1988) Accommodative spasm: a study of 17 cases. *J. Am. Optom. Assoc.* **59**, 527–538.

Sato, T. (1957) *The Causes and Prevention of Acquired Myopia.* (Self-published.)

Sato, T. (1981) Criticism of various accommodogeneous theories on school myopia. *Doc. Ophthalmol. Proc.*

Series No. 28 (H. C. Fledelius, P. H. Alsbirk and E. Goldschmidt, eds). Dr W. Junk, pp. 97–102.

Schaeffel, F., Glasser, A. and Howland, H. C. (1988) Accommodation, refractive error and eye growth in chickens. *Vis. Res.* **28**, 639–657.

Schaeffel, F., Troilo, D., Wallman, J. and Howland, H. C. (1990) Developing eyes that lack accommodation grow to compensate for imposed defocus. *Vis. Neurosci.* **4**, 177–183.

Schor, C. M. (1986) Adaptive regulation of accommodative vergence and vergence accommodation. *Am. J. Optom. Physiol. Opt.* **63**, 587–609.

Schor, C. M., Kotulak, J. C. and Tsuetaki, T. (1986) Adaptation of tonic accommodation reduces accommodative lag and is masked in darkness. *Invest. Ophthalmol. Vis. Sci.* **27**, 820–827.

Sethi, B. (1986) Vergence adaptation: a review. *Doc. Ophthalmol.* **63**, 247–263.

Simonelli, N. M. (1983) The dark focus of the human eye and its relationship to age and visual defect. *Human Factors* **25**, 85–92.

Slataper, F. J. (1950) Age norms of refraction and vision. *Arch. Ophthalmol.* **43**, 466–481.

Smith, G. (1983) The accommodative resting states, instrument accommodation and their measurement. *Optica Acta* **30**, 347–359.

Sollom, A. W. (1966) Unilateral spasm of accommodation and transient convergent squint due to an anxiety neurosis. *Br. Orthopt. J.* **23**, 118–119.

Sorsby, A. and Leary, G. A. (1970) *A Longitudinal Study of Refraction and its Components During Growth.* Medical Research Council Special Reports Series No. 309 HMSO.

Sorsby, A., Benjamin, B. and Sheridan, M. (1961) *Refraction and its Components During Growth of the Eye from the Age of Three.* Medical Research Council Special Reports Series No. 301. HMSO.

Stansbury F. C. (1948) Pathogenesis of myopia. *Arch. Ophthalmol.* **39**, 273–299.

Stenson, S. M. and Raskind, R. H. (1970) Pseudomyopia: etiology, mechanisms and therapy. *J. Ped. Ophthalmol.* **7**, 110–115.

Stenstrom, S. (1948) Investigation of the variation and correlation of the optical elements of human eyes (translated by D. Woolf). *Am. J. Optom. Arch. Am. Acad. Optom.* **48**, 340–350.

Stuart-Black Kelly, T. (1981) Myopia or expansion glaucoma. *Doc. Ophthalmol. Proc. Series* No. 28 (H. C. Fledelius, P. H. Alsbirk and E. Goldschmidt, eds). Dr W. Junk, pp. 109–116.

Suchoff, I. B. and Petito, G. T. (1986) The efficacy of visual therapy: accommodative disorders and non-strabismic anomalies of binocular vision. *J. Am. Optom. Assoc.* **57**, 119–125.

Suzuki, H. (1973) Observations on the intraocular changes associated with accommodation: an experimental study using radiographic technique. *Exp. Eye Res.* **17**, 119–128.

Suzumura, A. (1979) Accommodation in myopia. *J. Aichi. Med. Univ. Assoc.* **7**, 6–15.

Tait, E. F. (1951) Accommodative convergence. *Am. J. Ophthalmol.* **34**, 1093–1107.

Tokoro, T. (1988) The role of accommodation in myopia. *Acta Ophthalmol.* Suppl. 185, 153–155.

Tokoro, T., Funata, M. and Akazawa, Y. (1989) The role of intraocular pressure in elongation of the axial length. In: *Myopia: Pathogenesis, Prevention of Progression and Complications* (Proceedings of the International Symposium, Moscow). Health Ministry of the USSR, pp. 51–56.

Tomlinson, A. and Phillips, C. I. (1970) Applanation tension and axial length of the eyeball. *Br. J. Ophthalmol.* **54**, 548–553.

Troilo, D. (1990) Experimental studies of emmetropization in the chick. In: *Myopia and the Control of Eye Growth.* John Wiley & Sons, pp. 89–114.

Troilo, D. and Wallman, J. (1991) The regulation of eye growth and refractive state: an experimental study of emmetropization. *Vis. Res.* **31**, 1237–1250.

Tron, E. J. (1940) The optical elements of the refractive power of the eye. In: *Modern Trends in Ophthalmology* (F. Ridley and A. Sorsby, eds). Paul B. Hoeber, pp. 245–255.

Van Alphen, G. W. H. M. (1961) On emmetropia and ametropia. *Ophthalmologica* Suppl 142, 1–92.

Wallman, J., Xu, A., Wildsoet, C. *et al.* (1992) Moving the retina: a third mechanism of focusing the eye. *Invest. Ophthalmol. Vis. Sci.* (Suppl.) **33**, 1053.

Ward, P. A. and Charman, W. N. (1987) On the use of small artificial pupils to open-loop the accommodation system. *Ophthal. Physiol. Opt.* **7**, 191–193.

Weymouth, F. W. and Hirsch M. J. (1991) Theories, definitions, and classifications of refractive error. In: *Refractive Anomalies. Research and Clinical Applications* (T. Grosvenor and M. C. Flom, eds). Butterworth-Heinemann, pp. 1–14.

Whitefoot, H. and Charman, W. N. (1992) Dynamic retinoscopy and accommodation. *Ophthal. Physiol. Opt.* **12**, 8–17.

Wibaut, F. (1926) Emmetropization and origin of spherical anomalies of refraction. *Graefe's Arch. Aug.* **116**, 596–612.

Wick, B. and Currie, D. (1991) Dynamic demonstration of proximal vergence and proximal accommodation. *Optom. Vis. Sci.* **68**, 163–167.

Wildsoet, C. F. (1997) Active emmetropization– evidence for its existence and ramifications for clinical practice. *Ophthal. Physiol. Opt.* **17**, 279–290.

Wildsoet, C. and Wallman, J. (1995) Choroidal and scleral mechanisms of compensation for spectacle lenses in chicks. *Vis. Res.* **35**, 1175–1194.

Young, F. A. (1975) The development and control of myopia in human and subhuman primates. *Contacto* **19**, 16–31.

Young, F. A. (1981) Primate myopia. *Am. J. Optom. Physiol. Opt.* **58**, 560–566.

Young, F. A. and Leary, G. A. (1991) Accommodation and vitreous chamber pressure: a proposed mechanism for myopia. In: *Refractive Anomalies. Research and Clinical Applications* (T. Grosvenor and M. C. Flom, eds). Butterworth-Heinemann, pp. 301–309.

Zadnik, K. and Mutti, D. O. (1995) How applicable are animal myopia models to human juvenile onset myopia? *Vis. Res.* **35**, 1283–1288.

Zadnik, K., Mutti, D. O., Fusaro, R. E. and Adams, A. J. (1995) Longitudinal evidence of crystalline lens thinning in children. *Invest. Ophthalmol. Vis. Sci.* **36**, 1581–1587.

Zadnik, K., Satariano, W. A., Mutti, D. O. *et al.* (1994) The effect of parental history of myopia on children's eye size. *J. Am. Med. Assoc.* **271**, 1323–1327.

Autonomic correlates of near-vision in emmetropia and myopia

Bernard Gilmartin

6.1 Introduction

The autonomic nervous system (ANS) provides central and peripheral control processes which normally ensure the efficacy of sustained near vision in the young accommodating eye. The proposition that near vision might be a precursor to the development of myopia implies, therefore, that some anomaly of the ANS is a factor in producing the principal structural correlate of myopia, i.e. elongation of the vitreous chamber (Stenstrom, 1948; Sorsby and Leary, 1970; Bullimore *et al.*, 1992; Grosvenor and Scott, 1991; Jensen, 1991; McBrien and Adams, 1997). Whereas the likely source of such an anomaly is at present unclear, it is reasonable to adopt the working hypothesis that certain profiles of autonomic function could exacerbate an inherent genetic predisposition to myopia in the presence of appropriate environmental triggers.

The central thesis of this book, that excessive sustained near vision qualifies as a potent trigger has, however, to take account of the fact that the composite near response reflects well the inherent nature of autonomic control, that is, a profound mediation of central and peripheral processes to ensure homeostasis; an optimum balance between internal and external demands on the organism. Autonomic control thus requires complex responses and hence the descriptor near-vision complex is appropriate and comprises a variety of integrated peripheral elements, for example, accommodation, vergence, pupil constriction, cyclorotation and reduced intraocular pressure (IOP), each of which has central nervous system corollaries which are influenced by the cognitive demand of the task in hand (Figure 6.1).

To examine experimentally the association between myopia and near vision presents, therefore, special methodological difficulties which have constrained the majority of *in vivo* human investigations to the relatively simple expedient of pharmacological intervention with peripheral autonomic innervation of ciliary smooth muscle. That such an approach should be adopted is understandable as there are clear associations between accommodation and the development of myopia (*see* Chapter 5) and, further, the neuroeffector junction of ciliary muscle is accessible to a variety of topical pharmaceutical agents, the effects of which can be monitored straightforwardly by standard clinical procedures.

The majority of studies using parasympathetic blocking agents, such as, for example, atropine sulphate, have, however, been unsuccessful in the control of myopia onset and development (Goldschmidt and Jensen, 1987; Vogel, 1988; Jensen and Goldschmidt, 1991). The rationale of studies using these agents has invariably been to antagonize closed-loop accommodation. Of greater interest is pharmacological interference with processes of adaptation occurring during near vision as retention (or hysteresis) of a sustained accommodative response following prolonged near vision, an indicator of diminished adaptation, has been proposed by a number of workers to be a feasible precursor to the onset and development of myopia (Ebenholtz, 1983, 1988, 1991, 1992; Owens, 1991a; Gilmartin *et al.*, 1992; Rosenfield *et al.*, 1992; Gilmartin, 1997; Ong and Ciuffreda, 1997).

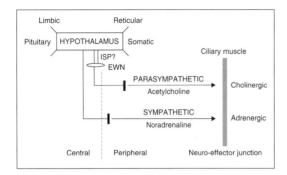

Figure 6.1 The source of autonomic innervation is the hypothalamus which has profound connections with all CNS areas. ISP represents a putative inhibitory sympathetic pathway between the hypothalamic centre and EWN, the Edinger–Westphal Nucleus. The first peripheral synapse occurs at the superior cervical and ciliary ganglia. (Adapted from Kaufman, 1992, Fig. 11.8, p. 397) Reproduced with permission from: Gilmartin, B. *et al.* (1992), Pharmacological effects on accommodative adaptation. *Optom. Vis. Sci.* **69**, 276–282. © The American Academy of Optometry, 1992.

In normal circumstances, the principal aim of autonomic homeostasis is to allow an organism to adapt to change in the environment by modulation of sensory, visceral, motor and neuroendocrine functions via centres in the hypothalamus and brain stem. Of particular relevance to this chapter is that the adaptive function of the ANS appears to reside principally in its sympathetic branch as its structural organization is such as to provide integration and dissemination of responses according to need; in contrast, the parasympathetic branch has a more focal response profile (Hamill, 1996).

Whereas there is incontrovertible evidence that the peripheral autonomic control of ocular accommodation is primarily due to parasympathetic innervation of the ciliary muscle and is mediated by muscarinic receptors, there is substantial evidence that the ciliary muscle also receives an inhibitory sympathetic innervation which is mediated by beta adrenoceptors (Gilmartin, 1986, 1998; Gilmartin *et al.*, 1992). The evidence has led to the proposal that the role of sympathetic innervation of the ciliary muscle may be to attenuate the retention of accommodation induced by periods of intense close work and thus reduce the risk of latent post-task transitory pseudomyopic changes. Without this attenuation a series of micro-adaptational processes may accumulate to a critical level, perhaps via an iterative ratchet-type response with regard to accommodative gain, which, when

exceeded, causes structural recalibration, that is, the increase in vitreous chamber length which is generally accepted as defining genuine myopia (Gilmartin and Winfield, 1995). Thus, in the context of adaptive responses to the environmental challenge of sustained near vision, an optimum level of sympathetic inhibition might provide the facility for an individual to maintain the emmetropic state whereas a deficit would predispose the individual to myopia.

This chapter will first comment on previous clinical studies on the use of autonomic agents to control myopia (*see also* Chapter 9). Evidence will then be presented in relation to the issue of dual innervation of the ciliary smooth muscle and will be set in the context of current views on the characteristics of autonomic innervation of the neuroeffector junction of ciliary muscle. An account will be given of laboratory work which has emanated from the suppositions outlined above concerning the possible aetiological role of sympathetic innervation in myopia. Attention will be drawn particularly to the category of myopia which appears typically in the late teens or early and middle twenties as it has no clear hereditary basis and is often reported as being directly linked to an occupational requirement for significant amounts of near-vision, or to a change in visual environment (for example an increase in the use of electronic displays). Finally, the putative mechanisms linking events in the anterior segment to structural changes in posterior sections of the globe will also be examined; that is, the links between accommodation, inherent ciliary and choroidal smooth muscle tone, scleral stretch and elongation of the posterior vitreous chamber.

6.2   Comment on previous clinical studies on the use of autonomic agents to manage myopia

The use of cycloplegic drugs to treat myopia was first suggested by Donders (1864), who attempted to treat pseudomyopia using atropine sulphate, although according to Curtin (1985) it is Wells (1811) who should be credited with first treating myopia with atropine. A variety of autonomic agents have been used in more recent times and include muscarinic antagonists, e.g. cycloplegic drugs such as atropine (Bedrossian, 1979; Yen *et al.*, 1989) and tropicamide (Curtin, 1970), adrenoceptor antagonists, e.g. timolol maleate (Jensen,

1991), and adrenoceptor agonists, e.g. phenylephrine (Kelly *et al.*, 1975) (*see* Chapter 9). Several reviews of the literature on the management of myopia with pharmaceutical agents (Goldschmidt and Jensen, 1987; Vogel, 1988; Jensen and Goldschmidt, 1991) have identified important limitations in terms of experimental design and methodology to the extent that there is no consensus as to their efficacy or otherwise. Of particular importance in this regard is that experimental masking is not usually possible, patient compliance is likely to be low, especially with relatively young children, and optimum matching of treatment and control groups is often weak. Repeated instillation of topical agents also carries some risk of systemic toxicity, together with the possibility of macular damage following prolonged mydriasis. Account also has to be taken of the significant effect of atropine on refractive and binocular performance at near given the uncertainty with regard to its efficacy in treating myopia (Goldschmidt, 1990).

Data from animal studies is also equivocal: atropine has been shown to arrest axial elongation produced by form deprivation in stumptail and pigtail macaque monkeys and in tree shrews (Young, 1965; McKanna and Casagrande, 1981; Raviola and Wiesel, 1990) but not in rhesus monkey following lid fusion (Raviola and Wiesel, 1990).

Furthermore, work on form-deprivation myopia in chick and tree shrew has suggested that non-selective muscarinic antagonists, which have been used in the majority of clinical studies on human myopia, may retard myopia not as a consequence of an effect on ciliary smooth muscle but as a local response of the retina or sclera (Stone *et al.*, 1991; Marzani *et al.*, 1994; Leech *et al.*, 1995) or choroidal blood flow (Reiner *et al.*, 1995).

The rationale adopted by the human studies cited above is invariably that myopia onset and development is principally associated with accommodative effort, intraocular pressure, or some interaction between the two. As indicated earlier, this chapter will approach the relationship from a different perspective: that the link between myopia and accommodation, in particular late-onset myopia, is more likely to be a failure of the accommodative system to adapt adequately to sustained near vision and that this adaptive facility is provided by optimum integration and augmentation of parasympathetic and sympathetic components of accommodative control (Rosenfield and Gilmartin, 1998).

6.3 Evidence for dual innervation of ciliary smooth muscle

The role of sympathetic innervation of the ciliary muscle in ocular accommodation has been reviewed elsewhere (Gilmartin, 1986) and is a topic that has attracted the attention in earlier years of physiologists (Helmholtz, 1909), ophthalmologists (Cogan, 1937) and optometrists (Morgan, 1946). A synopsis of more recent literature is given below.

6.3.1 Anatomical evidence

The ciliary muscle comprises longitudinal, reticular and circular muscle bundles, each of which has attracted interest in terms of differential autonomic innervation, distribution of sub-types of autonomic receptors and their relative contribution to regulation of aqueous outflow facility, the latter being an important function of ciliary muscle activity in relation to both trabecular and uveoscleral routes. The primate ciliary muscle is classified, however, as a fast, multi-unit smooth muscle which acts in a unified manner (Kaufman, 1992; Tamm and Lütjen-Drecoll, 1996). Although the ciliary muscle is innervated primarily by parasympathetic axons of the oculomotor nerve, the technique of histofluorescence has been used to identify adrenergic fluorescent terminals in the ciliary muscle of primates (Ehinger, 1966, 1971; Laties and Jacobowitz, 1966), although they were considered to be too few to provide an effective adrenergic innervation (Malmfors, 1965). This observation was supported by Ruskell (1973) who, by observing the absence of terminals with small granular vesicles (of a type known to be sympathetic) following superior cervical ganglionectomy, concluded that on average fewer than 1% of the terminal varicosities of monkey ciliary muscle were sympathetic although the incidence ranged from 0 to 2.5%. Furthermore, Ruskell (1973) noted that the sparseness of sympathetic terminals found in his study suggested that they were remote from many ciliary muscle fibres in monkeys. Ruskell considered that the large disparity between sympathetic and parasympathetic terminals cast doubt on the sympathetic terminals providing a useful function in the control of muscle contraction.

6.3.2 Physiological evidence

Of particular interest are the sympathetic nerve stimulation experiments carried out by Törnqvist (1966) on 13 young adult monkeys. He used a

Thorner optometer to measure refractive state on monkeys that were under general (pentobarbital) anaesthesia. All monkeys responded with a hyperopic change in refraction during stimulation of the cervical sympathetic nerve. It was found that the shifts could not be inhibited by alpha-adrenoceptor antagonists, even though these drugs significantly diminished the reduction in ciliary body volume that would follow the vasoconstriction effects of sympathetic stimulation (*see* section 6.5.2). Thus it appeared that the hypermetropic shifts were independent of vascular changes and were therefore associated with direct innervation of the ciliary muscle. In contrast, Törnqvist found that beta-receptor blocking drugs caused a complete elimination of the sympathetic stimulation response, even though the ciliary body volume changes proceeded as expected on sympathetic stimulation. Törnqvist postulated therefore that distance accommodation may be a consequence of sympathetic innervation of inhibitory beta-receptors present in ciliary smooth muscle.

An important observation by Törnqvist was that the magnitude and time course of accommodation changes induced by sympathetic stimulation were related to the prevailing level of cholinergic (i.e. parasympathetic or accommodative) tone. The hyperopic shifts associated with endogenous cholinergic tone amounted to around 0.50–1.0 D and took about 10 s to develop. An increase in cholinergic tone induced by the topical instillation of pilocarpine or physostigmine produced (for 6 eyes) responses that were two to four times greater for the same levels of sympathetic stimulation, but these took 20–40 s to develop. A deep block of cholinergic tone with atropine completely eliminated responses to sympathetic stimulation.

In a subsequent experiment on five young adult cynomolgus monkeys (*Macaca irus*), Törnqvist (1967) stimulated accommodation in a more physiological manner, i.e. by applying different stimulation frequencies to the oculomotor nerve and thus producing a background of electrically induced, rather than drug induced, parasympathetic activity. Törnqvist again found that, against this background of parasympathetic activity, the decrease in accommodation on cervical sympathetic nerve stimulation developed very slowly, with a maximal effect after 10–40 s. This would be too slow to provide an effective temporal response to the rapidly changing stimulus conditions of a normal visual environment. Conversely, it was found that the response to parasympathetic oculomotor nerve stimulation developed much more

quickly, with a maximal effect after 1–2 s. These findings with parasympathetic stimulation correlate with investigations on human accommodation response times which have shown that, after an initial latency of approximately 370 ms, accommodation stabilizes in about 1 s (Campbell and Westheimer, 1960). Törnqvist also noted that the degree of inhibitory sympathetic effect produced by sympathetic nerve stimulation (maintained at a constant five stimuli per second) varied according to the concurrent level of background parasympathetic activity. In the non-accommodating monkey (i.e., under general pentobarbital anaesthesia) the inhibitory effects gave an average hyperopia of 0.6 D, but when the parasympathetic level of activity was increased to give equivalent accommodation responses of 1.8, 3.1 and 7.1 D there was a proportionate increase in the inhibitory effects associated with the five stimuli per second rate, although the inhibitory effect was never greater than 1.5 D, even for very high levels of oculomotor stimulation (*see also* Hubbard *et al.*, 1998).

6.3.3　Pharmacological evidence

Van Alphen, Kern and Robinette (1965) used a range of adrenoceptor blocking drugs on strips of intraocular muscle dissected out from the enucleated eyes of cats, rabbits and monkeys. They found both alpha- and beta-adrenoceptors in cat ciliary muscle, with beta-receptors predominating. The receptors in rabbit ciliary muscle were predominantly alpha. Only beta-receptors could be demonstrated in the ciliary muscle of the monkey. The receptor distributions for each of the species were discussed in relation to whether the ciliary muscle participated in facilitation of aqueous outflow on administration of epinephrine but no comment was made regarding the accommodative significance of beta-receptors in monkey ciliary muscle.

One of Van Alphen's collaborators subsequently carried out an *in vitro* study on the presence, nature and distribution of the adrenoceptors of human intraocular muscles. Kern (1970) used dissected-out strips of sphincter, dilatator and ciliary muscle from 80 enucleated eyes. He used a range of adrenoceptor blocking agents to demonstrate that the ciliary muscle was almost exclusively populated by beta-adrenoceptors and that the action of catecholamines (e.g. noradrenaline) produced relaxation of the ciliary muscle. The dilatator pupillae muscle was found to have predominantly alpha-adrenoceptors whereas the sphincter pupillae presented alpha- and beta-receptors that were both inhibitory in nature and present in equal amounts. The receptor distributions found by Kern were equivalent to those found in monkeys in the earlier study of Van Alphen *et al.* (1965). Some years later, Van Alphen (1976) carried out work on human intraocular muscle and found similar receptor distributions to those reported by Kern (1970).

Hurwitz *et al.* (1972) modified the methodology adopted in Törnqvist's (1967) experiment. Using monkeys, they investigated the effects of stimulating and blocking ciliary muscle beta-receptors with subconjunctival injections of isoproterenol (a beta-adrenoceptor agonist) and propranolol (a beta-adrenoceptor antagonist), respectively, while simultaneously inducing monocular positive accommodation by electrical stimulation of the midbrain. They reached essentially the same conclusions as Törnqvist, that is, parasympathetic inhibition is a more important antagonist to positive accommodation than beta-sympathetic stimulation, and further that the inhibitory effects of isoproterenol were only significant when midbrain stimulation produced accommodation levels greater than 4 D, a response level which approximates to that exerted by young humans during sustained near vision. This conclusion concurs with Törnqvist's general observation that the level of sympathetic inhibition increases proportionately with concurrent levels of background parasympathetic activity.

Wax and Molinoff (1987) devised an assay technique that is appropriate for ocular structures and found that ciliary processes contained approximately 30% of the total number of beta-adrenoceptors in human iris/ciliary body preparations (dissected out shortly after death) whilst ciliary muscle and iris accounted for 40 and 30%, respectively. Furthermore, it was suggested that all of the receptors in the preparations were of the beta$_2$ subtype. These findings supported earlier work (Lograno and Reibaldi, 1986) and were confirmed by Zetterström and Hahnenberger (1988), who also noted the presence of a small population of inhibitory alpha$_1$ receptors.

6.3.4   Principal features of sympathetic innervation

It should be noted that the presence of an adrenoceptor population does not necessarily imply sympathetic control in functional terms, and the evidence for dual innervation has to be considered in the context of feasible integration of anatomical, physiological and pharmacological factors. Nevertheless, we can compile a picture of a predominant parasympathetic system interacting with a supplementary sympathetic system. The principal features of sympathetic input are that it is inhibitory, relatively small, probably no more than −2 D, and relatively slow; time courses range between 20 and 40 s compared with the 1 or 2 s for the parasympathetic system. Importantly, it appears that sympathetic inhibition is augmented by concurrent parasympathetic activity, that is, the inhibitory effects of a given level of sympathetic innervation will be enhanced by increasing levels of concurrent parasympathetic activity. Augmentation occurs on two counts: firstly, sympathetic inhibition will only become apparent when there is something to inhibit, and hence there is a baseline requirement for concurrent parasympathetic activity. Secondly, parasympathetic activity above this level appears to augment sympathetic input directly but not to an extent greater than −2 D even for very high parasympathetic levels. The majority of studies cited earlier also demonstrated variability in sympathetic facility, a feature which emerged from *in vivo* studies on human accommodation described later. Subsequent studies have also shown that an additional function of sympathetic inhibition is to attenuate positive shifts in accommodation induced by relatively high levels of cognitive demand (*see* section 6.5.4). It is clear that the properties of sympathetic innervation summarized above are able to fulfil the requirements of an adaptive facility which complements the fast reflexive nature of parasympathetic innervation.

6.4   The autonomic neuroeffector junction of ciliary smooth muscle: a summary

Peripheral neuroeffector activity in the ciliary muscle is mediated predominantly by the parasympathetic system via the action of the transmitter acetylcholine on muscarinic receptors (Kaufman, 1992). A general feature of ANS control is, however, dual innervation and, as indicated previously, there is evidence for a sympathetic input to the ciliary muscle in terms of the action of the transmitter noradrenaline on two subclasses of postsynaptic receptors: beta-adrenoceptors and alpha-adrenoceptors. It is clear, however, that both systems are not always mutually antagonistic, the final outcome of autonomic innervation depending

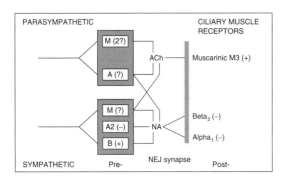

Figure 6.2 A schematic composite representation of the putative cross-linkages that might occur between parasympathetic and sympathetic transmitters and receptors at pre- and post-synaptic sites. The interactions highlight the complexity of mechanisms for modulation of transmitter release which are, to date, not fully understood. M = muscarinic receptor; A = alpha-adrenoceptor; B = beta-adrenoceptor; ACh = acetylcholine; NA = noradrenaline). Adapted from Figure 4.10, p. 67 in Ryall, R. W. (1989) *Mechanisms of Drug Action on the Nervous System*, 2nd edn. Cambridge University Press. Reproduced with permission from: Gilmartin, B. *et al.* (1992) Pharmacolological effects on accommodative adaptation. *Optom. Vis. Sci.* **69**, 276–282. © The American Academy of Optometry, 1992.

on, for example, the structure in question, quantitative and qualitative (i.e., inhibitory versus excitatory) features of parasympathetic and sympathetic supply and the nature and distribution of autonomic receptors and their subtypes. In recent years specific subtypes of autonomic receptors have been identified: muscarinic receptor subtype M_3 is concerned with contraction of ciliary smooth muscle (Pang *et al.,* 1994) and two subdivisions (1 and 2) of alpha- and beta-adrenoceptors have been linked to sympathetic inhibition of accommodation, that is, negative as opposed to positive accommodation (Figure 6.2).

6.4.1 Autoregulation in ANS innervation

It has, however, to be emphasized that autonomic neuroeffector junctions are not well defined simple synaptic structures: transmitter release is from mobile varicosities in extensive terminal branching fibres at variable distances from effector cells or bundles of smooth muscle cells which are in electrical contact with each other and which have a diffuse distribution of receptors (Hillarp, 1959; Burnstock, 1986a, 1992). Consequently, recent advances in autonomic physiology and pharmacology place more emphasis on the diversity of local

peripheral control mechanisms that occur prior to central control mechanisms (Burnstock, 1992).

It is also likely that the above major receptor subtypes are complemented by a variety of additional subtypes and further that autonomic nerves release more than one transmitter which subsequently combine to produce systems for chemical coding (Burnstock, 1990a). Account also has to be taken of the cross-linkage that can occur between cholinergic (i.e., parasympathetic) and adrenergic (i.e., sympathetic) transmitters and receptors at pre- and post-synaptic sites. The interactions create a complex mechanism for modulation of transmitter release which is, to date, not fully understood (Ryall, 1989; Starke *et al.,* 1989).

Furthermore, there are numerous neurotransmitter substances in autonomic nerves which include monoamines, purines and amino acids. Various neuropeptides (notably substance P) are known to have significant effects on ciliary muscle (Stone *et al.,* 1987) and reports have proposed that nitric oxide might have a role in negative accommodation and accommodative microfluctuations (Burnstock, 1986b; Tamm *et al.,* 1995). Importantly, it also appears that the autonomic nervous system exhibits plasticity in relation to the expression of transmitters and receptors during development and ageing and in response to hormones and growth factors (Burnstock, 1990b).

Clearly the above complexities of autonomic innervation make the functional consequences of dual innervation difficult to unravel in terms of accommodative adaptation to sustained visual tasks and moderate subsequent speculation on possible aetiological links between autonomic control, nearwork and the development of myopia.

6.5 Methodological considerations

Despite the complexities described, the approach adopted by most workers in this area has been to intervene with peripheral autonomic innervation at the ciliary muscle neuroeffector junction by blocking or stimulating respective cholinoceptors and adrenoceptors using topical instillation of various autonomic drugs (Gilmartin *et al.,* 1992). Whereas it would be valuable to intervene with the neuroeffector junction at both pre- and post-synaptic sites *in vivo*, work on humans imposes ethical constraints on agents and procedures that can be used, which means that normally only conventional topical agents may be employed. Unfortunately these agents are often inherently less specific in their receptor activity, which diminishes their value in experimental terms. Receptor specificity is also related to dose level at the receptor site which is subject to the vagaries of pharmacokinetics of drug absorption across the cornea. In addition, ocular effects can be confounded with central nervous system effects, as inevitably there will be some systemic absorption of topically instilled drugs.

6.5.1 Beta-adrenoceptor drug selectivity

Two widely available beta-adrenoceptor antagonists are timolol maleate (0.5%) and betaxolol HCl (0.5%). As beta$_2$-sympathetic receptors predominate in human ciliary smooth muscle, inhibition will occur with the predominantly non-selective (with regard to subtypes of receptor) beta-antagonist, timolol, but to a much lesser extent, if at all, with the predominantly beta$_1$-antagonist, betaxolol. Both agents will, however, reduce IOP by virtue of beta-adrenoceptor activity elsewhere in the eye, which is the principal reason for their clinical use in the treatment of chronic open-angle glaucoma. Reductions in IOP by as much as 4 mmHg in young normal subjects is common with topical beta-adrenoceptor drugs. Although the relationships between accommodation, IOP and myopia are ill-defined (*see* Chapter 5), it is expedient in terms of experimental design to use betaxolol, rather than saline, as a control for the potential interaction between accommodation and reduced IOP. Furthermore, the consensus is that neither agent will affect pupil size (Gilmartin *et al.*, 1984) or corneal curvature (Rosenfield and Gilmartin, 1987d).

6.5.2 Effects of topical ANS drugs on intraocular vasculature

Alpha-adrenoceptor agents are more likely to produce significant intraocular vascular effects than drugs which act on muscarinic or beta-adrenoceptors. These drugs produce their effects owing to the presence of alpha-receptors in the smooth muscle walls of intraocular blood vessels and thus make it difficult to isolate specific smooth muscle receptor effects, notably those at the ciliary muscle. There is, however, some potential for a specific ciliary muscle response as pharmacological work on excised human ciliary muscle has identified a small population of alpha$_1$-inhibitory receptors (Zetterström and Hahnenberger, 1988). Rosenfield *et al.* (1990) were unable to demonstrate any effects on tonic accommodation in a group of young subjects with the alpha$_1$-agonist phenylephrine HCl (10%) or the alpha$_1$-antagonist thymoxamine HCl (0.5%). In contrast alpha$_1$-receptor activity has significant effects on amplitude of accommodation which is likely to be linked to changes in ciliary body volume. For example, a decrease in volume will result from the vasoconstriction effect of the agonist phenylephrine which will increase ciliary collar diameter and hence produce a decrease in amplitude of accommodation of around 2 D in young subjects (Rosenfield *et al.*, 1990). Similar decreases in amplitude have been reported by a number of studies using both direct and indirect acting sympathomimetics (Biggs *et al.*, 1959; Stephens, 1985; Gimple *et al.*, 1994; Culhane and Winn, 1998).

6.5.3 Late-onset myopia

Although myopia often stabilizes around the age of 15 years, a significant number of individuals exhibit myopia for the first time later in life. Late- or adult-onset myopia appears typically in the late teens or early and middle twenties and has no clear hereditary basis (Goss and Winkler, 1983; Grosvenor, 1987; O'Neal and Connon, 1987; National Research Council, 1989; Baldwin *et al.*, 1991). Adult-onset myopia constitutes around 8% of all myopia, although an incidence of 25% has been proposed (Fledelius, 1995). It develops over a relatively short period and stabilizes at low dioptric levels of around 1.5 D. Nevertheless, levels of up to 4 D and more are not uncommon (Adams, 1987; Fledelius, 1995) and have allowed ocular biometric studies to demonstrate that the principal structural correlate for both early-onset myopia and late-onset myopia is elongation of the vitreous chamber depth (McBrien and Millodot, 1987; Bullimore *et al.*, 1992; Grosvenor and Scott, 1991, 1993; Fledelius, 1995; McBrien and Adams, 1997).

Attention has been drawn to late-onset myopia in many studies that have investigated sympathetic correlates of myopia as its association with near vision and accommodation is more clearly defined than in early-onset myopia. The incidence of late-onset myopia is often reported as being directly linked to an occupational requirement for significant amounts of near vision, or to a change in visual environment (for example an increase in the use of electronic displays). Further, a number of studies have reported differences in accommodative and oculomotor response profiles between late- and early-onset myopia and emmetropia

(Jiang, 1995, 1997; Abbott *et al.*, 1998; *see* Chapter 5). In experimental terms, the late-onset myopia group has special advantages in comparison with early-onset myopes: they are readily accessible to researchers (often being drawn from the student population), can participate effectively in relatively complex experimental procedures, and can comply more readily with the strictures of ethical requirements for ocular drug studies.

6.5.4   Cognitive factors

As near vision in modern visual environments often requires intensive periods of sustained processing of information, cognition is considered to be an important element in the link between near vision and myopia (Van Alphen, 1990; Birnbaum, 1993). Although the effects of psychological influences on components of the near-vision response have been reported (Westheimer, 1957; Miller and LeBeau, 1982; Matthews *et al.*, 1991; Winn *et al.*, 1991; Gray *et al.*, 1993), an area of contention is the effect of mental effort or cognitive demand on accommodation (Kruger, 1980; Malmstrom *et al.*, 1980; Bullimore and Gilmartin, 1987a). The relationship is particularly important when subjective methods of assessing accommodation are employed; for example, the difficult judgemental task of discriminating speckle motion in the laser optometer can produce overestimates of tonic accommodation (Post *et al.*, 1985; Bullimore *et al.*, 1986; Rosenfield and Ciuffreda, 1990). Consequently open-view objective infra-red optometers are the preferred method of measurement in most oculomotor laboratories.

Few studies, however, have directly tested the proposition that autonomic factors are involved in modulating the cognitive elements of the accommodative response. In the study by Bullimore and Gilmartin (1987a), a Canon (R-1) open-view objective infra-red optometer was used to investigate the effect of timolol 0.5% on shifts in dark room tonic accommodation. High and low levels of cognitive load were induced by using a reverse counting task. Twenty young emmetropes took part in a double-masked protocol against a saline control condition. Significant shifts in tonic levels found with mental effort (up to 1 D) were independent of sympathetic antagonism but only for individuals having initial tonic levels less than 1.2 D. For individuals with tonic levels greater than this ($n = 6$), sympathetic antagonism caused significant increases in shifts induced by the task. A

subsequent report (Bullimore and Gilmartin, 1987b) used a similar methodology to investigate the influence of cognitive demand on tonic accommodation for young emmetropes ($n = 15$) and late-onset myopes ($n = 15$). For low cognitive demand, tonic levels for the myopic group (0.81 D) were found to be significantly lower than those for the emmetropic group (1.14 D), a finding replicated in several subsequent studies (McBrien and Millodot, 1987; Rosenfield and Gilmartin, 1987c; Bullimore *et al.*, 1992). Of particular interest was the finding that cognitive demand produced in the myopes a mean shift in tonic levels of +0.35 D which was significantly greater than that for the emmetropic group (+0.07 D).

The experimental approach used in the two latter studies on tonic accommodation was subsequently applied to two further studies on closed-loop accommodation responses with stimulus levels of 1, 3 and 5 D (Bullimore and Gilmartin, 1988; Bullimore *et al.*, 1992). Twelve young emmetropes took part in the first study (Bullimore and Gilmartin, 1988). Mental effort was shown to induce a significant increase in mean response for the 1 D task, a response equivalent to the passive condition for the 3 D task and a significant reduction in response for the 5 D task. Sympathetic blocking with timolol only affected the accommodative level for the 5 D task in that it was significantly increased. The findings of the second study showed the same trend evident in the earlier study on tonic accommodation (Bullimore *et al.*, 1992): closed-loop responses of a group of late-onset myopes ($n = 14$) showed significant positive shifts with mental effort, although the shifts were found to be equal across all stimulus levels.

Unfortunately experiments on cognition and accommodation which combine refractive groups and sympathetic blocking drugs have yet to be undertaken but it is clear that account needs to be taken of the subtle and somewhat perplexing contribution of non-optical elements to the near-vision response. It also has to be appreciated that cognitive effects on the accommodation response are likely to have concomitant effects on pupil size which are mediated by autonomic activity (Matthews *et al.*, 1991).

6.5.5   Interactions between the cardiovascular system and accommodation

Tyrrell and his co-workers have identified interesting behavioural links between the oculomotor and vascular systems (Tyrrell *et al.*, 1995; Tyrrell *et al.*, 1998). The characteristics of systemic autonomic innervation profile can be quantified from electrocardiograms with reference to special autoregressive algorithms. The techniques can provide separate within-task indices of sympathetic and parasympathetic cardiac control. It was shown that when cardiac indices were used to discriminate between two subject groups in terms of autonomic control, the discrimination was also evident in concurrent measures of tonic accommodation and tonic vergence (Tyrrell *et al.*, 1995). A later study (Tyrrell *et al.*, 1998) considered whether a near visual task can influence cardiac behaviour. Reading text located at 15 cm for 20 minutes produced in a subset of subjects significant post-task adaptation of both accommodation and vergence which correlated with cardiovascular function, in particular a reduction in parasympathetic innervation to the heart. The implications of this work with regard to myopia development are at present unclear but the relationships found are intriguing given the systemic cardiovascular stasis which must inevitably accompany the enforced immobility of most prolonged near-vision tasks which involve a high cognitive demand.

6.6 Autonomic control of accommodation in emmetropia and myopia

The literature on pharmacological intervention with accommodation and its implications with regard to the relationship between myopia and near vision will be reviewed with reference to the three phases of accommodative response (Figure 6.3): the pre-task (or pre-adaptive) tonic level; within-task closed-loop responses; open-loop post-task regression towards the pre-task tonic level. The locus of these post-task regressions are stable and repeatable indexes (Strang *et al.*, 1994a) and can be used to deduce the nature of within-task accommodative adaptation. Type A, the most common, gives a very rapid regression to base-line levels, within 10 s, and occasionally a counter-adaptation, indicated by an initial negative component, may also be present. Type B gives a more monotonic regression and has a time-course of around 20–40 s. Type C only occurs occasionally and exhibits a retarded regression which can extend over several minutes.

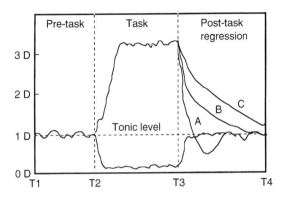

Figure 6.3 Schematic representation of three phases of accommodative response which can be used to assess the nature of within-task accommodative adaptation during sustained near vision: the pre-task (or pre-adaptive) open-loop tonic level; the within-task closed-loop response; open-loop post-task regression towards the pre-task tonic level. The locus of post-task regressions are stable and repeatable indexes and can be categorized as type A, the most common, which gives a very rapid regression to base-line levels, within 10 s, and occasionally a counter-adaptation, indicated by an initial negative component, may also be present; type B gives a more monotonic regression and has a time-course of around 20 s to 40 s; type C only occurs occasionally and exhibits a retarded regression which can extend over several minutes. Reproduced with permission from: Gilmartin, B. *et al.* (1992), Pharmacological effects on accommodative adaptation. *Optom. Vis. Sci.* **69**, 276–282. © The American Academy of Optometry, 1992.

6.6.1 Tonic accommodation

In recent years, tonic accommodation has figured in numerous studies of accommodation (Rosenfield *et al.*, 1993, 1994) and in particular its use as a reference level to assess the magnitude of post-task accommodative adaptation. The most consistent distinguishing feature in relation to myopia is that the resting or tonic level of accommodation is often, but not always, found to be lower in late-onset myopia than in emmetropia, that is, around 0.4 D lower when measured with an infra-red optometer (Ong and Ciuffreda, 1997; *see* Chapter 5).

Tonic accommodation exhibits significant inter-subject variation (Rosenfield *et al.*, 1993) and, given that parasympathetic innervation predominates in accommodation, it was clear from initial studies that the variation is due principally to parasympathetic innervation of the ciliary muscle (Gilmartin and Hogan, 1985). Using an He–Ne laser optometer, a range of approximately 0–2.5 D in tonic accommodation is illustrated in Figure 6.4

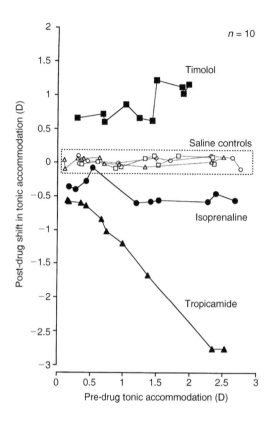

Figure 6.4 The effect of topical instillation of autonomic drugs on tonic accommodation with an He–Ne laser optometer in darkness. Data points represent the mean of five tonic accommodation measurements in dioptres (typical s.d. = 0.2) for each individual subject for each experimental condition. (Redrawn from Gilmartin and Hogan, 1985). Reprinted from: Rosenfield, M. *et al.* (1993) Tonic accommodation: a review I. Basic aspects. *Ophthal. Physiol. Opt.* **13**, 266–284. With permission from Elsevier Science.

for a group of ten young subjects. Topical instillation of the non-selective muscarinic receptor antagonist tropicamide (0.5%) caused a hyperopic shift in tonic accommodation which was directly proportional to its pre-drug level so that the inter-subject variation in tonic accommodation collapsed completely after 24 minutes.

Figure 6.4 also illustrates shifts in tonic levels with drugs that act on the sympathetic system. A significant mean hyperopic shift of 0.47 D was found following stimulation with the non-selective beta-adrenoceptor agonist isoprenaline sulphate (3%). The hyperopic shift varied little between subjects, which is consistent with the agonist action of isoprenaline, that is, it will simply add to

the prevailing level of sympathetic activity and thus produce a constant shift across tonic levels. In contrast, the non-selective beta-adrenoceptor antagonist timolol maleate (0.5%) produced a significant mean myopic shift of 0.87 D which showed a weak relationship with tonic accommodation. The shift increased from 0.6 D to 1.2 D as pre-drug tonic levels increased. Unlike isoprenaline, the antagonist action of timolol is such that its effect will depend on the prevailing level of sympathetic activity and if this varies then timolol's antagonist effect will vary. Figure 6.4 gives some indication that this was the case: beta-antagonism and hence sympathetic input increased as tonic levels increased.

As tonic levels are clearly determined by the prevailing level of parasympathetic activity, another way of interpreting the progressive myopic shift in tonic accommodation with timolol is that concurrent background parasympathetic or accommodative activity augments inhibitory sympathetic activity, an interpretation confirmed in later work (Gilmartin and Bullimore, 1987) and consistent with the functional role of sympathetic inhibition described by Törnqvist (1967) and Hurwitz *et al.* (1972), discussed earlier.

In a later study, Zetterström (1988) applied the results of her earlier *in vitro* pharmacological work (Zetterström and Hahnenberger, 1988) to the effects of various adrenoceptor drugs on accommodation and distance refraction in daylight and darkness. The study used a similar subjective laser optometer to that used by Gilmartin and Hogan (1985) but which differed in one important respect: the laser-speckle presentation time was 750 ms compared to 300 ms. Although this difference is highly likely to confound the measures (Hogan and Gilmartin, 1984). Zetterström's findings were nevertheless similar, although of lesser magnitude than those reported by Gilmartin and Hogan (1985): a myopic shift in tonic accommodation with timolol of 0.2 D (+/–0.1) and a hyperopic shift of +0.12 D (+/–0.07) with isoprenaline.

The much cited review on accommodation function by Toates (1972) concluded, from a theoretical bioengineering standpoint, that the tonic position represents the condition where there is no steady-state error between stimulus and response. Thus accommodation for objects closer than the tonic position is brought about by the combination of excitation of the parasympathetic system and inhibition of the sympathetic system; conversely, objects further than the tonic position require inhibition of the parasympathetic system accompanied by excitation of the sympathetic system. The notion, however, that tonic accommodation represents an equilibrium or fulcrum for parasympathetic and sympathetic innervation of the ciliary muscle does not hold, as Törnqvist's work and later studies (Gilmartin and Bullimore, 1987) have shown that the level of sympathetic input is a function of the concurrent level of parasympathetic activity. Thus it is incorrect to assume that the relatively low tonic levels reported for late-onset myopia imply that the condition is a consequence of weak or deficient sympathetic innervation.

6.6.2   Within-task accommodative response

Steady-state accommodation

The range of accommodation responses to natural stimuli in young eyes is best represented by the well-known stimulus–response curve whose principal components are accommodative lag for near targets, a lead of accommodation for low demands and a linked intermediate quasi-linear stimulus–response relationship (Ciuffreda, 1991). These components have been used to provide indices of accommodative function such as the amplitude of accommodation and estimates of the accuracy of accommodation (derived from the gradient of the linear portion) and tonic accommodation (derived from the intersection of the linear plot with the unit-ratio line). It is unlikely, however, that the latter holds and hence the corollary, that stimulus demands higher than the tonic level are mediated by the parasympathetic system and lower stimulus demands are mediated by the sympathetic system is invalid owing to the need, outlined earlier, for a substantial concurrent level of parasympathetic activity to augment sympathetic input.

Nevertheless, a systematic investigation of the effect of topical adrenergic agents on the stimulus–response curve using new methods of analysis (Chauhan and Charman, 1995) would be of interest, particularly as there is evidence of a difference in response curves between refractive groups, notably late-onset myopia (McBrien and Millodot, 1986a; Jiang, 1997; Abbott *et al.*, 1998). However, it is worthwhile noting that the passive condition used by Bullimore and Gilmartin (1987b) in their study on cognitive factors in emmetropia and myopia (*see* section 6.5.4) could not differentiate differences in steady-state levels of accommodation between the groups, albeit for a restricted range of accommodative stimuli. In any event, the efficacy of closed-loop measures of

accommodation is likely to mask the relatively small contribution from the sympathetic system which may account for the inability to demonstrate significant effects of beta-adrenoceptor agents on amplitude of accommodation (Gilmartin *et al.*, 1984). The latter finding is unfortunate as significant differences in amplitude between refractive groups have been reported (McBrien and Millodot, 1986b). Pupil size and concomitant effects on depth-of-focus are, of course, crucial to all of the above measures; to date, none of the beta-adrenoceptor agents employed in accommodation studies has been shown to have a significant effect on pupil size (Gilmartin *et al.*, 1984).

Accommodative microfluctuations

The accommodative response to a specific stimulus involves microfluctuations of accommodation and these deserve attention owing to proposals that they may monitor the accuracy of steady-state accommodation and in addition possess the potential for autonomic control (Winn and Gilmartin, 1992). There is no evidence to date of a direct relationship between accommodative microfluctuations and myopia. It appears that the complex waveform of microfluctuations is more likely to be a consequence of inherent rhythmic variation in IOP and choroidal blood flow rather than neurological control of steady-state accommodation. Simultaneous measurements of accommodation and systemic arterial pulse have shown that the location of the high frequency components is significantly correlated with arterial pulse (Winn *et al.*, 1990) and that the low-frequency components are correlated with respiration (Collins *et al.*, 1995). Furthermore, whereas betaxolol and timolol have been shown to affect microfluctuations significantly, the results reflect principally their systemic cardioselective characteristics (related to their beta$_1$-adrenoceptor action) in that a reduction in heart rate and hence arterial pulse reduces correspondingly the peak frequency of the higher frequency components of ocular microfluctuations (Owens *et al.*, 1991; Strang *et al.*, 1994b).

Accommodation–convergence interactions

Investigating the effects of autonomic drugs when eyes both accommodate and converge is an appropriate experimental route as the principal synergistic elements of the near-vision response are retained. The hypothesis would be that sympathetic agonists would enhance the inhibitory input of the sympathetic system with the result, for a given accommodative response, of greater net

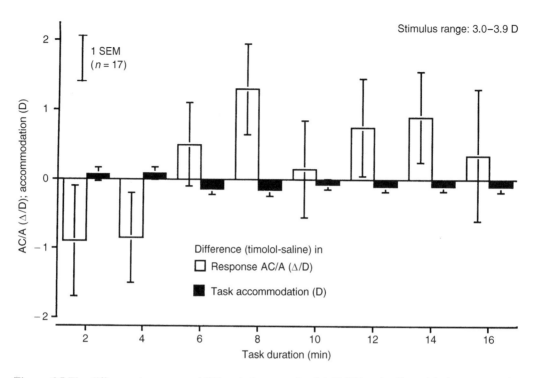

Figure 6.5 The difference in response AC/A ratio between timolol (0.5%) and saline trials for a group of 17 young emmetropes. There was no significant difference in level of accommodation during the task for either trial. Reprinted from: Rosenfield, M. and Gilmartin, B. (1987) Oculomotor consequences of beta-adrenoceptor antagonism during sustained near-vision. *Ophthal. Physiol. Opt.* **7**, 127–130. With permission from Elsevier Science.

drive from the parasympathetic system and hence an increase in the response AC/A. Conversely, sympathetic antagonists would inhibit sympathetic input and result in a reduced net drive from the parasympathetic system and hence a decrease in the response AC/A.

Stephens (1985) showed that hydroxyamphetamine hydrobromide (1%), a predominantly indirect-acting alpha- and beta-adrenoceptor agonist, produced a significant increase in AC/A whereas phenylephrine HCl (10%), a direct acting alpha-adrenoceptor agonist, produced a small but insignificant rise in AC/A. By subtracting the effects of each agent, Stephens concluded that pharmacologically induced beta-adrenoceptor activity was responsible for the net increase in AC/A. However, the mixed pharmacological profile of the sympathomimetic agents used, especially in relation to vascular effects (*see* section 6.5.2), and the subjective methods of measurement employed for a small (*n* = 8) sample of subjects, limit the value of these observations.

Nevertheless, the study prompted Rosenfield and Gilmartin (1987b) to consider the more direct

effects of the beta-antagonist timolol on response AC/A for a group of 17 young emmetropes. The hypothesis outlined above received support: a significant drop in AC/A occurred with timolol which subsided after the first 4 minutes of the 16 minute near task and then tended to increase over the course of the task (Figure 6.5).

A subsequent study (Rosenfield and Gilmartin, 1987d) took account of reports which suggested that lower tonic accommodation in late-onset myopes may, compared with other refractive groups, be a consequence of reduced sympathetic innervation to the ciliary muscle. For this to be the case, the reduction in accommodative convergence found in the earlier study for emmetropes would be of a significantly lower magnitude in late-onset myopia. The study examined the effect of timolol on accommodative-convergence for three refractive groups (each comprising 20 subjects): emmetropes, early- and late-onset myopes. Accommodative convergence was derived from accommodation stimuli of 3.3, 4.1 and 4.8 D and concomitant changes in heterophoria were assessed with a Maddox rod and tangent scale.

Timolol produced a significant reduction in accommodative convergence in the emmetropic group but not for either the early- or late-onset groups. Thus a deficit in sympathetic innervation was not shown to be a specific feature of late-onset myopia, a finding which was to receive some support from experiments conducted almost a decade later (Gilmartin and Winfield, 1995). There is clearly scope for further work in this area given the possible links between vergence and myopia advanced in Chapter 7 and the availability of a beta$_1$-adrenoceptor antagonist as a more appropriate control agent (*see* section 6.5.1).

The uncoupling of accommodation and vergence during sustained near vision was advanced some years ago by Skeffington (1991) as a precursor to myopia onset and development and has been adopted by a cohort of practitioners as a method of clinical management. A detailed account is given elsewhere (*see* Chapter 8) but it is of note that Skeffington considered the uncoupling to be partly attributable to general and interactive anomalies of autonomic and endocrine function, citing as reference sources the work of Cannon (1929) and Seyle (1956).

Within-task dynamic measures of accommodation
An important feature of sympathetic inhibition to emerge from the animal work of Törnqvist was its temporal characteristics in relation to parasympathetic activity; that is, a slow adaptive function compared to a fast reflex system. Weber and his associates (1989) examined these properties in relation to the effect of timolol on the amplitude and dynamics of accommodation. High-resolution A-scan echography was used to measure changes in crystalline lens thickness as a function of time-constants with subjects in a prone position. A small 10 MHz ultrasound transducer was attached to a haptic lens in one eye while the fellow eye was presented simultaneously with accommodation stimulus levels of 2, 4, 6 and 8 D. The data on seven young subjects indicated a significant effect of timolol on accommodation responses but only when subjects accommodated from far-to-near, which the authors interpreted as being consistent with the inhibitory nature of sympathetic innervation.

Direct measures of dynamic accommodation have also been made using the Canon R-1 objective infra-red optometer (Winn *et al.*, 1993). Accommodation responses were recorded continuously to sinusoidal Maltese Cross target movement within a Badal optical system over a stimulus range from 2 to 4 D. The target frequency was varied from 0.05 to 0.5 Hz. It was hypothesized that if rate of change of background parasympathetic activity is a significant factor in dual innervation, then the lower frequencies would induce a combined parasympathetic/sympathetic response as there is sufficient time for the parasympathetic system to trigger the slower inhibitory sympathetic system and thus produce an optimum response. Conversely, for the higher frequencies, the faster parasympathetic system would predominate in providing an optimum response owing to insufficient time being available to induce sympathetic activity. For the hypothesis to be valid only the lower frequency responses should be susceptible to the blocking effects of timolol, as it blocks the inhibitory beta$_2$-receptors. Betaxolol responses should match the saline control over the whole frequency range, as its selective beta$_1$-receptor antagonism restricts its principal effects to the lowering of the IOP.

Preliminary data have provided some support for the hypothesis (Owens, 1991b; Strang, 1995; Culhane and Winn, 1997): reduced gain was found at lower frequencies when beta$_2$-adrenoceptors were blocked with timolol whereas the betaxolol gain matched that of saline. No difference in gain was evident between any of the treatments at the faster frequencies as the conditions were not conducive to inhibitory sympathetic activity. Whereas these tracking experiments provided some insight into the temporal properties of autonomic control of accommodation, the results on both gain and phase measurements (and related step responses) were inconclusive. Although potentially a fruitful area of research, it appears that to date no studies have been fully reported on whether, firstly, the dynamics of accommodation differ between refractive groups and, secondly, whether the groups can be differentiated with regard to autonomic control of temporal responses (Winn and Culhane, 1998).

6.6.3   Post-task measures of accommodative adaptation

Accommodative hysteresis and dark focus
It was the prescient study of Ebenholtz (1983) which posed the question as to whether near-task-induced shifts in accommodation could act as a precursor to induced myopia. He suggested that positive and negative shifts in post-task accommodation are determined by the relationship

between task position and initial pre-task dark focus (or tonic accommodation). Using a subjective laser optometer, it was shown that after an 8 minute fixation period the post-task dark focus of 12 emmetropes either increased by 0.34 D or relaxed by 0.21 D depending upon whether fixation was at the near- or far-point of accommodation, respectively. No significant shifts in adaptation occurred when the fixation target was placed at the subject's original tonic position. Ebenholtz noted, however, that the far-point of accommodation target was on average 0.98 D beyond the original tonic accommodation position and produced a −0.21 D shift, whereas the near-point of accommodation target was on average 5.12 D closer than the original tonic accommodation position, but only produced a +0.34 D shift. Ebenholtz suggested that the non-linearity of these accommodative hysteresis effects can be attributed to independent subsystems governing accommodative increase and relaxation. Using similar methodologies, his subsequent studies (Ebenholtz, 1988, 1991,1992) presented further evidence that dark focus was an important metric for assessing the magnitude of accommodative hysteresis and considered that the long duration (i.e., approximately 30 minutes) non-monotonic post-task shifts in dark focus may reflect differences in parasympathetic and sympathetic near-target hysteresis.

Nearwork-induced transient myopia
Nearwork-induced transient myopia has been defined as the short-term myopic shift in far point of around, on average, 0.25 D which occurs immediately following a sustained near visual task and persists for up to 30 s. The changes are measured directly with objective infra-red optometers under experimental conditions which closely match natural viewing conditions. Following their comprehensive review of the phenomenon, Ong and Ciuffreda (1995, 1997) speculated that these shifts may provide sufficient retinal defocus to trigger the development of myopia if allowed to accumulate over a prolonged period (*see* Chapters 5 and 10). Of special interest is their view that nearwork-induced transient myopia may result from inefficient processing of retinal blur and/or computational delay in conjunction with a deficiency in sympathetic inhibition. It would be of interest to investigate the effect of autonomic agents on this form of pseudomyopia for a variety of test paradigms, although again the efficacy of closed-loop accommodation and factors pertaining

to depth-of-focus may mask the relatively small adrenergic contribution.

6.6.4 Post-task measures of accommodative regression

Post-task measures of accommodative regression (*see* Figure 6.3) are of particular value as investigating the nature of autonomic control while a task is in progress presents methodological difficulty owing to the inherent closed-loop nature of near-vision responses. The assumption is that the characteristics of ciliary muscle innervation operating during the task will contribute to slow within-task accommodative adaptation processes which, on termination of the task, determine the locus or pattern of regression of accommodation towards the pre-task tonic position. For example, it may be that within-task sympathetic inhibition could contribute to the rapid Type A response or that a deficit in inhibition could lead to the retarded Type C response. It should be emphasized that tonic accommodation is an inherently non-transient element of the accommodation system and as such provides a valuable reference against which to assess the nature of post-task accommodative hysteresis (Rosenfield and Gilmartin, 1989; Hung, 1992; Rosenfield *et al.*, 1993, 1994; Hung *et al.*, 1996).

Sustained near vision augments sympathetic innervation
Gilmartin and Bullimore (1987) measured accommodative adaptation in a group of young emmetropes ($n = 15$) with reference to pre- and post-task tonic accommodation using a Canon R-1 objective infra-red optometer. Post-task tonic accommodation was measured under darkroom conditions immediately after a 10 minute counting task and at 1 second intervals over a period of 90 seconds; the task was located at 0.3 D and 5 D. Timolol was used to block beta-receptors and produced significant differences between far and near regression patterns during the 50 seconds immediately following the task. The mean differences were found to be positively correlated with pre-task tonic values such that they were negative or slightly positive for subjects with pre-task tonic levels less than 0.75 D ($n = 7$) but predominantly positive for subjects with pre-task tonic levels greater than 0.75 D ($n = 8$). For the latter group mean shifts in tonic levels of approximately 0.5 D occurred over the 50 second recording period (Figure 6.6).

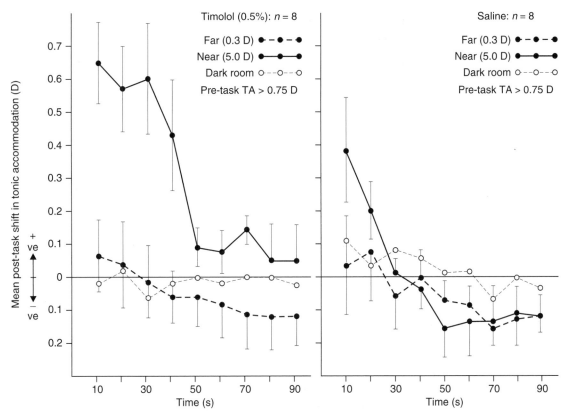

Figure 6.6 Mean post-task shift in darkroom accommodative level against time for each experimental condition combining drug and task accommodation (TA) treatments for the group of 8 subjects having pre-task tonic levels > 0.75 D. Error bars represent +/−1 SEM. (NB: The *y*-axis, originally referred to as post-task shift in tonic accommodation, is now more correctly described as post-task accommodative adaptation, *see* section 6.6.4). Reprinted from: Gilmartin, B. and Bullimore, M. A. (1987) Sustained near-vision augments sympathetic innervation of the ciliary muscle. *Clin. Vis. Sci.* **1**, 197–208. With permission from Elsevier Science.

Thus topical instillation of timolol demonstrated that inhibitory sympathetic innervation of the ciliary muscle provides the facility to attenuate the magnitude and duration of post-task accommodative adaptation induced by the 5 D task; no equivalent effect occurred for the 0.3 D task. It was *deduced* that sympathetic innervation of ciliary smooth muscle was augmented by concurrent parasympathetic (i.e., accommodative) activity, thus supporting Törnqvist's work on the monkey, and that emmetropes with relatively low pre-task tonic levels may prove more susceptible to enhanced post-task hysteresis effects following relatively high levels of accommodative demand by virtue of them not having access to an inhibitory facility.

The experimental approach adopted by Gilmartin and Bullimore (1987) was used to investigate the additional finding that emerged from Törnqvist's experiments that, being a slow adaptive component,

sympathetic inhibition required 20–40 seconds to develop. Rosenfield and Gilmartin (1989) varied the duration time of a 3 D letter detection task to intervals of 15, 30 and 45 seconds. They showed a significant post-task counter-adaptation for the 45 s task (i.e., a negative regression compared to pre-task tonic levels) for a group of late-onset myopes (*n* = 10). Neither the counter-adaptation nor the variation in post-task adaptation with task duration was evident in a matched group of emmetropes (*n* = 10), which led the authors to speculate that the myopic group had a specific sympathetic inhibitory facility. The experiment was consequently repeated on eight of the original group of myopes following instillation of timolol and for a 45 second task duration. The original post-task counter-adaptation responses were eliminated by timolol such that post-task regression matched those found originally for the emmetropic group. The conclusion that late-

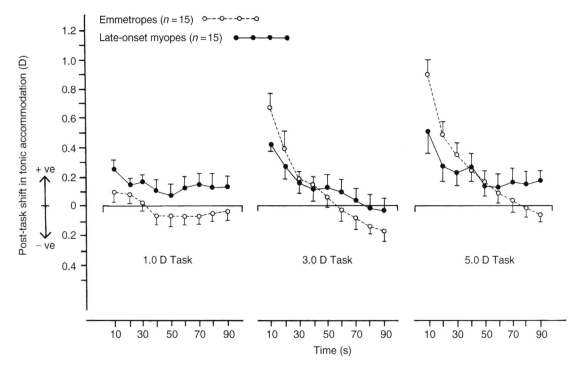

Figure 6.7 Mean post-task shift in darkroom accommodative level against time following a 10 min task at stimulus distances equivalent to 1, 3 and 5 D for a group of young late-onset myopes ($n = 15$) and a group of young emmetropes ($n = 15$). Error bars represent +/–1 SEM. (NB: The y-axis, originally referred to as post-task shift in tonic accommodation, is now more correctly described as post-task accommodative adaptation, *see* section 6.6.4). Reproduced with permission from: Gilmartin, B. and Bullimore, M. A. (1991) Adaptation of accommodation to sustained visual tasks in emmetropia and late-onset myopia. *Optom. Vis. Sci.* **68**, 22–26. © The American Academy of Optometry, 1991.

onset myopes are not deficient in sympathetic input was supported in later work (Gilmartin and Winfield, 1995).

Accommodative regression in emmetropia and myopia

McBrien and Millodot (1988) investigated differences in post-task adaptation in emmetropia, early- and late-onset myopia and hyperopia. Using the same type of optometer as that employed by Gilmartin and Bullimore (1987), the data showed significant positive shifts in adaptation level for the myopes ($n = 10$) following 15 minute tasks located at 37 and 20 cm when compared with emmetropes ($n = 16$). Mean shifts of around +0.35 D were evident at the first 1 minute data point and were maintained and somewhat enhanced, at the subsequent 7 and 15 minute data points. In addition, they found that post-task adaptation changes were negatively correlated, albeit weakly, with pre-task tonic levels at each distance.

A subsequent study by Gilmartin and Bullimore (1991) considered whether the differences reported by McBrien and Millodot (1988) were a sequel to enhanced differences occurring prior to their 1 minute recording point. The same experimental method adopted by Gilmartin and Bullimore (1987) was employed and compared accommodative responses associated with a 10 minute task located at 1, 3 and 5 D for a group of young emmetropes ($n = 15$) and a group of late-onset myopes ($n = 15$). In view of the distinction in post-task regression patterns identified by Gilmartin and Bullimore (1987) for emmetropes with pre-task tonic levels greater than 0.75 D, an attempt was made to ensure that tonic levels exceeded this for both refractive groups. The results show that significant differences in rates of post-task accommodative regression to pre-task tonic levels occur between emmetropes and late-onset myopes as accommodative demand is increased (Figure 6.7). The differences in the rate of post-task regressions could not be attributed to variations in within-task accommodative response or to pre-task tonic accommodation levels: the former was clearly equivalent for each refractive group; the latter reflected the lower values for late-onset myopes reported in previous literature but the differences were not consistent.

A further study (Strang *et al.*, 1994a) investigated the inter-trial variability of post-task regression patterns following a 3 minute near task set at 3 D above pre-task tonic levels for 10 emmetropic subjects and 10 late-onset myopes. Post-task measurements of accommodation were taken at 2 second intervals using the Canon R-1 optometer. Based on three successive trials separated by at least one day, the study was able to show regression patterns to be repeatable stable measures of post-task accommodative adaptation and furthermore was able to replicate the differences found between emmetropes and myopes in the study of Gilmartin and Bullimore (1991).

Beta-adrenoceptor antagonism in emmetropia and myopia

A number of methodological issues unresolved in previous work were addressed and incorporated into the study of Gilmartin and Winfield (1995). The work investigated the effect of topical instillation of timolol, betaxolol and saline on post-task regression patterns following a 3 minute fixation of a far task set at 0.2 D and a near task which was set at 4 D above the actual response level found for the far task. Accommodation responses were again measured with the Canon R-1 optometer and sampled in single-shot mode at 1.5 second intervals over a 60 s post-task period. The experiment was double-blind throughout and had a 2 day washout between drug instillations. Eighteen undergraduate subjects were used, aged between 19 and 23. The subjects were drawn from three refractive groups: emmetropes, early-onset myopes and late-onset myopes (that is, myopia onset after 16 years of age; the mean age of onset for the group was just under 19 years).

Raw data for subject EW, a late-onset myope, is illustrated in Figure 6.8A and compares post-task regressions for timolol and betaxolol trials. The betaxolol regression matched that of its respective saline control, that is, a rapid type A regression to the mean tonic level following both far and near tasks (*see* Figure 6.3). Similar results were found for timolol following the far task although an overshoot was found in the later stages of recording; the reasons as to what it might represent were

unclear. Of particular note for subject EW was the retarded regression to the tonic level following the near task in the timolol trial.

To condense the data, the far and near regression plots were subtracted and the difference expressed as a percentage of the mean difference between far and near accommodation levels occurring during the final 15 seconds of the task period. This was carried out for each of the seven mean-sphere readings located symmetrically about each 10 second data point. The positive shift with timolol (relative to betaxolol) found for subject EW indicates a retardation or attenuation of regression from which it was deduced that sympathetic inhibition is present (Figure 6.8B). EW was one of six subjects making up the late-onset myope group, and whilst she was representative of those members of the group showing a timolol effect, a range of response profiles was found across the late-onset myope group.

The overall profile of response to the drug treatments was found not to differ significantly between each of the refractive groups used; examples of clear effects were counter-balanced by subjects without effects. For example, a positive shift with timolol relative to betaxolol was found for emmetrope KP (Figure 6.9A) but not for subject OW (Figure 6.9B). Similar examples of the diversity of response could be drawn from the early-onset myopia group.

Support for these findings has come from work by Otsuka *et al.* (1998). The investigation used an objective quasi-static recording technique to assess accommodative adaptation by comparing pre- and post-task stimulus-response plots. Using topical instillation of timolol the work demonstrated, for a sample of 52 subjects, induced adaptative effects which are approximately equivalent in magnitude and time course to the attenuation effects shown by Gilmartin and Winfield (1995). Although the sample was not classified into different refractive groups, the inter-subject variation in response profile appeared to be similar to that found by Gilmartin and Winfield (1995) and importantly showed significant counter-adaptive effects with the nonselective beta-agonist isoprenaline.

6.7 Putative mechanisms linking ANS, accommodation and myopia

6.7.1 Sympathetic deficit as a precursor to myopia

The finding by Gilmartin and Winfield (1995) that certain individuals have less sympathetic facility

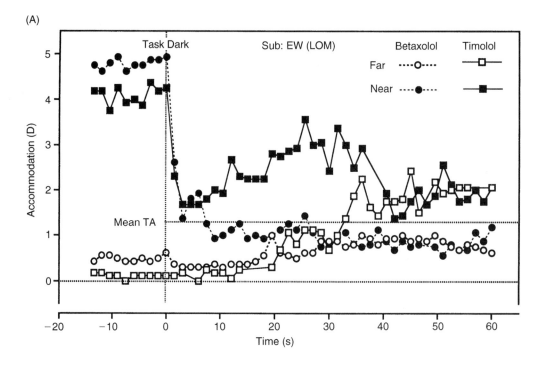

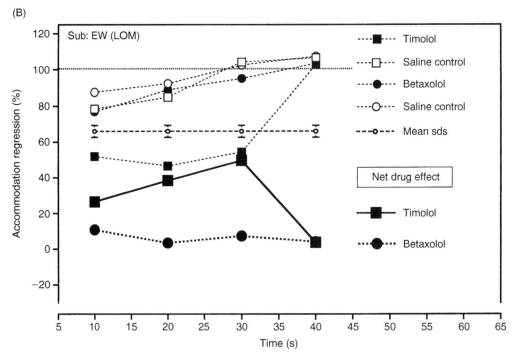

Figure 6.8 (A) Post-task regression patterns (raw data) for late-onset myope EW for timolol and betaxolol trials. (B) Condensed data for subject EW. The top plots show the summarized data for each drug and saline trials. Error bars represent, for each time period, the mean standard deviation (derived from each set of seven data points) for all conditions. In the bottom plots account has been taken of the respective saline controls and the net drug effect is shown as the relative differences in regression between timolol and betaxolol. Reprinted from: Gilmartin, B. and Winfield, N. R. (1995) The effect of topical β-adrenoceptor antagonists on accommodation in emmetropia and myopia. *Vis. Res.* **35**, 1305–1312. With permission from Elsevier Science.

(A)

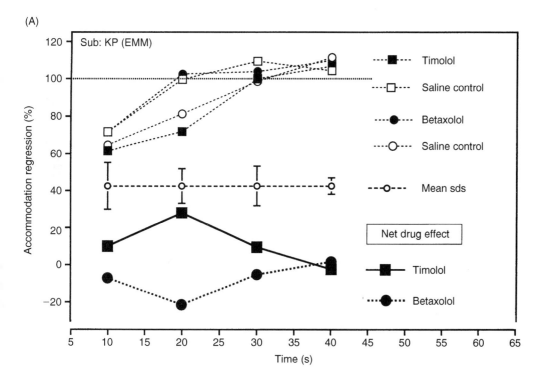

(B)

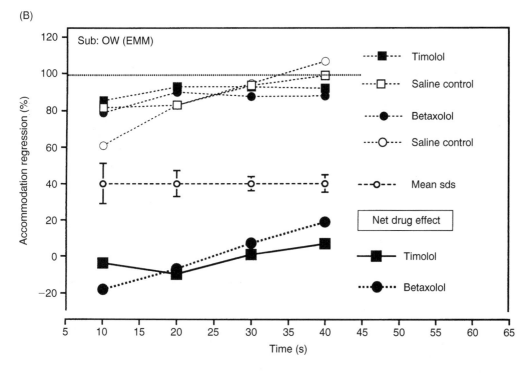

Figure 6.9 Condensed data for post-task regression patterns of two subjects drawn from the emmetropic group: (A) data for subject KP; (B) data for subject OW. *See* Figure 6.8 for details of plot. Reproduced with permission from: Gilmartin, B. (1998) Pharmacology of accommodative adaptation. In *Accommodative/Vergence Mechanisms in the Visual System*, Franzén, O. and Richter, H. (Eds). Berkhauser Ferlag, Stockholm (in press).

has led to the hypothesis that myopia, and in particular late-onset myopia (as it has a more well-defined link with sustained accommodation), may result from a progressive sequence. Firstly, there is diminished augmentation of sympathetic inhibition of ciliary smooth muscle which would normally accompany sustained near vision; the deficit may have an hereditary basis and be exacerbated by high levels of cognitive demand. Secondly, the sympathetic deficit alters the near oculomotor autonomic response profile and triggers a series of *latent* within-task micro-adaptational processes; these processes could be driven by subperceptual retinal blur processes linked to enhanced accommodative lag at near or to uncoupling of normal accommodative-vergence interactions. Thirdly, the adaptational processes accumulate to a critical level (perhaps via an iterative ratchet-type response with regard to accommodative gain) where structural recalibration takes place, that is, elongation of the vitreous chamber.

The extent to which the above processes could produce the *manifest* changes in visual performance at near (for example perceived blur and reduced accommodative facility) noted in some reports (Gwiazda *et al.*, 1993, 1995; Held, 1998; Ong and Ciuffreda, 1995, 1997) requires further work. In any event, it does appear from the studies described earlier that the initial stages of the process, that is a propensity to accommodative hysteresis, can be effectively exposed by analysing the loci of open-loop post-task regressions of accommodation to pre-task tonic levels following sustained near vision.

Of note is that the work of Gilmartin and Winfield (1995) indicates that if a link between a deficit in sympathetic inhibition and the onset and development of myopia is induced by near-work in young adults, then it should occur across refractive groups rather than being restricted to the late-onset myopia group. There is epidemiological evidence that this is in fact the case. O'Neal and Connon (1987) found substantial myopic shifts in a group of approximately 1000 young US Air Force cadets after 2.5 years of their training course which involved very extensive close work. The shifts occurred in all three of the refractive groups analysed: hyperopes, emmetropes and myopes. Those cadets who were myopic on entry were most vulnerable: 70% were shown to have increased myopia of around 1 D on average. Importantly significant myopic shifts were also evident in

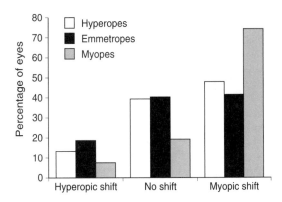

Figure 6.10 Distribution of refractive change in a group of US Air Force cadets following 2.5 years of very extensive close work. Whilst those cadets who were myopic on entry were most vulnerable, significant myopic shifts occurred for all ametropic groups. Reproduced with permission from: O'Neal, M. R. and Connon, T. R. (1987) Refractive error change at the United States Air Force Academy–class of 1985. *Am. J. Opt. Physiol. Opt.* **62**, 344–354. © The American Academy of Optometry, 1987.

40% of the emmetropes and hyperopes examined (Figure 6.10).

6.7.2 Continuity of ciliary muscle-choroidal tone

In his comprehensive and much cited monograph on aspects of emmetropia and ametropia, Van Alphen (1961) proposed that the ciliary muscle-choroid layer behaved as a single functional unit which could act physiologically like a continuous elasto-musculous sheet of smooth muscle surrounding the eye. He speculated that the resistance offered by this ciliary-choroid capsule emanated directly from the tone of the ciliary muscle and that, by mediating the effects of IOP, could regulate the effect of IOP on the sclera. Van Alphen assumed that the net level of IOP was the chief determinant of the degree of scleral stretch. His second assumption was that optimum ciliary tone, that is, the tonus which achieves and maintains the emmetropic state, was determined by the efficacy of input to the Edinger–Westphal nucleus from cortical and subcortical pathways. It is well known that visual degradation can induce substantial levels of ametropia and as the nucleus receives most of its afferent connections from the reticular formation there is the potential at least for its output to be modulated by autonomic activity. Interestingly, Van Alphen suggested that variations in this latter source of control could account for the variability in degree of induced myopia resulting from lid suture in monkeys.

Van Alphen and his associates have provided evidence that, rather than being a fragile structure, the choroid has a modulus of elasticity more than 10% greater than the modulus of the sclera (Graebel and Van Alphen, 1977; Van Alphen, 1986, 1990; Van Alphen and Graebel, 1991). This would be sufficient to provide a reduction of pressure (relative to IOP) in the suprachoroidal space of the cat of 2 mmHg (Van Alphen, 1961) and presumably the reduction of 3.7 mmHg found subsequently in the cynomolgus monkey by Emi *et al.* (1989). Further evidence of the continuity of the ciliary–choroidal capsule was evident from work on enucleated human eyes which were partly denuded by removing all of the sclera behind the equator (Van Alphen, 1986). Saline infusion of the eyes induced axial elongation rather than overall radial expansion, a feature evident in later work on computed retinal contours in anisomyopia (Logan *et al.*, 1995). The use of markers and histological controls after fixation with the eye under pressure indicated that the elongation emanated from ciliary muscle stretch.

Of special relevance to the theme of this book is Van Alphen's insistence that it is *inherent* ciliary muscle tonus that ultimately determines scleral stretch rather than stimulus-evoked contraction of the ciliary muscle. The degree to which measures of tonic accommodation genuinely reflect inherent choroidal tonus has yet to be resolved, but it is reasonable to assume that some extrapolation could be devised. Van Alphen also considered that a cardinal factor in juvenile-onset myopia could be subcortical processes related to cognitive stress associated with learning. He proposed that the autonomic nervous system may be more important than the visual cortex in the origin of school myopia. Despite his earlier experiments on ciliary muscle adrenoceptors it appears that Van Alphen considered central processes to predominate and did not directly address the issue of whether inhibitory sympathetic input to the ciliary muscle could contribute to ciliary–choroidal tone, although he has not dismissed the possibility of a putative link (Van Alphen, 1990).

6.7.3 Animal studies of myopia

An overview on the use of autonomic agents to alter experimentally induced myopia in animals has been given earlier (*see* section 6.2). There is increasing evidence from animal studies in support of the concept of an active emmetropization mechanism that may be linked to accommodation (McBrien, 1998; Wildsoet, 1997). The contribution of autonomic factors to induction of myopia in animals has, however, not been widely discussed in terms of physiological control of near-vision responses. Interestingly, although chicks have striated rather than smooth ciliary muscle, they do appear to have a facility for sympathetic inhibition of accommodation mediated by beta-adrenoceptors (Troilo *et al.*, 1993; Francis *et al.*, 1998). Chicks have been most widely used in animal myopia work but, to date, it is not clear how the characteristics of form-deprivation myopia in this species extend our understanding of juvenile and adult-onset myopia. Wallman *et al.* (1987) have, however, suggested that printed text may constitute a form-deprivation stimulus for the human retina. Chapter 4 reviews work on the induction of refractive error in animals which includes chick, tree shrew and monkey. Of special interest to clinicians is the finding of Hung, Crawford and Smith (1995) concerning the ability of infant monkeys to compensate for imposed interocular differences in refraction by altering ocular growth patterns (*see* Wildsoet, 1997 for review).

Of relevance to this chapter, and to the earlier comments concerning choroidal function, is the potential facility for choroidal accommodation found in studies on chick and tree shrew. Chicks can use choroidal accommodation to compensate, in part, for focusing errors such that compensation for imposed myopia and hyperopia can be achieved by increasing and decreasing respectively the thickness of the choroid. The choroidal changes occur rapidly, are transitory and can account for up to one half of the early compensation to myopic defocus in young chicks. There is, however, a complementary slower mechanism by which the growth of the sclera is regulated to produce long-term changes in eye size (Wildsoet and Wallman, 1995; Wildsoet, 1997).

It has been reported that myopic eye growth in the chick induced by form degradation leads to a marked reduction in choroidal blood flow (Reiner *et al.*, 1995). The reduction appeared, however, to be a consequence of eye enlargement and the authors suggested therefore that choroidal blood flow *per se* does not play a role in eye growth whether induced experimentally or naturally occurring. In addition, the results of experiments on the relationship between accommodation and experimentally induced myopia were found to be consistent with those reported in previous literature on the chick; that is, accommodation is unnecessary for most forms of induced myopia.

Of particular interest and relevance to this chapter are the results of supplementary experiments carried out by Reiner *et al.* (1995). The experiments considered the effect of *chronic* accommodation on eye growth in chicks. Sub-conjunctival daily 50 μl injections of 15% nicotine were given to eight 4-day-old chicks for a period of 2 weeks. Chick ciliary muscle is striated and hence an increase in accommodation will result from the agonist action of nicotine on nicotinic receptors. The above dose was found to produce accommodation levels of between 1 and 2 D that lasted for a duration of 4–6 hours. The authors believed that this regimen might reasonably match the duration and magnitude of accommodative effort that occur when humans undertake intense close work on a daily basis. The induced accommodation yielded a slight but significant myopic shift in refractive error of −0.75 D when the treated eye was compared to the non-treated eye; the shift was associated with a concomitant increase in axial length of the treated eye. The authors concluded that the findings appeared to provide some tentative support for the idea that sustained accommodation can promote myopia and ocular enlargement.

6.7.4   Choroidal function in humans

Choroidal blood flow accounts for approximately 90% of total ocular blood flow in humans and may supplement its main functions of retinal nutrition and retinal heat dissipation (Langham *et al.*, 1989) by modulating the integration of smooth muscle activity between anterior and posterior segments of the globe. The objective of such an integrative process may be to maintain optimum stretch-inducing forces on the sclera or perhaps to regulate in some way the biochemistry of scleral extracellular matrix. This division of function may be of particular significance as it has been observed that elastic stretching of the sclera accounts for less than 20% of the observed difference in axial length between myopia and contralateral control eyes in tree shrews monocularly deprived of form vision (Phillips and McBrien, 1995).

Cheng *et al.* (1992) used *in vivo* high-resolution magnetic resonance imaging to show that significant thinning of both the choroid and the sclera occurred in the posterior segment of the globe of myopes when compared to both emmetropes and hyperopes. On average the choroid was 0.4 mm thinner in the myopic group, which comprised 7

eyes with errors ranging from −3.00 to −9.50 D. The associated standard deviation of choroidal measurements in Cheng *et al.* (1992) was relatively low (around 0.1), which suggests that thinning occurred for both low and high refractive errors. The amplitude of intraocular pressure pulse and pulsatile ocular blood flow (caused by the systolic bolus of blood entering the choroidal circulation) also correlates significantly with axial length (James *et al.*, 1991).

The degree to which the ANS contributes to the above processes, and their significance with regard to the development of myopia, is at present obscure but autonomic control of choroidal function may prove to be crucial to our understanding of the genesis of myopia, whether it be derived from transmission of inherent smooth muscle tonus from the ciliary muscle, and hence sustained accommodative effort at near, or from intraocular blood flow, retinal nutrition and associated growth factors.

Whatever regulatory systems operate to determine eye size will, however, have to account for the mechanical forces on the sclera evident during convergence at near. Greene (1991) notes that the peak force exerted by the ciliary muscle is 0.6 g, significantly less than the 150 g exerted by the medial rectus muscle during convergence. In particular, the oblique muscles can exert significant amounts of localized tensile stress on the posterior sclera and Greene and McMahon (1979) consider that this, together with the increase in vitreous pressure associated with convergence, is sufficient to distort permanently the sclera. A different interpretation has been presented, however, by Ong and Ciuffreda (1997), who point out that typical operational extraocular forces are generally less, of the order of 40 g, and that for the posterior attachments of the oblique muscle, forces are unlikely to exceed a modest 4 g. In any event it appears that vitreous forces are likely to be distributed throughout the whole of the posterior chamber rather than confined to the posterior segment (Goss and Wickham, 1995).

6.7.5   Late-adult-onset myopia

Although the chapter has centred on events occurring at the neuro-effector junctions of ciliary smooth muscle there are other sites which have the potential for autonomic control, notably where the ciliary muscle is attached anteriorly by means of tendons to the scleral spur and trabecular meshwork and posteriorly to the elastic network of

Bruch's membrane of the choroid (Tamm *et al.*, 1991). To date, the pharmacology of these areas is not well defined but pharmacological intervention with the restraining force provided by the posterior anchoring ligaments in relation to the forward movement of the ciliary muscle on contraction may prove to be of special relevance to presbyopia.

It is possible that these anchoring sites may also be important in relation to the development of myopia associated with sustained near vision in the older eye. This is a feasible proposition as it appears that these posterior attachments are in turn linked to the scleral canal such that the whole accommodative plant is linked to the posterior sections of the globe (Kaufman, 1992). Preliminary work on the epidemiology of myopia onset and development which occurs during the incipient phase of presbyopia indicates that around 15% of individuals show a mean myopic shift of around 0.75 D during this time, which could expose some intriguing links between near vision, myopia and possibly uveoscleral aqueous outflow mechanisms (Gilmartin, 1995). It also appears that these myopic changes are likely to be axial as McBrien and Adams (1997) have shown significant myopic changes, all axial, to occur in a group of 78 clinical microscopists engaged in intense histological inspection work over a 2-year period. The mean age of the group was 30.83 years and would have included incipient presbyopes as the range extended from 21 to 61 years of age.

6.8 Amelioration of myopia

6.8.1 Pharmacological intervention

The use of various pharmacological agents to manage myopia has been outlined earlier and an account appears in Chapter 9. The results of the majority of studies to date have been equivocal and insufficient to offset the ethical considerations of adverse and toxic reactions attendant with prolonged instillation of pharmaceutical agents in either adults or children.

Attention will be drawn, however, to Jensen's comprehensive monograph on myopia progression in young schoolchildren (Jensen, 1991). The study included the topical use of timolol maleate (0.5%) over a 2-year period with examinations every 6 months. The rationale for the use of timolol was based on its ocular hypotensive effect properties

rather than on its ability to antagonize the inhibitory beta$_2$-adrenoceptors present on ciliary smooth muscle. Strict criteria were used to select treatment and control groups such that the initial screening of nearly 9000 Danish schoolchildren (7–12 years old) generated a sample of 159 myopic children all with myopia of at least −1.25 D. Each examination was carried out by the same investigator, under the same conditions and the children were randomly assigned to one of three groups: a control group, a group wearing bifocal lenses, and a group undergoing timolol instillation.

Timolol was found to reduce the rate of myopia development in children allocated to the group designated as having high risk of myopia development, but the reduction was not statistically significant. In contrast, children allocated to the low risk group showed an *increase* in myopia progression with timolol which Jensen considered might be due to an increase in ciliary muscle tone. The observation is of interest as, based on the accommodative regression work cited earlier, it is more likely that myopia progression would be controlled with a beta-adrenoceptor *agonist* (e.g. isoprenaline sulphate). This may also account for why Hosaka (1988) failed to find any significant effects on myopia progression in an earlier study which used topical instillation of the non-selective beta-antagonist timolol and the mixed alpha- and beta-antagonist labetalol.

Accordingly, application of timolol over an extended period for medical purposes (e.g. topical therapy for open-angle glaucoma) might predispose the recipient to myopia. To date, no consistent changes in accommodative or refractive state have been reported although, of course, the majority of patients receiving treatment for glaucoma would be post-presbyopic. The report by Van Buskirk (1980) is, however, of interest. Using data from the US National Registry, 547 reports of adverse effects associated with topical timolol therapy were analysed. Visual disturbance was indicated in 52 of the reports, 7 of which noted myopia of between 1.5 and 3.0 D; the myopia reversed on discontinuation of the drug.

A study on cynomolgus monkeys is also of interest (Lütjen-Drecoll and Kaufman, 1986a, 1986b). Monkeys were treated twice daily in one eye with timolol (180 µl) or epinephrine (adrenaline) (540–600 µl) for around a 6-month period in order to assess adverse morphological changes. The timolol-treated animals ($n = 6$) were found to be significantly more myopic, by approximately

2.0 D, than the epinephrine-treated ($n = 2$) or the control animals ($n = 11$). The authors concluded that the increase in myopia could either be mediated solely by ciliary muscle beta-adrenergic blockade or linked to pathophysiological changes in the trabecular meshwork and ciliary muscle.

6.8.2   Aspects of operant conditioning (biofeedback)

The rapid development in electronic technology has, in recent years, extended greatly the facility to monitor biological activity and has stimulated and renewed interest in whether the extent to which we can exercise control over nominally involuntary autonomic functions has clinical utility in the treatment of certain psychological and medical disorders. Operant conditioning (or biofeedback) has, however, yet to gain general acceptance in the medical fraternity even though recent work has striven to resolve the methodological limitations of early investigations. Ophthalmic applications of biofeedback have achieved varying levels of success with regard to the correction of oculomotor anomalies (e.g. strabismus, nystagmus and amblyopia), control of intraocular pressure and suppression of blepharospasm (Abadi *et al.*, 1981; Rotberg and Surwit, 1981; Ciuffreda and Goldrich, 1983; Halperin and Yolton, 1986).

Myopia therapy using accommodation biofeedback is one of the few non-invasive methods of myopia treatment available and is based principally on the work of Trachtman (1987; *see* Gilmartin *et al.*, 1991 for review). The principal aim is to train patients to gain greater control over voluntary accommodation in order to ameliorate functional myopia, although it is claimed that the facility can also be used to treat early presbyopia and latent hyperopia. Trachtman defines functional myopia as: myopia less than 2 D (although it is proposed that patients with up to 4 D of myopia can participate in training successfully); a significant difference between subjective refraction and static retinoscopy; a history of prolonged close work; a high negative relative accommodation; an onset of myopia in the late teens or early twenties and an absence of ocular pathology. It is suggested that patients can anticipate improvement of unaided visual acuity to 6/9 or 6/6 with a commensurate reduction in myopia of 2 D to 3 D. Of relevance to this chapter is that Trachtman (1987) also speculates that up to 2 D of myopia reduction occurs in the initial stage of training from a relaxation of

parasympathetic-induced spasm of accommodation and that subsequent myopia reduction emanates from patient control of sympathetic-induced negative accommodation.

There does not yet appear to be a body of clinical and experimental literature substantial enough to endorse myopia therapy using accommodation biofeedback techniques as a prescriptive method of clinical management of myopia. Although there are reports that the technique can induce up to a 3 D reduction in myopia, the claims are of limited value owing to the lack of objective data, for example pre- and post-training cycloplegic refraction. The pre- and post-training measures of subjective letter acuity used by many studies are, with repeated trials, particularly vulnerable to individual differences in the ability to learn how to discriminate and interpret blurred images. More comprehensive clinical trials are needed before accommodation biofeedback can qualify as an established method of clinical treatment of myopia (Gilmartin *et al.*, 1991).

6.9   Concluding remarks

Progress towards a fuller understanding of autonomic correlates of near vision in emmetropia and myopia will emanate from the integration of data from human and animal research into myopia (Zadnik and Mutti, 1995). The former requires experimental paradigms which can manage adequately the complexities of the psychophysiology of near vision; the latter a consensus on the most appropriate species on which to model myopia development. Sympathetic innervation of ciliary smooth muscle has been advanced in this chapter as a potential mechanism for adaptation to sustained accommodative effort but it is still unclear how, or whether, this facility can modulate to any extent the myopic structural changes that occur in the posterior segment of the globe. Longitudinal studies designed to test the correlation between autonomic response profiles and ametropic status, the former being indexed by accommodative responses as described in this chapter or by other general tests of autonomic function, would be of great interest.

Should it transpire that pharmacological management of myopia in humans becomes feasible, the ability to predict the incidence and likely development of myopia using techniques with high sensitivity and specificity will be a crucial aspect in respect of sample selection and experimental design (Mutti and Zadnik, 1995). Further, an analysis of cases of autonomic dysfunction such as, for example, Horner's syndrome, would be profitable. Finally, identifying aspects of structure and function of the choroid relevant to the development of myopia deserves special attention as they may prove to be the bridge between human and animal work.

Whilst for most individuals near vision would appear to be an innocuous part of everyday life, it represents, for the researcher a perplexing process in terms of how an organism interacts with the visual environment. The contribution of the ANS to this process will inevitably prove to be elusive, as is evident from the elegant description of ANS function by Bernard (1878): 'Nature thought it prudent to remove the important phenomena which it controls from the caprice of an ignorant will.'

Acknowledgements

I am especially indebted to the following individuals for their contributions to the studies described in this chapter: Mark Bullimore, Lyle Gray, Rob Hogan, Helen Owens, John Pugh, Mark Rosenfield, Niall Strang, Barry Winn and Nicola Winfield.

References

Abadi, R. V., Carden, D. and Simpson, J. (1981) Listening for eye movements. *Ophthal. Physiol. Opt.* **1**, 19–27.

Abbott, M. L., Schmid, K. L. and Strang, N. C. (1998) Differences in the accommodation stimulus response curves of adult myopes and emmetropes. *Ophthal. Physiol. Opt.* **18**, 13–20.

Adams A. J. (1987) Axial length elongation, not corneal curvature, as a basis of adult onset myopia. *Am. J. Optom. Physiol. Opt.* **64**, 150–151.

Baldwin, W. R., Adams, A. J. and Flattau, P. (1991) Young adult myopia. In: *Refractive Anomalies: Research and Clinical Applications* (T. Grosvenor and M. C. Flom, eds). Butterworth-Heinemann, pp. 104–120.

Bedrossian, R. H. (1979) The effect of atropine on myopia. *Ophthalmology* **86**, 713–717.

Bernard, C. (1878) *La Science Experimentale.* Bailliere, p. 150.

Biggs, R. D., Alpern, M. and Bennett, D. R. (1959) The effect of sympathomimetic drugs upon the amplitude of accommodation. *Am. J. Ophthalmol.* **48**, 169–171.

Birnbaum, M. H. (1993) *Optometric Management of Nearpoint Vision Disorders.* Butterworth-Heinemann.

Bullimore, M. A. and Gilmartin, B. (1987a) Tonic accommodation, cognitive demand and ciliary muscle innervation. *Am. J. Optom. Physiol. Opt.* **64**, 45–50.

Bullimore, M. A. and Gilmartin, B. (1987b) Aspects of tonic accommodation in emmetropia and late-onset myopia. *Am. J. Optom. Physiol. Opt.* **64**, 499–503.

Bullimore, M. A. and Gilmartin, B. (1988) The accommodative response, refractive error and mental effort. 1. The sympathetic nervous system. *Doc. Ophthalmol.* **69**, 385–397.

Bullimore, M. A., Gilmartin, B. and Hogan, R. E. (1986) Objective and subjective measurement of tonic accommodation. *Ophthal. Physiol. Opt.* **6**, 57–62.

Bullimore, M. A., Gilmartin, B. and Royston, J. M. (1992) Steady-state accommodation and ocular biometry in late-onset myopia. *Doc. Ophthalmol.* **80**, 143–155.

Burnstock, G. (1986a) Autonomic neuromuscular junctions: current developments and future directions. *J. Anat.* **146**, 1–30.

Burnstock, G. (1986b) The changing face of autonomic neurotransmission. (The first Von Euler Lecture in Physiology.) *Acta Physiol. Scand.* **126**, 67–91.

Burnstock, G. (1990a) Cotransmission. The Fifth Heymans Lecture. *Int. Pharmacodyn. Ther.* **304**, 7–33.

Burnstock, G. (1990b) Changes in expression of autonomic nerves in aging and disease. *J. Autonom. Nerv. Syst.* **30**, 525–534.

Burnstock, G. (1992) Autonomic neuroeffector mechanisms. In: *The Autonomic Nervous System*, Vol. 1 (G. Burnstock and C. H. V. Hoyle, eds). Harwood Academic Publishers.

Campbell, F. W. and Westheimer, G. (1960) Dynamics of accommodation responses of the human eye. *J. Physiol. Lond.* **151**, 285–295.

Cannon, W. B. (1929) *Bodily Changes in Pain, Hunger, Fear and Rage: an Account of Relevant Researches into the Function of Emotion.* Appleton.

Chauhan, K. and Charman, W. N. (1995) Single figure indices for the steady-state accommodative response. *Ophthal. Physiol. Opt.* **15**, 217–221.

Cheng, H. M., Singh, O. S., Kwong, K. K. *et al.* (1992) Shape of the myopic eye as seen with high-resolution magnetic resonance imaging. *Optom. Vis. Sci.* **69**, 698–701.

Ciuffreda, K. J. (1991) Accommodation and its anomalies. In: *Visual Optics and Instrumentation* (W. N. Charman, ed.), Vol. 1: *Vision and Visual Dysfunction* (general ed. J. Cronly-Dillon). Macmillan, ch. 11, pp. 231–279.

Ciuffreda, K. J. and Goldrich, S. G. (1983) Oculomotor biofeedback therapy. *Int. Rehabil. Med.* **5**, 111–117.

Cogan, D. G. (1937) Accommodation and the autonomic nervous system. *Arch. Ophthalmol.* **18**, 739–766.

Collins. M. J., Davis, B. and Wood, J. M. (1995) Microfluctuations of steady-state accommodation and the cardiopulmonary system. *Vis. Res.* **35**, 2491–2512.

Culhane, H. M. and Winn, B. (1997) Modulation of temporal closed-loop accommodation response by sympathetic innervation. *Invest. Ophthalmol. Vis. Sci.* (Suppl.) **38**, S984.

Culhane, H. M. and Winn, B. (1998). Accommodation responses with α ₁-adrenoceptor stimulation. *Invest. Ophthalmol. Vis. Sci. (suppl.)*, **39**, S1049.

Curtin, B. J. (1970) Myopia: a review of its aetiology, pathogenesis and treatment. *Surv. Ophthalmol.* **15**, 1–17.

Curtin, B. J. (1985) *The Myopias: Basic Science and Clinical Management.* Harper & Row.

Donders, F. C. (1864) *On the Anomalies of Accommodation and the Refraction of the Eye* (translated by W. D. Moore). The New Sydenham Society, pp. 579–580.

Ebenholtz, S. M. (1983) Accommodative hysteresis: a precursor for induced myopia? *Invest. Ophthalmol. Vis. Sci.* **24**, 513–515.

Ebenholtz, S. M. (1988) Long term endurance of adaptive shifts in tonic accommodation. *Ophthal. Physiol. Opt.* **8**, 427–431.

Ebenholtz, S. M. (1991) Accommodative hysteresis: fundamental asymmetry in decay role after near and far focusing. *Invest. Ophthalmol. Vis. Sci.* **32**, 148–153.

Ebenholtz, S. M. (1992) Accommodation hysteresis as a function of target–dark focus position. *Vis. Res.* **32**, 925–929.

Ehinger, B. (1966) Adrenergic nerves to the eye and to related structures in man and in the cynomolgos monkey (*Macaca irus*). *Invest. Ophthal. Vis. Sci.* **5**, 42–52.

Ehinger, B. (1971) A comparative study of the adrenergic nerves to the anterior segment of some primates. *Z. Zellforsch. Mikrosk. Anat.* **116**, 157–177.

Emi, K., Pederson, J. E. and Carol, B. T. (1989) Hydrostatic pressure of the suprachoroidal space. *Invest. Ophthal. Vis. Sci.* **30**, 233–238.

Fledelius, H. C. (1995) Adult-onset myopia–oculometric features. *Acta Ophthalmol.* **73**, 397–401.

Francis, E. L., Troilo, D. and Wildsoet, C. F. (1998). Time course of cycloplegia in chicks: relationship to mydriasis and effect of timolol. *Invest. Ophthalmol. Vis. Sci. (suppl.)*, **39**, S506.

Gilmartin, B. (1986) A review of the role of sympathetic innervation of the ciliary muscle in ocular accommodation. *Ophthal. Physiol. Opt.* **6**, 23–37.

Gilmartin, B. (1995) The aetiology of presbyopia: a summary of the role of lenticular and extralenticular structures. *Ophthal. Physiol. Opt.* **15**, 431–437.

Gilmartin, B. (1998) Pharmacology of accommodative adaptation. In: *Accommodative/Vergence Mechanisms in the Visual System* (O. Franzén and H. Richter, eds). Berkhauser Ferlag (in press).

Gilmartin, B. and Bullimore, M. A. (1987) Sustained near-vision augments sympathetic innervation of the ciliary muscle. *Clin. Vis. Sci.* **1**, 197–208.

Gilmartin, B. and Bullimore, M. A. (1991) Adaptation of accommodation to sustained visual tasks in emmetropia and late-onset myopia. *Optom. Vis. Sci.* **68**, 22–26.

Gilmartin, B. and Hogan, R. E. (1985) The relationship between tonic accommodation and ciliary muscle innervation. *Invest. Ophthal. Vis. Sci.* **26**, 1024–1029.

Gilmartin, B. and Winfield, N.R. (1995) The effect of topical β-adrenoceptor antagonists on accommodation in emmetropia and myopia. *Vis. Res.* **35**, 1305–1312.

Gilmartin, B., Bullimore, M. A., Rosenfield, M. *et al.* (1992) Pharmacological effects on accommodative adaptation. *Optom. Vis. Sci.* **69**, 276–282.

Gilmartin, B., Gray, L. S. and Winn, B. (1991) The amelioration of myopia using accommodation biofeedback: a review. *Ophthal. Physiol. Opt.* **11**, 304–313.

Gilmartin, B., Hogan, R. E. and Thompson, S. M. (1984) The effect of timolol maleate on tonic accommodation, tonic vergence and pupil diameter. *Invest. Ophthal. Vis. Sci.* **25**, 763–771.

Gimple, G., Doughty, M. J. and Lyle, W. M. (1994) A large sample study of the effects of phenylephrine 2.5% eyedrops on the amplitude of accommodation in man. *Ophthal. Physiol. Opt.* **14**, 123–128.

Goldschmidt, E. (1990) Myopia in humans: can progression be arrested? In: *Myopia and the Control of Eye Growth.* Ciba Foundation Symposium No. 155. Wiley, pp. 222–234.

Goldschmidt, E. and Jensen, H. (1987) Pharmaceutical agents in the control of myopia. *Res. Clin. Forums* **9**, 43–51.

Goss, D. A. and Wickham, M. G. (1995) Retinal-image mediated ocular growth as a mechanism for juvenile onset myopia and for emmetropization. *Doc. Ophthalmol.* **90**, 341–375.

Goss, D. A. and Winkler, R. L. (1983) Progression of myopia in youth: age of cessation. *Am. J. Optom. Physiol. Opt.* **60**, 651–658.

Graebel, W. P. and Van Alphen, G. W. H. M. (1977) The elasticity of sclera and choroid of the human eye and its implications on scleral rigidity and accommodation. *J. Biomech. Eng.* **99**, 203–208.

Gray, L. S., Winn, B., Gilmartin, B. and Eadie, A. S. (1993) Objective concurrent measures of open-loop accommodation and vergence under photopic conditions. *Invest. Ophthal. Vis. Sci.* **34**, 2996–3003.

Greene, P. R. (1991) Mechanical considerations in myopia. In: *Refractive Anomalies: Research and Clinical Applications* (T. Grosvenor and M. C. Flom, eds). Butterworth-Heinemann, pp. 287–300.

Greene, P. R. and McMahon, T. A. (1979) Scleral creep vs temperature and pressure *in vitro*. *Exp. Eye Res.* **29**, 527–537.

Grosvenor, T. (1987) Review and a suggested classification system for myopia on the basis of age-related prevalence and age of onset. *Am. J. Optom. Physiol. Opt.* **64**, 545–554.

Grosvenor, T. and Scott, R. (1991) A comparison of refractive components in youth-onset and early adult-onset myopia. *Optom. Vis. Sci.* **68**, 204–209.

Grosvenor, T. and Scott, R. (1993) Three-year changes in refraction and its components in youth-onset and early adult-onset myopia. *Optom. Vis. Sci.* **70**, 204–209.

Gwiazda, J., Bauer, J., Thorn, F. and Held, R. (1993) Myopic children show insufficient accommodative response to blur. *Invest. Ophthalmol. Vis. Sci.* **34**, 690–694.

Gwiazda, J., Bauer, J., Thorn, F. and Held, R. (1995) A dynamic relationship between myopia and blur-driven accommodation in school-aged children. *Vis. Res.* **35**, 1299–1304.

Halperin, E. and Yolton, R. L. (1986) Ophthalmic applications of biofeedback. *Am. J. Optom. Physiol. Opt.* **63**, 985–998.

Hamill, R.W. (1996) In: *Primer on the Autonomic Nervous System* (D. Robertson, P. A. Low and R. J. Polinsky, eds). Academic Press, pp. 12–25.

Held, R. (1998) The accommodative response to blur in myopic children. In: *Accommodative/Vergence Mechanisms in the Visual System* (O. Franzén and H. Richter, eds). Berkhauser Ferlag (in press).

Helmholtz, H. (1909) In: *Handbuch der Physiologischen Optik*, 3rd edn (J. P. C. Southall, ed. and trans.), Vol. I. Dover Publications.

Hillarp, N. Å. (1959) The construction and functional organisation of the autonomic innervation apparatus. *Acta Physiol. Scand.* Suppl. 157, **46**, 1–38.

Hogan, R. E. and Gilmartin, B. (1984) The choice of laser speckle exposure duration in the measurement of tonic accommodation. *Ophthal. Physiol. Opt.* **4**, 365–368.

Hosaka, A. (1988) The role of pharmaceutical agents. Japanese studies. *Acta Ophthalmol.* Suppl. 185, 65–68.

Hubbard, W. C., Robinson, J. C., Schmidt, K., Rohen, J. W., Tamm, E. R. and Kaufman, P. L. (1998). Superior cervical ganglionectomy in monkeys: effects on refraction and intraocular pressure. *Invest. Ophthalmol. Vis. Sci. (suppl.)*, **39**, S869.

Hung, G. K. (1992) Adaptation model of accommodation and vergence. *Ophthal. Physiol. Opt.* **12**, 319–326.

Hung, G. K., Ciuffreda, K. J. and Rosenfield, M. (1996) Proximal contribution to a linear static model of accommodation and vergence. *Ophthal. Physiol. Opt.* **16**, 31–41.

Hung, L.-F., Crawford, M. L. J. and Smith, E. L. (1995) Spectacle lenses alter eye growth and the refractive status of young monkeys. *Nature Med.* **1**, 761–765.

Hurwitz, B. S., Davidowitz, J., Chin, N. B. and Breinin, G. B. (1972) The effects of the sympathetic nervous system on accommodation: 1. Beta sympathetic nervous system. *Arch. Ophthalmol.* **87**, 668–674.

James, B., Trew, D. R., Clark, K. and Smith, S. E. (1991) Factors influencing the ocular pulse–axial length. *Graefe's Arch. Clin. Exp. Ophthalmol.* **229**, 341–344.

Jensen, H. (1991) Myopia progression in young school children. *Acta Ophthalmol.* **200** (Suppl.), 1–79.

Jensen, H. and Goldschmidt, E. (1991) Management of myopia: pharmaceutical agents. In: *Refractive Anomalies: Research and Clinical Applications* (T. Grosvenor and M. C. Flom, eds). Butterworth-Heinemann, pp. 371–383.

Jiang, B.-C. (1995) Parameters of accommodative and vergence systems and the development of late-onset myopia. *Invest. Ophthalmol. Vis. Sci.* **36**, 1737–1742.

Jiang, B.-C. (1997) Integration of a sensory component into the accommodation model reveals differences between emmetropia and late-onset myopia. *Invest. Ophthalmol. Vis. Sci.* **38**, 1511–1516.

Kaufman, P. L. (1992) Accommodation and presbyopia: neuromuscular and biophysical aspects. In: *Adler's Physiology of the Eye*, 9th edn (M. H. Hart Jr, ed.). Mosby-Year Book, pp. 406–407.

Kelly, T. S.-B., Chatfield, C. and Tustin, T. (1975) Clinical assessment of the arrest of myopia. *Br. J. Ophthalmol.* **59**, 529–538.

Kern, R. (1970) Die adrenergischen Receptoren der intra-ocularen Muskeln des Menschen. *Graefe's Arch. Ophthalmol.* **180**, 231–248.

Kruger, P. B. (1980) The effect of cognitive demand on accommodation. *Am. J. Optom. Physiol. Opt.* **57**, 440–445.

Langham, M. E., Farrell, R. A., O'Brien, V. *et al.* (1989) Blood flow in the human eye. *Acta Ophthalmol.* **67**, 9–13.

Laties, A. M. and Jacobowitz, D. (1966) A comparative study of the autonomic innervation of the eye in monkey, cat and rabbit. *Anat. Rec.* **156**, 383–389.

Leech, E. M., Cottriall, C. L. and McBrien, N. A. (1995) Pirenzepine prevents form-deprivation myopia in a dose dependent manner. *Ophthal. Physiol. Opt.* **15**, 351–356.

Logan, N. S., Gilmartin, B. and Dunne, M. C. M. (1995) Computation of retinal contour in anisomyopia. *Ophthal. Physiol. Opt.* **15**, 363–366.

Lograno, M. D. and Reibaldi, A. (1986) Receptor responses in fresh human ciliary muscle. *Br. J. Pharmacol.* **87**, 379–385.

Lütjen-Drecoll, E. and Kaufman, P. L. (1986a) Long-term timolol and epinephrine in monkeys. 1. Functional morphology of the ciliary processes. *Trans. Ophthalmol. Soc. UK* **105**, 180–195.

Lütjen-Drecoll, E. and Kaufman, P. L. (1986b) Long-term timolol and epinephrine in monkeys. 2. Morphological alterations in trabecular meshwork and ciliary muscle. *Trans. Ophthalmol. Soc. UK* **105**, 196–207.

Malmfors, T. (1965) The adrenergic innervation of the eye as demonstrated by fluorescence microscopy. *Acta Physiol. Scand.* **65**, 259–267.

Malmstrom, F. V., Randle, R. J., Bendix, J. S. and Weber, R. J. (1980) The visual accommodation response during concurrent mental activity. *Percept. Psychophys.* **28**, 440–448.

Marzani, D., Lind, G. J., Chew, S. J. and Wallman, J. (1994) The reduction of myopia by muscarinic antagonists may involve a direct effect on scleral cells. *Invest. Ophthalmol. Vis. Sci.* (Suppl.), **35**, 1801.

Matthews, G., Middleton, W., Gilmartin, B. and Bullimore, M. A. (1991) Pupillary diameter and cognitive load. *J. Psychophysiol.* **5**, 265–271.

McBrien, N. A. (1998) The role of accommodation in the control of ocular growth and myopia. In: *Accommodative/Vergence Mechanisms in the Visual System* (O. Franzén and H. Richter, eds). Berkhauser Ferlag. (In press.)

McBrien, N. A. and Adams, D. W. (1997) A longitudinal investigation of adult-onset and adult progression of myopia in an occupational group. *Invest. Ophthalmol. Vis. Sci.* **38**, 321–333.

McBrien, N. A. and Millodot, M. (1986a) The effect of refractive error on the accommodation response gradient. *Ophthal. Physiol. Opt.* **6**, 145–149.

McBrien, N. A. and Millodot, M. (1986b) Amplitude of accommodation and refractive error. *Invest. Ophthalmol. Vis. Sci.* **27**, 1187–1190.

McBrien, N. A. and Millodot, M. (1987) Biometric investigation of late-onset myopic eyes. *Acta Ophthalmol.* **65**, 461–468.

McBrien, N. A. and Millodot, M. (1988) Differences in adaptation of tonic accommodation with refractive state. *Invest. Ophthalmol. Vis. Sci.* **29**, 460–469.

McKanna, J. A. and Casagrande, V. A. (1981) Atropine affects lid-suture myopia development: experimental studies of chronic atropinization in tree shrews. *Doc. Ophthalmol. Proc. Ser.* No. 28 (H. C. Fledelius, P. H. Alsbirk and E. Goldschmidt, eds). Dr W. Junk, pp. 187–192.

Miller, R. J. and LeBeau, R. C. (1982) Induced stress, situationally-specific trait anxiety, and dark focus. *Psychophysiology* **19**, 260–265.

Morgan, M. W. (1946) A new theory for the control of accommodation. *Am. J. Physiol.* **23**, 99–110.

Mutti, D. O. and Zadnik, K. (1995) The utility of three predictors of childhood myopia: a Bayesian analysis. *Vis. Res.* **35**, 1345–1352.

National Research Council (1989) *Myopia: Prevalence and Progression.* National Academy Press.

O'Neal, M. R. and Connon, T. R. (1987) Refractive error change at the United States Air Force Academy–class of 1985. *Am. J. Opt. Physiol. Opt.* **62**, 344–354.

Ong, E. and Ciuffreda, K. J. (1995) Nearwork-induced transient myopia. *Doc. Ophthalmol.* **91**, 57–85.

Ong, E. and Ciuffreda, K. J. (1997) *Accommodation, Near Work and Myopia.* Optometric Extension Program Foundation.

Otsuka, N., Tsuchiya, K., Ukai, K., Yoshitomi, T. and Ishikawa, S. (1998) Adrenoceptors affect accommodation by modulating cholinergic activity. *Jap. J. Ophthal.* **42**, 66–70.

Owens, D. A. (1991a) Near work, accommodative tonus and myopia. In: *Refractive Anomalies: Research and Clinical Applications* (T. Grosvenor and M. C. Flom, eds). Butterworth-Heinemann, pp. 318–344.

Owens, H. (1991b) The effect of beta-adrenergic receptor antagonists on the temporal accommodative response. PhD Thesis, University of Aston, Birmingham, UK, pp. 157–162.

Owens, H., Winn, B., Gilmartin, B. and Pugh, J. R. (1991) The effect of topical beta-adrenergic antagonists on the dynamics of steady-state accommodation. *Ophthal. Physiol. Opt.* **11**, 99–104.

Pang, I. H., Matsumoto, S., Tamm, E. and DeSantis, L. (1994) Characterization of muscarinic receptor involvement in human ciliary muscle cell function. *J. Oc. Pharmacol.* **10**, 125–136.

Phillips, J. R. and McBrien, N. A. (1995) Form deprivation myopia: elastic properties of sclera. *Ophthal. Physiol. Opt.* **15**, 357–362.

Post, R. B., Johnson, C. A. and Owens, D. A. (1985) Does performance of tasks affect the resting focus of accommodation? *Am. J. Opt. Physiol. Opt.* **62**, 533–537.

Raviola, E. and Wiesel, T. N. (1990) Neural control of eye growth and experimental myopia in primates. In: *Myopia and the Control of Eye Growth.* Ciba Foundation Symposium No. 155 (G. R. Bock and K. Widdows, eds). Wiley, pp. 22–44.

Reiner, A., Shih, Y.-F. and Fitzgerald, M. E. C. (1995) The relationship of choroidal blood flow and accommodation to the control of ocular growth. *Vis. Res.* **35**, 1227–1245.

Rosenfield, M. and Ciuffreda, K. J. (1990) Proximal and cognitively-induced accommodation. *Ophthal. Physiol. Opt.* **10**, 252–256.

Rosenfield, M., Ciuffreda, K. J. and Gilmartin, B. (1992) Factors affecting accommodative adaptation. *Optom. Vis. Sci.* **69**, 270–275.

Rosenfield, M. and Gilmartin, B. (1987a) Synkinesis of accommodation and vergence in late-onset myopia. *Am. J. Optom. Physiol. Opt.* **64**, 929–937.

Rosenfield, M. and Gilmartin, B. (1987b) Oculomotor consequences of beta-adrenoceptor antagonism during sustained near vision. *Ophthal. Physiol. Opt.* **7**, 127–130.

Rosenfield, M. and Gilmartin, B. (1987c) Effect of a near-vision task on the response AC/A of a myopic population. *Ophthal. Physiol. Opt.* **7**, 225–233.

Rosenfield, M. and Gilmartin, B. (1987d) Beta-adrenergic receptor antagonism in myopia. *Ophthal. Physiol. Opt.* **7**, 359–364.

Rosenfield, M. and Gilmartin, B. (1989) Temporal aspects of accommodative adaptation. *Optom. Vis. Sci.* **66**, 229–234.

Rosenfield, M. and Gilmartin, B. (1998). Accommodative adaptation during sustained near-vision reduces accommodative error. *Invest. Ophthalmol. Vis. Sci. (suppl.)*, **39**, S1049.

Rosenfield, M., Ciuffreda, K. J., Hung, G. K. and Gilmartin, B. (1993) Tonic accommodation: a review I. Basic aspects. *Ophthal. Physiol. Opt.* **13**, 266–284.

Rosenfield, M., Ciuffreda, K. J., Hung, G. K. and Gilmartin, B. (1994) Tonic accommodation: a review II. Accommodative adaptation and clinical aspects. *Ophthal. Physiol. Opt.* **14**, 265–277.

Rosenfield, M., Gilmartin B., Cunningham, E. and Dattani, N. (1990) The influence of alpha-adrenergic antagonists on tonic accommodation. *Curr. Eye Res.* **9**, 267–272.

Rotberg, M. H. and Surwit, R. S. (1981) Biofeedback techniques in the treatment of visual and ophthalmologic disorders. *Biofeed. Self Reg.* **6**, 375–388.

Ruskell, G. L. (1973) Sympathetic innervation of the ciliary muscle in monkeys. *Exp. Eye Res.* **16**, 183–190.

Ryall, R. W. (1989) *Mechanisms of Drug Action on the Nervous System*, 2nd edn. Cambridge University Press, pp. 43–79.

Seyle, H. (1956) *The Stress of Life.* McGraw-Hill.

Skeffington, A. M. (1991) Practical Applied Optometry. In: *Optometric Extension Programme* 83 (A. Hendrickson, ed.). Optometric Extension Program Foundation.

Sorsby, A. and Leary, G. A. (1970) *A Longitudinal Study of Refraction and Its Components During Growth.* Medical Research Council Special Reports Series No. 309. HMSO.

Starke, K., Gothert, M. and Kilbinger, H. (1989) Modulation of neurotransmitter release by presynaptic autoreceptors. *Physiol. Rev.* **69**, 864–989.

Stenstrom, S. (1948) Investigation of the variation and the correlation of the optical elements of human eyes. *Am. J. Optom. Arch. Am. Acad. Optom.* **58**, 1–71.

Stephens, K. G. (1985) Effect of the sympathetic nervous system on accommodation. *Am. J. Optom. Physiol. Opt.* **62**, 402–406.

Stone, R. A., Kuwayama, Y. and Laties, A. M. (1987) Regulatory peptides in the eye. *Experientia* **43**, 791–800.

Stone, R. A., Lin, T. and Laties, A. M. (1991) Muscarinic antagonist effects on experimental chick myopia. *Exp. Eye Res.* **52**, 755–758.

Strang, N. C. (1995) Modulation of foveal image quality in myopia: investigation of spatiotopic and retinotopic factors. PhD Thesis. Glasgow Caledonian University, Glasgow, UK, pp. 108–119.

Strang, N. C., Winn, B. and Gilmartin, B. (1994a) Repeatability of post-task regression of accommodation in emmetropia and late-onset myopia. *Ophthal. Physiol. Opt.* **14**, 88–91.

Strang, N. C., Winn, B., Gilmartin, B. and Brosnahan, D. (1994b) Assessment of ocular response to topical β-adrenoceptor antagonists using accommodative microfluctuations. *Ophthal. Physiol. Opt.* **14**, 293–297.

Tamm, E. and Lütjen-Drecoll, E. (1996) Ciliary body. *Micros. Res. Tech.* **33**, 390–439.

Tamm, E. R., Flügel-Koch, C., Mayer, B. and Lütjen-Drecoll, E. (1995) Nerve cells in the human ciliary muscle: ultrastructural and immunocytochemical characterization. *Invest. Ophthalmol. Vis. Sci.* **36**, 414–426.

Tamm, E., Lütjen-Drecoll, E., Jungkuntz, W. and Rohen, J. W. (1991) Posterior attachment of the ciliary muscle in young, accommodating old, presbyopic rhesus monkeys. *Invest. Ophthalmol. Vis. Sci.* **32**, 1678–1692.

Toates, F. M. (1972) Accommodation function of the human eye. *Physiol. Rev.* **52**, 828–863.

Törnqvist, G. (1966) Effect of cervical sympathetic stimulation on accommodation in monkeys. *Acta Physiol. Scand.* **67**, 363–372.

Törnqvist, G. (1967) The relative importance of the parasympathetic and sympathetic nervous systems for accommodation in monkeys. *Invest. Ophthalmol. Vis. Sci.* **6**, 612–617.

Trachtman, J. N. (1987) Biofeedback of accommodation to reduce myopia: a review. *Am. J. Optom. Physiol. Opt.* **64,** 639–643.

Troilo, D., Li, T. and Howland, H. C. (1993) Negative accommodation occurs in the chick and may be mediated by sympathetic input. *Invest. Ophthalmol. Vis. Sci.* (Suppl.), **34**, 1310.

Tyrrell, R. A., Pearson, M. A. and Thayer, J. F. (1998) Behavioural links between the oculomotor and cardiovascular systems. In: *Accommodative/Vergence Mechanisms in the Visual System.* (O. Franzén and H. Richter, eds). Berkhauser Ferlag. (In press.)

Tyrrell, R. A., Thayer, J. F., Friedman *et al.* (1995) A behavioural link between the oculomotor and cardiovascular systems. *Int. Physiol. Behav. Sci.* **30**, 46–67.

Van Alphen, G. W. H. M. (1961) On emmetropia and ametropia. *Ophthalmologica* **142** (Suppl.), 1–92.

Van Alphen, G. W. H. M. (1976) The adrenergic receptors of the intraocular muscles of the human eye. *Invest. Ophthalmol. Vis. Sci.* **15**, 502–505.

Van Alphen, G. W. H. M. (1986) Choroidal stress and emmetropization. *Vis. Res.* **26**, 723–734.

Van Alphen, G. W. H. M. (1990) Emmetropization in the primate eye. In: *Myopia and the Control of Eye Growth.* Ciba Foundation Symposium No. 155 (G. R. Buck and K. Widdows, eds). Wiley, pp. 115–125.

Van Alphen, G. W. H. M. and Graebel, W. P. (1991) Elasticity of tissues involved in accommodation. *Vis. Res.* **31**, 1417–1438.

Van Alphen, G. W. H. M., Kern, R. and Robinette, S. L. (1965) Adrenergic receptors of the intraocular muscles. *Arch. Ophthalmol.* **74**, 253–259.

Van Buskirk, E. M. (1980) Adverse reactions from timolol administration. *Ophthalmology* **87**, 447–450.

Vogel, R. (1988) Pharmaceutical agents and the prevention or reduction of progressive myopia. *Acta Ophthalmol.* **185** (Suppl.), 134–139.

Wallman, J., Gottlieb, M. D., Rajaram, V. and Fugate-Wentzek, L. A. (1987) Local retinal regions control local eye growth and myopia. *Science* **237**, 73–77.

Wax, M. B. and Molinoff, P. B. (1987) Distribution and properties of β-adrenergic receptors in human iris-ciliary body. *Invest. Ophthalmol. Vis. Sci.* **28**, 420–430.

Weber, J., Tuinenburg, A. E. and Van der Heijde, G. L. (1989) Effect of timolol on the amplitude and dynamics of accommodation. *Doc. Ophthalmol.* **72**, 341–347.

Wells, W. C. (1811) *Philosophical Transactions* (cited by Curtin, 1985).

Westheimer, G. (1957) Accommodation measurements in empty visual fields. *J. Opt. Soc. Am.* **47**, 714–718.

Wildsoet, C. (1997) Active emmetropization—evidence for its existence and ramifications for clinical practice. *Ophthal. Physiol. Opt.* **17**, 279–290.

Wildsoet, C. and Wallman, J. (1995) Choroidal and scleral mechanisms of compensation for spectacle lenses in chicks. *Vis. Res.* **35**, 1175–1194.

Winn, B. and Culhane, H. M. (1998). Autonomic control of accommodation. *Invest. Ophthalmol. Vis. Sci. (suppl.)*, **39**, S1049.

Winn, B. and Gilmartin, B. (1992) Current perspective on accommodative microfluctuations. *Ophthal. Physiol. Opt.* **12**, 252–256.

Winn, B., Gilmartin, B., Mortimer L. C. and Edwards, N. R. (1991) The effect of mental effort on open- and closed-loop accommodation. *Ophthal. Physiol. Opt.* **11**, 335–339.

Winn, B., Gilmartin, B. and Strang, N. C. (1993) Temporal closed-loop measures of accommodation show that sustained accommodation augments sympathetic innervation of ciliary muscle. *Invest. Ophthalmol. Vis. Sci.* (Suppl.), **34**, 1310.

Winn, B., Pugh, J. R., Gilmartin, B. and Owens, H. (1990) Arterial pulse modulates temporal response characteristics of accommodation. *Curr. Eye Res.* **9**, 971–975.

Yen, M., Liu, J., Kao, S. and Shiao, C. (1989) Comparison of the effect of atropine and cyclopentolate on myopia. *Ann. Ophthalmol.* **21**, 180–187.

Young, F. A. (1965) The effect of atropine on the development of myopia in monkeys. *Am. J. Optom. Arch. Am. Acad. Optom.* **42**, 439–449.

Zadnik, K. and Mutti, D. O. (1995) How applicable are animal myopia models to human juvenile onset myopia? *Vis. Res.* **35**, 1283–1288.

Zetterström, C. (1988) Effects of adrenergic drugs on accommodation and distant refraction in daylight and darkness. *Acta Ophthalmol.* **66**, 58–64.

Zetterström, C. and Hahnenberger, R. (1988) Pharmacological characterization of human ciliary muscle adrenoceptors *in vitro*. *Exp. Eye Res.* **46**, 421–430.

7

Vergence and myopia

David A. Goss and Mark Rosenfield

The reported association between myopia and nearwork leads one to consider which aspects of near visual function might be associated with refractive error development. The two primary oculomotor responses that occur during nearwork include changes in the output of ocular accommodation and convergence. The possible relationship between ocular accommodation and the development of myopia was reviewed in Chapter 5; this chapter will examine the hypothesis that the characteristics of ocular vergence during sustained near vision may be involved in the aetiology of myopia.

7.1 Historical introduction

Stansbury (1948) cited Von Graefe (1854) as being the earliest to indicate that the actions of the medial and lateral rectus muscles may cause stretching and distension of the eyes during periods of sustained near vision. Later, Donders (1864) also stated that a potential cause of myopia was the pressure of the extraocular muscles on the eyeball during strong convergence of the visual axes. Additionally, in the 1909 appendices to Helmholtz's *Treatise on Physiological Optics* (Southall, 1924), Gullstrand noted that during convergence for close work, 'steady fixation involving exertion on the part of all the external muscles, together with the customary knitting of the eyebrows as in sickness, may have a tendency to elongate the axis of the eye'.

A number of possible mechanisms whereby the actions of the vergence system could be associated with myopia development were proposed in the early literature. For example, Von Arlt (1876) postulated that the pressure of the extraocular muscles during convergence impeded blood outflow through the vortex veins, leading to congestion and increased intraocular tension. Alternatively, Stilling (1891) proposed that the action of the superior oblique muscle may be responsible for myopia development. He stated that myopia varied with the anatomical position of the trochlea, with a low (presumably meaning inferior) pulley position leading to globe compression. However, subsequent studies (*see* Stansbury, 1948) were unable to verify the theory that refractive error varied with the position of the trochlea in the orbit.

Jackson (1931) reported that 'excessive convergence in the majority of cases starts the myopia and keeps it progressive'. In an attempt to verify Jackson's statement, Luedde (1932) investigated the effect of monocular cycloplegia (atropine) on myopia progression. It was argued that monocular cycloplegia would effectively dissociate the two eyes, thereby minimizing the demand upon fusional vergence. Luedde reported a reduction in myopia progression in both eyes, and claimed that this provided evidence for the role of vergence in the development of myopia. Interestingly, the effect of monocular atropine was also examined by Bedrossian (1979), who confirmed the observation of reduced myopic progression in the cyclopleged eye. However, their interpretation of similar results differed, Luedde claiming that atropine reduced the effect of excessive vergence, whereas Bedrossian suggested that atropine inhibited myopic progression by reducing the accommodative response.

Luedde's findings that monocular cycloplegia appeared to retard myopic progression in both eyes might appear to support the vergence hypothesis, although no values for amplitude of accommodation or pupillary diameter were provided. These data would be valuable in order to determine whether any systemic absorption of atropine occurred, which would produce an effect in the contralateral, non-treated eye.

Both Donders (1864) and Linder (1946) observed a lower incidence of myopia in watch-makers than might have been predicted in view of the amount of near vision required by this occupation. Donders suggested that the reduced incidence of myopia may be related to the use of monocular loupes which would reduce the vergence demand. It should be noted, however, that the magnifying effect of the loupe might also lower the accommodative stimulus. In a more recent review of the early literature concerning the relationship between myopia and heterophoria, Curtin (1985) indicated that authorities such as von Graefe, Landolt and Pascal had all observed that uncorrected myopia was associated with exophoria. This reduced vergence response is likely to have resulted from the decreased output of accommodative convergence in uncorrected myopia.

7.2   Myopia and the vergence response

The earliest published data linking myopia with the magnitude of the vergence response appears to be that of Snell (1936). He examined distance (6 m) heterophoria findings in more than 1000 myopic patients from his practice. Snell noted that the majority of myopes (55.3%) were esophoric, while only 30.4% were exophoric. Additionally, the average near point of convergence for 100 myopes was 16.8 meter angles (MA), whereas Snell reported an average value for all normal subjects of 15 MA, with 10.5 MA representing the minimum value found in normals. Only 6 myopes had a near point of convergence below this minimum normal level, whereas 67 of the 100 myopes had values greater than 15 MA. Work in the second half of the twentieth century has also suggested that the onset and greater progression of myopia tend to be associated with a more convergent ocular posture, when the myopia is corrected. It should be stressed that the association of esophoria with myopia occurs in corrected myopia, whereas exophoria is

quite common in uncorrected myopia due to the reduced output of accommodative convergence.

Birnbaum (1979, 1981) suggested that before myopia becomes clinically manifest, an incipient stage could be identified when patients have either very low amounts of hyperopia, emmetropia, or up to 0.25 D of myopia. One might also consider whether the inception of myopia may be related to variations in:

1 near heterophoria;
2 vergence ranges;
3 positive relative accommodation;
4 accommodative convergence;
5 vergence adaptation.

Each of these possibilities will be discussed below.

7.2.1   Near heterophoria and myopia

Goss (1991) collected private practice patient data for a group of children who had optometric examinations before and after the onset of myopia, and for a group of children who remained emmetropic at all examinations (minimum of two) between 6 and 15 years of age. The 'became myopic' group were emmetropic at an initial examination at 6 years of age or older, and became myopic prior to 15 years of age, and no more than 1 year after the last examination at which emmetropia was found. The 'remained emmetropic' group and the 'became myopic' group were matched in terms of practice location, gender and age. The data from the last examination before becoming myopic in the 'became myopic' group were compared with the age-matched examination data for the 'remained emmetropic' group. The mean near-point heterophoria through the distance refractive correction for the 'became myopic' and 'remained emmetropic' groups was 1.0Δ eso (SEM = 0.8, $n = 61$) and 2.0Δ exo (SEM = 0.8, $n = 61$), respectively. This difference was significant.

A similar study was performed by Drobe and de Saint-André (1995). Patients were classified as stable emmetropes or pre-myopes based upon the refractive error at their second examination, which was conducted less than 2 years after the initial testing. The mean near lateral heterophoria for the pre-myopic and stable emmetropic groups was 0.6Δ eso (SEM = 1.4, $n = 23$) and 2.3Δ exo (SEM = 0.9, $n = 23$), respectively. This difference was not significant, possibly due to the relatively small sample size. However, the magnitude of the mean

Table 7.1 Prevalence of near heterophorias in children who either became myopic or remained emmetropic in the Goss and Jackson (1996b) prospective study

	Became myopic	Remained emmetropic
More than 4Δ of exophoria	13 (44.8%)	17 (29.3%)
Between 3Δ exo- and 1Δ esophoria	9 (31.0%)	32 (55.2%)
More than 2Δ of esophoria	7 (24.1%)	9 (15.5%)

difference in heterophorias between the two groups (2.9Δ) was very similar to that reported earlier by Goss (1991). Further, Drobe and de Saint-André observed that the risk for myopia onset was significantly greater for patients having either esophoria or orthophoria at near when compared with exophoric subjects.

Subsequently, Goss and Jackson (1996a, 1996b) conducted a prospective study to examine clinical optometric findings prior to the onset of myopia in children. Initially emmetropic children were examined at 6-monthly intervals over a 3-year period. The 'remained emmetropic' individuals were defined as those children who were still emmetropic 1 year after their third study visit. Data at the last examination before becoming myopic for children in the 'became myopic' group were compared with the data at the third study visit for children in the 'remained emmetropic' group, since this visit yielded the closest mean age for the two groups. The mean heterophoria for the 'became myopic' and 'remained emmetropic' groups was 2.3Δ exo (SEM = 0.9, n = 29) and 1.5Δ exo (SEM = 0.6, n = 58), respectively. This difference was not significant. However, the distribution of near heterophorias in the 'remained emmetropic' group had significant positive kurtosis, whereas the distribution for the 'became myopic' group did not show kurtosis. Furthermore, there were proportionately more 'remained emmetropic' subjects in the mid-range of heterophorias (i.e., 3Δ exo to 1Δ eso) than 'became myopic' subjects (*see* Table 7.1). The near heterophoria cutoffs for the prediction of myopic onset are given in Table 7.2. In both the Goss (1991) and Drobe and de Saint-André (1995) retrospective studies, orthophoria and esophoria at near were risk factors for myopia. Additionally, in the Goss and Jackson (1996b) prospective study, near heterophorias outside the range of 3Δ exo to

1Δ eso were risk factors for myopia. It is unclear why high exophorias were risk factors in the latter study. However, one possible explanation was that there may have been more subjects with pseudo convergence insufficiency in the prospective study (Goss and Jackson, 1996b), i.e., exophoria at near secondary to an abnormally high lag of accommodation (Scheiman and Wick, 1994; Goss, 1995). Such an explanation for the higher number of exophoric patients in the prospective study would be consistent with the theory that retinal image focus acts as a feedback signal to direct the rate of ocular posterior segment enlargement (Goss and Wickham, 1995; Hung *et al.*, 1995; Wallman and McFadden, 1995) (*see* section 5.9.1). Furthermore, the mean heterophorias were similar in the two retrospective studies (Table 7.3).

Adams and McBrien (1992) examined 251 clinical microscopists who ranged from 21 to 63 years of age (median age, 29.7 years). Forty-nine per cent of the subjects had a self-reported onset or progression of myopia in adulthood after entry into the clinical microscopy profession. Median near heterophorias measured with the Maddox wing were orthophoria in the subjects who had reported previous myopic changes and 1Δ exophoria in subjects who did not exhibit myopic changes. Whilst this difference was statistically significant, it is smaller than the degree of repeatability of most subjective heterophoria measurement techniques (Schroeder *et al.*, 1996). More recently, Goss and Jackson (1996b) analysed the changes in near heterophoria in both the prospective study data and in the retrospective private practice data from Goss (1991), as shown in Figures 7.1 to 7.4. In both data sets, there was a convergent shift in the near heterophoria of 3–4Δ over an approximate 2-year period, beginning before the onset of myopia. Thus more convergent near heterophorias tend to be associated with myopia onset, and furthermore, near heterophorias appear to shift to a more convergent position around the time of myopia onset.

Relation of near heterophoria to rate of childhood myopia progression

Roberts and Banford (1963, 1967) reported myopia progression data for patients refracted at least twice before 17 years of age. Data were reported for 231 females and 165 males, all of whom wore single-vision lenses. The mean rate of myopia progression was greatest amongst those patients having esophoria at near (0.48 D/yr; n = 167), while

Table 7.2 Cut-offs for predicting myopia onset and the chi-square statistics for distribution within the 'became myopic' group and 'remained emmetropic' group according to those cut-offs

Study	Cut-off for predicted myopia	Chi-square	Statistical significance
Goss (1991)	Orthophoria or any esophoria	3.97	*P*<0.05
Drobe and de Saint-André (1995)	Orthophoria or any esophoria	4.29	*P*<0.05
Goss and Jackson (1996b)	3Δ exo- to 1Δ esophoria	4.52	*P*<0.05

Table 7.3 Mean near heterophorias (Δ) and positive relative accommodation (D) associated with myopia onset and continuing emmetropia. Plus and minus phorias indicate eso- and exophoria, respectively

	Became myopic			Remained emmetropic			Statistical significance
	n	Mean	SD	*n*	Mean	SD	
Near phorias							
Goss (1991)	61	+1.0	6.0	61	−2.0	6.0	*P* < 0.001
Drobe and de Saint-André (1995)	23	+0.6	6.7	23	−2.3	4.2	*P* = 0.08
Goss and Jackson (1996b)	29	−2.3	4.5	58	−1.5	4.6	*P* = 0.43
Positive relative accommodation							
Goss (1991)	32	−2.53	0.98	32	−3.16	1.03	*P* < 0.02
Drobe and de Saint-André (1995)	20	−2.84	1.89	24	−4.02	1.95	*P* = 0.04
Goss and Jackson (1996a)	29	−1.46	0.92	58	−2.04	1.11	*P* = 0.02

the lowest progression rates were found in those individuals having near heterophoria between ortho- and 4Δ exophoria (mean myopia progression = 0.39 D/yr; *n* = 105). The results from this study are illustrated in Figure 7.5. Unfortunately, Roberts and Banford did not state whether the differences between groups were significant.

Similar findings were reported by Goss (1990) (*see* Figure 7.6). For patients with habitual near heterophorias within Morgan's (1944) normal range of ortho to 6Δ exo, the mean rate of myopia progression was 0.39 D/yr, while the mean rate for patients with esophoria was 0.50 D/yr. Patients with habitual near exophoria greater than 6Δ had a mean progression rate of 0.45 D/yr. The difference between these three groups was significant. These results indicate that children with esophoria at near through their refractive corrections have higher rates of myopia progression than children with orthophoria or exophoria. Rates were lowest when the heterophoria was in the range of orthophoria to low exophoria.

7.2.2   Positive relative accommodation (PRA)

Goss (1991) observed significant differences in mean PRA findings between the 'became myopic' and 'remained emmetropic' groups, with mean values of −2.53 D (SEM = 0.17, *n* = 32) and −3.16 D (SEM = 0.18, *n* = 32), respectively, being recorded. This difference was significant. Similarly, both Drobe and de Saint-André (1995) and Goss and Jackson (1996a) also reported significantly lower PRA values in the pre-myopic population, when compared with the stable emmetropic group. During PRA testing, the introduction of minus lenses under binocular conditions stimulates an increase in blur-driven accommodation which is accompanied by increased accommodative convergence (AC). The increased output of AC necessitates negative fusional vergence in order to maintain clear and binocular single-vision (Rosenfield, 1997a). Accordingly, the lower PRA finding observed in pre-myopes could either reflect an inability to increase blur-driven accommodation or a failure to exert adequate negative fusional

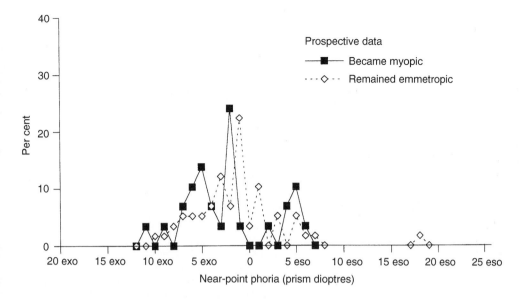

Figure 7.1 Frequency distribution of near phorias in the prospective study by Goss and Jackson (1996b). The solid squares and solid lines depict the frequency in the 'became myopic' group. The open diamonds and dashed lines indicate the frequency in the 'remained emmetropic' group. (From Goss and Jackson, 1996b)

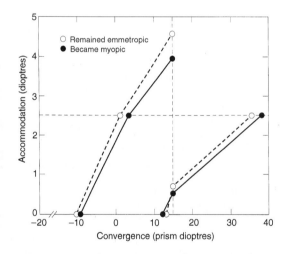

Figure 7.2 Zones of clear single binocular vision for the 'became myopic' group (solid circles) and the 'remained emmetropic' group (filled circles) in the Goss and Jackson (1996a) study. In order of increasing accommodative stimulus, the points on the left side of the zone are 4 m base-in break, 40 cm base-in blur, and positive relative accommodation. On the right side of the zone, the plotted points are the 4 m base-out blur, negative relative accommodation, and the 40 cm base-out blur. (From Goss and Jackson, 1996a)

vergence at near. Since the base-in and base-out fusional ranges were reported to be equivalent for

'became myopic' and 'remained emmetropic' groups (Goss and Jackson, 1996a; *see* section 7.2.3), this would suggest that the reduced PRA finding in myopic individuals may have been due to an inability to increase blur-driven accommodation (*see* section 5.5.4).

A way of assessing whether the PRA was lower in the 'became myopic' group because of negative fusional vergence would be to predict the PRA by extrapolating from the base-in blur values to the 2.5 MA vergence stimulus adopted for clinical testing at near. Adopting this procedure, Goss and Jackson (1996a) observed that the difference in the magnitude of extrapolated values between the two refractive groups was similar to the difference in measured PRA. This finding suggests that the lower PRA in the 'became myopic' group may be secondary to the shift in the zone of clear and single binocular vision to a more convergent position at near.

7.2.3   Vergence ranges

Goss and Jackson (1996a) reported that the mean values of base-in and base-out fusional vergence ranges were equivalent for the 'became myopic' and 'remained emmetropic' groups. However, the zone of clear single binocular vision (Hofstetter, 1983) appeared to be more convergent in the became myopic group (Figure 7.7). For example,

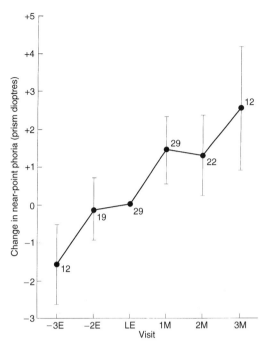

Figure 7.3 Change in near phoria with time in the 'became myopic' group in the Goss and Jackson (1996b) prospective study. The change in phoria plotted on the *y*-axis is the mean difference in the phorias at the visits indicated on the *x*-axis from the phorias taken at the last examination before the child became myopic. The error bars represent one standard error. The interval between visits was about 6 months. The numbers next to the plotted points indicate the number of subjects. −3E, third examination to the last before becoming myopic; −2E, second examination to the last before becoming myopic; LE, last examination before becoming myopic; 1M, first examination at which myopia was observed; 2M, second examination after onset of myopia; 3M, third examination after onset of myopia. (From Goss and Jackson, 1996b)

the midpoint of the near fusional vergence range was more convergent in the 'became myopic' group (mean = 5.8Δ, SEM = 0.6, *n* = 29) when compared with the 'remained emmetropic' group (mean = 3.2Δ, SEM = 0.5, *n* = 58), a difference which was significant.

7.2.4 Accommodative convergence and myopia

Several studies have reported differences in accommodative convergence (AC) between populations of myopes and non-myopes. For example, Manas (1955) selected random patient records for groups of myopes and hyperopes (each comprising

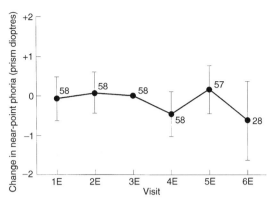

Figure 7.4 Change in near phoria with time in the 'remained emmetropic' group in the Goss and Jackson (1996b) prospective study. Plotted on the *y*-axis is the mean difference from the near phoria measurement at the third study examination. Error bars represent one standard error. The interval between study visits was approximately 6 months. The visit designations 1E, 2E, . . . , 6E on the *x*-axis indicate the first, second, . . . , sixth study visits, with the letter E indicating that emmetropia was found at each of the visits. The numbers next to the plotted points indicate the numbers of persons. (From Goss and Jackson, 1996b)

n = 100) and observed mean stimulus AC/A ratios of 5.1Δ/D (SEM = ±0.2) and 4.0Δ/D (SEM = ±0.2), respectively. This difference was statistically significant. Ogle and Martens (1957) used a fixation disparity procedure to determine the stimulus AC/A ratio in 104 subjects. While the mean AC/A ratio for the whole group was 3.4Δ/D, only 2 of the 15 myopes tested had AC/A ratios lower than the mean value, whereas the hyperopes tended to have lower than average AC/A ratios. Later, Rosenfield and Gilmartin (1987a,b) assessed accommodative convergence in populations of emmetropes, early- and late-onset myopes. In the first study (Rosenfield and Gilmartin, 1987a), the early onset myopes demonstrated significantly greater amounts of accommodative convergence and higher response AC/A ratios than the other two groups. In the second investigation (Rosenfield and Gilmartin, 1987b), both groups of myopes showed greater amounts of accommodative convergence than the emmetropes.

In a longitudinal investigation, Jiang (1995) monitored 44 college students over a 2–3-year period. Initially 33 of the subjects were emmetropic, with spherical equivalent refractive corrections ranging from −0.25 to +0.37 D in both eyes. Seven out of the 11 myopes had increases in myopia during the experimental period, and six of the

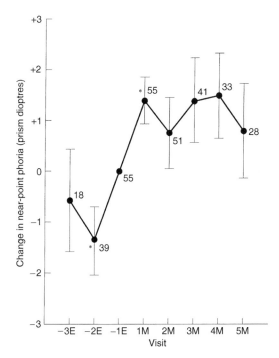

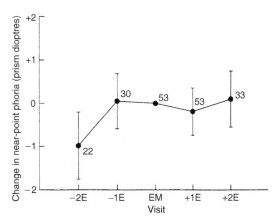

Figure 7.6 Change in near phoria with time in the 'remained emmetropic' group in the private practice data originally described by Goss (1991). The values on the y-axis are the mean differences in near phoria from the near phoria found at the examination used for match to the 'became myopic' group (EM). The −1E visit was the examination just before EM, and −2E was just before −1E. The +1E visit was the one just after EM, and +2E was just after +1E. The letter E indicates that emmetropia was found at each visit. The mean interval between visits was about 1 year. (From Goss and Jackson, 1996b)

Figure 7.5 Change in near phoria with time in the 'became myopic' group in the private practice data originally described by Goss (1991). Plotted on the y-axis is the mean difference in near phoria from that found at the last examination before the onset of myopia. The error bars are one standard error. The asterisks indicate means which are significantly different from zero. On the x-axis, −1E is the last exam before myopia onset; otherwise, the symbols on the x-axis are as in Figure 7.2. The average time between visits was about 1 year. The numbers next to the plotted points indicate the number of patients. (From Goss and Jackson, 1996b)

emmetropic subjects developed myopia during the study. The response AC/A ratio in the group of progressing myopes was significantly higher than for the stable emmetropes. Additionally, the response AC/A ratio was higher in those emmetropes who became myopic when compared with emmetropes who stayed emmetropic. These studies indicate that a higher AC/A ratio may be associated with myopic development.

7.2.5 Vergence adaptation in myopes

Flom and Takahashi (1962) observed a shift in heterophoria after the correction of myopia in previously uncorrected or undercorrected subjects. These observations were made on 28 consecutive myopic patients. The amount of undercorrection varied between 0.12 and 2.69 D, with 11 of the 28

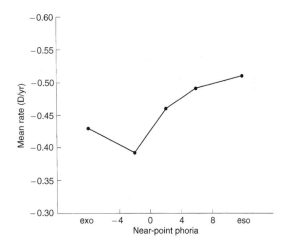

Figure 7.7 Mean rate of childhood myopia progression as a function of near-point phoria in single-vision lens wearers in the Roberts and Banford study (1963, 1967). (From Goss, 1994)

patients being undercorrected by at least 1.00 D. They observed that previously uncorrected or undercorrected myopes tended to be esophoric at near through their full refractive correction. However, if the full correction was worn for a week, then the mean near heterophoria shifted by 2Δ in the exophoric direction. Flom and Takahashi concluded that when myopia is uncorrected there is a reduction in the accommodative stimulus, and thus in the accommodative response, with an associated decrease in accommodative convergence. In order to maintain bifixation at the reading distance, accommodative convergence is supplemented by positive fusional convergence which may stimulate vergence adaptation, i.e., the onset of slow fusional vergence (Rosenfield, 1997b). The sustained output of slow fusional vergence may still be manifest when the new stronger lenses are first worn, thereby changing the heterophoria in the eso direction. However, with continued wearing of the full refractive correction, the output of slow fusional vergence will decline, with the heterophoria then shifting in the exo direction.

One might suggest that the heterophoria shifts associated with myopia onset in youth reported by Goss and Jackson (1986b) occurred for the same reason as the changes reported by Flom and Takahashi (1962), i.e., due to the sustained output of slow fusional vergence. However, the eso shift observed by Goss and Jackson took place before the onset of myopia, so it was not due to an uncorrected refractive error. Furthermore, even when myopia appeared in the subjects in the Goss and Jackson study, the amount of uncorrected myopia was much less than that reported by Flom and Takahashi. Additionally, the subjects used by Flom and Takahashi were older than those included in the Goss and Jackson (1996b) study. It may be that exo shifts in near heterophoria are less likely to occur until after childhood myopia progression has either slowed or stopped. Indeed, an analysis of private practice records suggests that an exo shift in near heterophoria may also be associated with the cessation of childhood myopia progression (Goss and Wolter, paper in preparation).

North *et al.* (1989) compared vergence adaptation in groups of emmetropes, early- and late-onset myopes. Prism adaptation was measured in response to 6Δ base-in and base-out prisms at both distance and near. No significant differences in the magnitude of vergence adaptation were observed between the three refractive groups for any of the four adapting conditions. Thus vergence adaptation may not differ as a function of refractive status in young adults.

7.3   Summary of results

The results of studies analysing vergence responses in myopia have been fairly consistent, and can be summarized as follows:

1 Near heterophorias are more convergent in children who become myopic when compared with those who remain emmetropic. Further, the onset of myopia in children is associated with either any esophoria, or high (>6Δ) amounts of exophoria at near.
2 Children with esophoria or high (>6Δ) amounts of exophoria at near tend to have higher rates of myopia progression.
3 A more convergent near fusional vergence range midpoint and lower PRA was reported in children who developed myopia.
4 Myopic adults had significantly higher stimulus and response AC/A ratios.
5 Equivalent magnitudes of vergence adaptation were observed for both myopic and emmetropic young adults.

7.4   Near heterophoria and the control of childhood myopia progression with bifocals

Bifocal lenses have often been used in an attempt to retard myopic progression in children (Goss, 1994). As described by Grosvenor in Chapter 9, this procedure has achieved somewhat mixed success. Variability in study outcomes could be due to a number of factors including proper alignment and adjustment of the spectacles, subject inclusion criteria, patient compliance, type and power of the reading additions, data analysis methodologies and patient characteristics.

Few investigations of myopia control with bifocals have examined their results as a function of patient characteristics. However, Roberts and Banford (1963, 1967) reported rates of childhood myopia progression as a function of near-point heterophoria and AC/A ratio for patients seen in their practice. For patients who had orthophoria or exophoria at near, the mean rates of myopia progression were 0.41 D/yr (*n* = 181) for single-vision lens wearers and 0.38 D/yr (*n* = 17) for bifocal lens wearers. The mean progression rates for patients with esophoria at near were 0.48 D/yr (*n* = 167) for single-vision lens wearers and 0.28 D/yr (*n* = 65) for bifocal lens wearers. Roberts and Banford did not provide standard deviations or report whether

Table 7.4 Mean rates of myopic progression (D/yr) as a function of stimulus AC/A ratios calculated from distance and near heterophorias

Stimulus AC/A ratio	Single-vision lens wearers		Bifocal lens wearers	
	n	Mean	*n*	Mean
0–4.9	84	0.44	8	0.41
5–6.9	138	0.42	29	0.34
7–8.9	81	0.46	27	0.34
≥9.0	39	0.59	19	0.31

From Roberts and Banford, 1963, 1967

any of these differences were statistically significant. The data from Roberts and Banford also indicated that the success of bifocal control of myopia varied with the stimulus AC/A ratio, as shown in Table 7.4. The reduction in progression rates with bifocals increased with the stimulus AC/A ratio. The difference between single-vision and bifocal lenses was only 0.03 D/yr for patients with stimulus AC/A ratios of up to 4.9Δ/D, but 0.28 D/yr for patients with AC/A ratios of 9.0Δ/D or greater.

Goss (1986) used data from three optometry practices to examine whether a relationship existed between near heterophoria and the ability of bifocals to retard myopic progression in children between 6 and 15 years of age. For those patients having near heterophorias greater than 6Δ exophoria, the mean progression rates for the single-vision and bifocal lens wearers were 0.47 D/yr (SEM = 0.11, *n* = 9) and 0.48 D/yr (SEM = 0.16, *n* = 3), respectively. The mean progression rates for patients whose near heterophorias lay between orthophoria and 6Δ eso for the single-vision and bifocal lens wearers were 0.43 D/yr (SEM = 0.04, *n* = 27) and 0.45 D/yr (SEM = 0.07, *n* = 18), respectively. These were obviously minimal and not statistically significant differences. However, for esophoric subjects, bifocal wearers had significantly lower progression rates (0.32 D/yr, SEM = 0.03, *n* = 35) than single-vision lens wearers (0.54 D/yr, SEM = 0.10, *n* = 10).

Subsequently, Goss and Grosvenor (1990) re-analysed data from the Houston myopia control study (Young *et al.*, 1985; Grosvenor *et al.*, 1987) in terms of the near heterophoria. The mean myopia progression rates for the few patients with near exophoria greater than 6Δ were 0.50 D/yr (SEM = 0.13, *n* = 5) in the single-vision lens wearers and 0.43 D/yr (SEM = 0.10, *n* = 6) in the bifocal wearers. For patients with near heterophorias in the

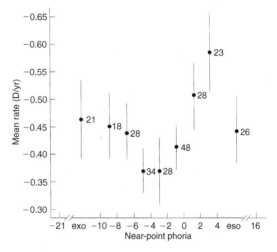

Figure 7.8 Mean rates of childhood myopia progression as a function of near-point phoria through habitual near-point prescription, from Goss (1990). The error bars indicate one standard error, and the numbers indicate the numbers of patients. (From Goss, 1994)

normal range of ortho to 6Δ exophoria, the mean rates of progression for the single-vision and bifocal lens wearers were 0.43 D/yr (SEM = 0.07, *n* = 20) and 0.42 D/yr (SEM = 0.04, *n* = 41), respectively. Patients with esophoria at near had mean rates of 0.51 D/yr (SEM = 0.09, *n* = 7) in the single-vision group and 0.31 D/yr (SEM = 0.08, *n* = 18) in the bifocal group. The difference in progression rates for esophores in the single-vision and bifocal groups was not statistically significant. However, the 0.2 D/yr difference is very similar to the findings of both Roberts and Banford (1963, 1967) and Goss (1986). The similarity of these findings is illustrated in Figure 7.8.

Jensen (1991) conducted a prospective study of myopia control with bifocals which included cover

Table 7.5 Mean rates of myopic progression (D/yr) as a function of near heterophoria

	Single-vision wearers	Bifocal wearers
Exophoria	0.56 ($n = 31$)	0.44 ($n = 28$)
Orthophoria	0.53 ($n = 10$)	0.45 ($n = 13$)
Esophoria	0.69 ($n = 8$)	0.62 ($n = 10$)

From Jensen, 1991.

test heterophorias with patient fixation at a working distance of 30 cm. The mean findings are shown in Table 7.5. The differences between the single-vision lens group and the bifocal group were not statistically significant. The reduction of myopia progression with bifocals in esophores observed by Jensen (1991) was less than that reported by Roberts and Banford (1963, 1967), Goss (1986) and Goss and Grosvenor (1990). In these three studies, heterophoria measurements were taken subjectively using the von Graefe method with a near-point test card at 40 cm. In contrast, Jensen (1991) measured objective heterophorias by the cover test with patient fixation at a working distance of 30 cm. Some of the subjects categorized by Jensen as orthophoric might have been found to be esophoric on the von Graefe test for a number of reasons. Firstly, the minimum deviation observable with the cover test may be only 2–4Δ (von Noorden, 1980), whereas the subjective von Graefe test can detect smaller magnitudes of deviation. Secondly, the accommodative response, and thus accommodative convergence, may be reduced during the cover test if the target does not constitute an adequate accommodative stimulus. Unfortunately, Jensen did not specify the cover test fixation target. Thirdly, a greater proximal vergence response may occur during the von Graefe test due to the physical presence of the phoropter (Schroeder *et al.*, 1996) when compared with a cover test performed in free space. The supposition that some of the orthophores in Jensen's study might have exhibited esophoria during von Graefe testing might also be supported by the observation that Jensen had the lowest percentage of subjects with esophoria of any of the aforementioned studies: Roberts and Banford, 232 out of 430 (54%); Goss, 45 out of 102 (44%); Goss and Grosvenor, 25 out of 97 (26%); Jensen, 25 out of 145 (17%).

Both Roberts and Banford (1963, 1967) and Goss (1986) observed that bifocals were more

effective in reducing the rate of myopic progression in patients demonstrating a larger lag of accommodation with the binocular dynamic cross-cylinder test (Rosenfield, 1997a). This test determines the near addition lens required to equalize the accommodative stimulus and response. Esophoria at near is often associated with higher lags of accommodation as the negative fusional vergence necessary to compensate for the esophoria will produce lower convergent accommodation and therefore a reduced aggregate accommodative response. Goss and Uyesugi (1995) supplemented the findings presented by Goss (1986) with data from three additional locations to examine whether both heterophoria and binocular cross-cylinder measurements were independently related to the bifocal control of myopia. The results from Goss and Uyesugi (1995) indicated that the reduced rate of progression found in esophoric patients was independent of the binocular dynamic cross-cylinder findings (*see* Table 7.6).

More recently, Fulk and Cyert (1996) conducted an 18-month prospective study to examine myopia progression in children with esophoria at near. They followed 28 esophoric subjects (14 wearing single-vision lenses and 14 wearing bifocals) for 18 months. The mean rates of myopia progression for the bifocal and single-vision lens wearers was 0.39 D/yr (SEM = 0.12) and 0.57 D/yr (SEM = 0.11), respectively. This difference was not statistically significant, possibly due to the limited sample size. However, the magnitude of the difference was very similar to that observed previously by Roberts and Banford (1963, 1967), Goss (1986) and Goss and Grosvenor (1990). The rates of myopia progression during the 6-monthly examination intervals adopted by Fulk and Cyert are provided in Table 7.7. The first and third periods ran from Autumn to Spring. The second 6-monthly interval went from Spring to Autumn, and thus included the school summer vacation. A repeated-measure analysis of variance indicated that the effect of time of year on progression rate was significant, and that this effect varied between the two treatment groups. These results suggest that the effect of bifocals on myopia control may take some time to become apparent because a difference in progression rates was not observed until the third 6-month period of the study. Additionally, myopia control with bifocals may be less effective during the time when school work is reduced, as suggested by the negligible difference in progression rates during the second 6-month period of the study.

Table 7.6 Mean rates of childhood myopia progression (D/yr) as a function of prescribed lens type, near heterophoria group, and binocular dynamic cross-cylinder (DCC) findings

	Single-vision wearers			Bifocal wearers			
Phoria, DCC	*n*	Mean	SD	*n*	Mean	SD	Statistical significance
ortho and exo, low DCC	72	0.42	0.26	18	0.34	0.19	*P* = 0.22
ortho and exo, high DCC	26	0.42	0.27	32	0.43	0.21	*P* = 0.90
eso, low DCC	26	0.65	0.38	23	0.26	0.21	*P* = 0.0001
eso, high DCC	25	0.54	0.24	35	0.34	0.17	*P* = 0.0004

High DCC group: median dynamic cross-cylinder finding greater than +1.00. Low DCC group: median dynamic cross-cylinder finding of +1.00 or less.
From Goss and Uyesugi, 1995.

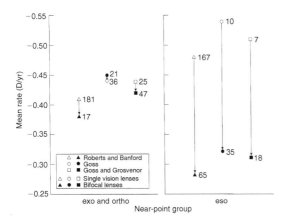

Figure 7.9 Mean rates of childhood myopia progression as a function of spectacle correction type and near-point phoria. The data are from the studies of Roberts and Banford (1963, 1967), Goss (1986) and Goss and Grosvenor (1990). Near-point phorias were measured by the von Graefe method through the subjective refraction. The numbers indicate numbers of patients. (From Goss, 1994)

7.4.1 Relation of distance heterophoria to bifocal control of childhood myopia progression

In another examination of the effectivity of bifocals for myopia control, Miles (1962) also published distance heterophoria measurements. Goss (1994) estimated progression rates from Miles' data. The progression rates for children who wore single-vision lenses were: distance exophoria, 0.35 D/yr (*n* = 18); distance orthophoria, 0.27 D/yr (*n* = 31); and distance esophoria, 0.51 D/yr (*n* = 54). Among bifocal wearers with orthophoria or exophoria (*n* = 18), the rates of myopia progression were 0.77 D/yr before bifocal wear and 0.51 D/yr

with bifocals. The rates for bifocal wearers with distance esophoria (*n* = 30) were 0.73 D/yr before bifocal wear and 0.38 D/yr with bifocals. However, bifocals were often prescribed for those individuals whose myopia was progressing fastest.

From these estimates of progression rate, it appears that myopia control with bifocals was somewhat more effective in patients with distance esophoria when compared with those having distance orthophoria or exophoria. However, Roberts and Banford (1963, 1967) observed little change in bifocal effectivity as a function of distance heterophorias. Their mean rates of progression are shown in Table 7.8. It appears that myopia progression rates are somewhat lower with bifocals in all distance heterophoria categories. However, no statistical analysis was included in this study.

These results suggest that bifocals may be more effective in controlling myopic progression in children with esophoria at near through their refractive corrections. However, no clear distinction can be made based on the distance heterophoria finding. The results of both the bifocal studies and differences in vergence responses will now be considered with respect to possible mechanisms for the aetiology of myopia.

7.5 How might ocular vergence be associated with the aetiology of myopia?

In attempting to link myopia development with ocular vergence, four possible theories appear to exist, namely:

1 The extraocular muscles act directly on the posterior segment of the globe, thereby stretching the sclera and producing an increase in the axial length.

Table 7.7 Mean rates of myopia progression (D/yr) assessed at 6-monthly intervals in esophoric subjects examined by Fulk and Cyert (1996)

	Single-vision ($n = 14$)		Bifocals ($n = 14$)	
	Mean	SEM	Mean	SEM
1st 6 months, during school year	0.68	0.12	0.61	0.15
2nd 6 months, including summer vacation	0.26	0.09	0.32	0.12
3rd 6 months, during school year	0.80	0.17	0.37	0.18

Table 7.8 Mean rates of myopia progression (D/yr) as a function of distance heterophoria in the Roberts and Banford study (1963, 1967)

	Single-vision		Bifocal	
Distance phoria	n	Mean	n	Mean
>2.5 exo	40	0.54	3	0.45
0.6–2.5 exo	109	0.43	14	0.37
0.5 exo–0.5 eso	141	0.42	35	0.28
0.6–2.5 eso	60	0.45	26	0.34
>2.5 eso	28	0.46	8	0.35

2 The extraocular muscles impose mechanical forces upon the sclera such that the intraocular pressure is increased, which in turn stretches the sclera and elongates the eye.

3 Esophoria is produced by excessive accommodative convergence, which might result from an increased accommodative response with either a normal or high accommodative convergence to accommodation (AC/A) ratio. The increased accommodative response is actually the primary cause for myopic development.

4 Esophoria necessitates negative fusional vergence under associated conditions. The latter may produce a decreased aggregate accommodative response due to the reduced output of convergent accommodation. The decreased accommodative response is actually the primary cause for myopic development.

The evidence for and against each of these hypotheses will be considered in turn: (1) and (2) will be grouped under mechanical effects of vergence and myopia (section 7.5.1), while hypotheses (3) and (4) will be combined under esophoria and myopia (section 7.5.2).

7.5.1 Mechanical effects of vergence and myopia development

As noted in section 7.1, many theories have been proposed whereby the mechanical forces exerted by the extraocular muscles on the sclera could produce axial elongation. However, more recently, Greene (1980, 1991) applied engineering principles to the mechanical forces which could possibly alter the structure of the eye. He noted that the physical changes producing axial elongation generally only occur in the posterior portion of the globe, with the myopic eye becoming a prolate spheroid with a thinner posterior sclera. Greene suggested that these changes may either be due to a mechanical weakness in the posterior region of the eye, or that the deforming forces are concentrated in that area. Alternatively, these two factors may occur concurrently.

Greene (1980) stated that extension of the posterior portion of the globe could result from the action of the oblique muscles, since these are the only extraocular muscles which insert into the posterior half of the globe. Furthermore, the entrance of the optic nerve through the sclera would augment the stress at the edge of the entrance hole, although the lamina cribrosa would provide some internal reinforcement. Greene stated that the peak force capabilities of the extraocular muscles were 250 times greater than that of the ciliary muscle, indicating that vergence must mechanically dominate accommodation. However, alternative calculations by Ong and Ciuffreda (1997) suggested that the mechanical stresses imposed by the contraction of a single oblique muscle may actually only be around 1 to 10 times that of the ciliary muscle (although these forces would be approximately doubled when both oblique muscles contracted simultaneously). Nevertheless, further experimental evidence is required to confirm that the forces generated by the extraocular muscles can indeed deform the human sclera. Curtin (1969) attempted to produce permanent deformation on strips of human and pig sclera by imposing loads equivalent to 100 mmHg, yet the specimens returned to their original length when the load was removed. Interestingly, Phillips and McBrien (1995) observed that elastic stretching of the sclera accounted for less than 20% of the observed difference in axial length between myopia and contralateral control eyes in tree shrews monocularly deprived of form vision. Other factors such as temperature and the cumulative effects of time may also have significant effects on rate of deformation (Maurice and Mushin, 1966; Tokoro, 1970; Mohan *et al.*, 1977; Greene and McMahon, 1979).

In addition to the extraocular muscles exerting forces directly on the sclera, they may also impose indirect stresses via changes in intraocular pressure (IOP). Coleman and Trokel (1969) observed sustained increases in IOP of 5–10 mmHg during levoversion. However, Moses *et al.* (1982) reported approximate increases for two eyes of only 1.8 and 1.9 mmHg, respectively on nasal gaze, although increases of 3.18 and 3.74 mmHg were observed on temporal gaze. Thus the changes in IOP during convergence appear to be relatively small, especially when compared with the effects of either lid blinking (increases of 5–10 mmHg) or lid squeezing (increases of approximately 80 mmHg) (Coleman and Trokel, 1969). Small changes in IOP may also result from downward head posture (Tokoro *et al.*, 1989) and accommodation (Young, 1975).

Accordingly, it is unclear whether these IOP changes would be sufficient to produce axial elongation. The pressure changes are relatively small, and presumably would have to be maintained for prolonged periods of time in order to affect the sclera, i.e., the most rigid tunic of the eye (Bell, 1978). Furthermore, a recent longitudinal study by Edwards and Brown (1996) demonstrated an increase in IOP *after* the development of myopia. However, they had a relatively small sample size (only 13 children developed myopia) and indeed stated that the findings need to be confirmed in a larger population. However, it is conceivable that the small increases in IOP could supplement those forces exerted directly upon the sclera during contraction of the extraocular muscles.

7.5.2 Near esophoria and myopia development

As previously described, several studies have demonstrated that myopia is frequently associated with esophoria at near (Goss, 1991; Goss and Jackson, 1996a, 1996b). While this oculomotor deviation could result from an increased accommodative response producing excess accommodative convergence, patients with near-point esophoria more typically exhibit a higher lag of accommodation, i.e., a reduced accommodative response (Scheiman and Wick, 1994).

An esophoric patient will need to exert negative fusional vergence under associated conditions in order to maintain binocular single vision. The lower fusional vergence response will be accompanied by reduced convergent accommodation. A decreased aggregate accommodative response may subsequently result from this decline in convergent accommodation and it is this increased lag of accommodation, with the resulting hyperopic defocus, which might ultimately stimulate axial elongation due to the retinal image being located beyond the retina (Goss and Zhai, 1994; Goss and Wickham, 1995; Hung *et al.*, 1995; Norton and Siegwart, 1995; Wallman and McFadden, 1995) (*see* Chapters 3 and 10).

This near esophoria may be produced by vergence adaptation stimulated during prolonged near fixation (Carter, 1963; Schor, 1983). For example, 30 minutes of critical viewing in a stereoscope produced a mean convergent shift in heterophoria of 1.3Δ (Stenhouse-Stewart, 1945). Additionally, Forrest (1960) reported eso shifts in heterophoria after 5 minutes of reading that was deemed to be 'visually stressful', while Ehrlich (1987) noted that 2 hours of a visual search task with binocular fixation at 20 cm resulted in a shift of the 33 cm heterophoria of 1.6Δ in the eso direction. Convergent shifts in heterophoria have also been observed during repeated measurement of dissociated heterophorias (Birnbaum, 1985; Christenson *et al.*, 1990). Therefore, one might speculate that the sequence of events leading to myopia development could be:

1 nearwork induces esophoria due to vergence adaptation;
2 esophoria leads to an increased lag of accommodation due to negative fusional vergence producing a lower output of convergent accommodation;
3 the higher lag of accommodation produces hyperopic defocus when viewing a near object leading ultimately to axial elongation.

Longitudinal studies of myopia development are required to verify the precise sequence of events over time.

References

Adams, D. W. and McBrien, N. A. (1992) Prevalence of myopia and myopic progression in a population of clinical microscopists. *Optom. Vis. Sci.* **69**, 467–473.

Bedrossian, R. H. (1979) The effect of atropine on myopia. *Ophthalmol.* **86**, 713–717.

Bell, G. R. (1978) A review of the sclera and its role in myopia. *J. Am. Optom. Assoc.* **49**, 1399–1403.

Birnbaum, M. H. (1979) Management of the low myopia pediatric patient. *J. Am. Optom. Assoc.* **50**, 1281–1289.

Birnbaum, M. H. (1981) Clinical management of myopia. *Am. J. Optom. Physiol. Opt.* **58**, 554–559.

Birnbaum, M. H. (1985) An esophoric shift associated with sustained fixation. *Am. J. Optom. Physiol. Opt.* **62**, 732–735.

Carter, D. B. (1963) Effects of prolonged wearing of prism. *Am. J. Optom. Arch. Am. Acad. Optom.* **40**, 265–273.

Christenson, G. N., Korth, C. J. and Marolivio, M. (1990) An investigation of the 'esophoric shift' and its relationship to parameters of the fixation disparity curve. *J. Behav. Optom.* **1**, 179–182.

Coleman, D. J. and Trokel, S. (1969) Direct-recorded intraocular pressure variations in a human subject. *Arch. Ophthalmol.* **82**, 637–640.

Curtin, B. J. (1969) Physiopathologic aspects of scleral stress-strain. *Trans. Am. Ophthalmol. Soc.* **67**, 417–461.

Curtin, B. J. (1985) *The Myopias: Basic Science and Clinical Management.* Harper & Row, pp. 104–106, 182–183, 293.

Donders, F. C. (1864) *On the Anomalies of Accommodation and Refraction of the Eye* (translated by W. D. Moore). The New Sydenham Society, p. 343.

Drobe, B. and de Saint-André, R. (1995) The premyopic syndrome. *Ophthal. Physiol. Opt.* **15**, 375–378.

Edwards, M. H. and Brown, B. (1996) IOP in myopic children: the relationship between increases in IOP and the development of myopia. *Ophthal. Physiol. Opt.* **16**, 243–246.

Ehrlich, D. L. (1987) Near vision stress: vergence adaptation and accommodative fatigue. *Ophthal. Physiol. Opt.* **7**, 353–357.

Flom, M. C. and Takahashi, E. (1962) The AC/A ratio and undercorrected myopia. *Am. J. Optom. Arch. Am. Acad. Optom.* **39**, 305–312.

Forrest, E. B. (1960) A modern philosophy of vision. IV. The story of stress. *Optom. Weekly* **51**, 332–334, 732–735.

Fulk, G. W. and Cyert, L. A. (1996) Can bifocals slow myopia progression? *J. Am. Optom. Assoc.* **67**, 749–754.

Goss, D. A. (1986) Effect of bifocal lenses on the rate of childhood myopia progression. *Am. J. Optom. Physiol. Opt.* **63**, 135–141.

Goss, D. A. (1990) Variables related to the rate of childhood myopia progression. *Optom. Vis. Sci.* **67**, 631–636.

Goss, D. A. (1991) Clinical accommodation and heterophoria findings preceding juvenile onset of myopia. *Optom. Vis. Sci.* **68**, 110–116.

Goss, D. A. (1994) Effect of spectacle correction on the progression of myopia in children–a literature review. *J. Am. Optom. Assoc.* **65**, 117–128.

Goss, D. A. (1995) *Ocular Accommodation, Convergence, and Fixation Disparity: A Manual of Clinical Analysis*, 2nd edn. Butterworth-Heinemann.

Goss, D. A. and Grosvenor, T. (1990) Rates of childhood myopia progression with bifocals as a function of nearpoint phoria: consistency of three studies. *Optom. Vis. Sci.* **67**, 637–640.

Goss, D. A. and Jackson, T. W. (1996a) Clinical findings before the onset of myopia in youth: 2. Zone of clear single binocular vision. *Optom. Vis. Sci.* **73**, 263–268.

Goss, D. A. and Jackson, T. W. (1996b) Clinical findings before the onset of myopia in youth: 3. Heterophoria. *Optom. Vis. Sci.* **73**, 269–278.

Goss, D. A. and Uyesugi, E. F. (1995) Effectiveness of bifocal control of childhood myopia progression as a function of near point phoria and binocular cross-cylinder. *J. Optom. Vis. Dev.* **26**, 12–17.

Goss, D. A. and Wickham, M. G. (1995) Retinal-image mediated ocular growth as a mechanism for juvenile onset myopia and for emmetropization–a literature review. *Doc. Ophthalmol.* **90**, 341–375.

Goss, D. A. and Zhai, H. (1994) Clinical and laboratory investigations of the relationship of accommodation and convergence function with refractive error–a literature review. *Doc. Ophthalmol.* **86**, 349–380.

Greene, P. R. (1980) Mechanical considerations in myopia: relative effects of accommodation, convergence, intraocular pressure, and the extraocular muscles. *Am. J. Optom. Physiol. Opt.* **57**, 902–914.

Greene, P. R. (1991) Mechanical considerations in myopia. In: *Refractive Anomalies. Research and Clinical Applications* (T. Grosvenor and M. C. Flom, eds). Butterworth-Heinemann, pp. 287–309.

Greene, P. R. and McMahon, T. A. (1979) Scleral creep vs. temperature and pressure in vitro. *Exp. Eye Res.* **29**, 527–537.

Grosvenor, T., Perrigin, D. M., Perrigin, J., *et al.* (1987) Houston myopia control study: a randomized clinical trial. Part II. Final report by the patient care team. *Am. J. Optom. Physiol. Opt.* **64**, 482–498.

Hofstetter, H. W. (1983) Graphical analysis. In: *Vergence Eye Movements: Basic and Clinical Aspects* (C. M. Schor and K. J. Ciuffreda, eds). Butterworths, pp. 439–464.

Hung, L.-F., Crawford, M. L. J. and Smith, E. L. (1995) Spectacle lenses alter eye growth and the refractive status of young monkeys. *Nature Med.* **1**, 761–765.

Jackson, E. (1931) Norms of refraction. *Trans. Sec. Ophthalmol. Am. Med. Assoc.* pp. 174–190.

Jensen, H. (1991) Myopia progression in young school children. A prospective study of myopia progression and the effect of a trial with bifocal lenses and beta blocker eye drops. *Acta Ophthalmol.* Suppl. 200 (Monograph).

Jiang, B.-C. (1995) Parameters of accommodative and vergence systems and the development of late-onset myopia. *Invest. Ophthalmol. Vis. Sci.* **36**, 1737–1742.

Linder, K. (1946) Ueber den einfluss von umwelt und vererbung auf die entstehung der schulmyopie. *Graefe's Arch. Ophthal.* **146**, 336–376 (cited by Curtin, 1985).

Luedde, W. H. (1932) Monocular cycloplegia for the control of myopia. *Am. J. Ophthalmol.* **15**, 603–609.

Manas, L. (1955) The inconstancy of the ACA ratio. *Am. J. Optom. Arch. Am. Acad. Optom.* **32**, 304–315.

Maurice, D. M. and Mushin, A. S. (1966) Production of myopia in rabbits by raised body-temperature and increased intra-ocular pressure. *Lancet* **ii**, 1160–1162.

Miles, P. W. (1962) A study of heterophoria and myopia in children some of whom wore bifocal lenses. *Am. J. Ophthalmol.* **54**, 111–114.

Mohan, M., Rao, V. A. and Dada, V. K. (1977) Experimental myopia in the rabbit. *Exp. Eye Res.* **25**, 33–38.

Morgan, M. W. (1944) Analysis of clinical data. *Am. J. Optom. Arch. Am. Acad. Optom.* **21**, 477–491.

Moses, R. A. (1981) Accommodation. In: *Adler's Physiology of the Eye. Clinical Application* (R. A. Moses, ed.). C. V. Mosby, pp. 304–325.

Moses, R. A., Lurie, P. and Wette, R. (1982) Horizontal gaze position effect on intraocular pressure. *Invest. Ophthalmol. Vis. Sci.* **22**, 551–553.

North, R. V., Sethi, B. and Owen, K. (1989) Adaptation ability of subjects with different refractive errors. *Optom. Vis. Sci.* **66**, 296–299.

Norton, T. T. and Siegwart, J. T. Jr (1995) Animal models of emmetropization: matching axial length to the focal plane. *J. Am. Optom. Assoc.* **66**, 405–414.

Ogle, K. N. and Martens, T. G. (1957) On the accommodative convergence and the proximal convergence. *Arch. Ophthalmol.* **57**, 702–715.

Ong, E. and Ciuffreda, K. J. (1997) *Accommodation, Nearwork and Myopia.* Optometric Extension Program, pp. 152–161.

Phillips, J. R. and McBrien, N. A. (1995) Form deprivation myopia: elastic properties of sclera. *Ophthal. Physiol. Opt.* **15**, 357–362.

Roberts, W. L. and Banford, R. D. (1963) Evaluation of bifocal correction technique in juvenile myopia. O. D. dissertation, Massachusetts College of Optometry.

Roberts, W. L. and Banford, R. D. (1967) Evaluation of bifocal correction technique in juvenile myopia. *Optom. Weekly* **58**(38), 25–28, 31; **58**(39), 21–30; **58**(40), 23–28; **58**(41), 27–34; **58**(43), 19–24, 26.

Rosenfield, M. (1997a) Accommodation. In: *The Ocular Examination. Measurement and Findings* (K. Zadnik, ed.). Saunders, pp. 87–121.

Rosenfield, M. (1997b) Tonic vergence and vergence adaptation. *Optom. Vis. Sci.* **74**, 303–328.

Rosenfield, M. and Gilmartin, B. (1987a) Effect of a near vision task on the response AC/A of a myopic population. *Ophthal. Physiol. Opt.* **7**, 225–233.

Rosenfield, M. and Gilmartin, B. (1987b) Beta-adrenergic receptor antagonism in myopia. *Ophthal. Physiol. Opt.* **7**, 359–364.

Scheiman, M. and Wick, B. (1994) *Clinical Management of Binocular Vision–Heterophoric, Accommodative, and Eye Movement Disorders.* Lippincott.

Schor, C. M. (1983) Fixation disparity and vergence adaptation. In: *Vergence Eye Movements: Basic and Clinical Aspects* (C. M. Schor and K. J. Ciuffreda, eds). Butterworths, pp. 465–516.

Schroeder, T. L., Rainey, B. B., Goss, D. A. and Grosvenor, T. P. (1996) Reliability of and comparisons among methods of measuring dissociated phoria. *Optom. Vis. Sci.* **73**, 389–397.

Snell, A. C. (1936) A statistical study of functional muscle tests in axial myopia. *Trans. Sect. Ophthalmol. Am. Med. Assoc.* 49–64.

Southall, J. P. C. (1924) *Helmholtz's Treatise on Physiological Optics* (translated from the 3rd German edn). Dover Publications, pp. 379–380.

Stansbury, F. C. (1948) Pathogenesis of myopia. A new classification. *Arch. Ophthalmol.* **39**, 273–299.

Stenhouse-Stewart, D. D. (1945) Some observations on a tendency to near-point esophoria, and possible contributory factors. *Br. J. Ophthalmol.* **29**, 37–42.

Stilling, J. (1891) Ueber das wachsthum der orbita und dessen beziehungen zur refraction. *Arch. Augenheilkd* **22**, 47–60 (cited by Stansbury, 1948).

Tokoro, T. (1970) Experimental myopia in rabbits. *Invest. Ophthalmol.* **9**, 926–934.

Tokoro, T., Funata, M. and Akazawa, Y. (1989) The role of intraocular pressure in elongation of the axial length. In: *Myopia: Pathogenesis, Prevention of Progression and Complications* (Proceedings of the International Symposium, Moscow). Health Ministry of the USSR, pp. 51–56.

Von Arlt (1876) *Ueber die Ursachen und die Entstehung der Kurzsichtigkeit.* Wilhelm Braumüller, Vienna (cited by Stansbury, 1948).

von Noorden, G. K. (1980) *Burian–von Noorden's Binocular Vision and Ocular Motility–Theory and Management of Strabismus*, 2nd edn. Mosby, p. 187.

Wallman, J. and McFadden, S. (1995) Monkey eyes grow into focus. *Nature Med.* **1**, 737–739.

Young, F. A. (1975) The development and control of myopia in human and subhuman primates. *Contacto* **19**, 16–31.

Young, F. A., Leary, G. A., Grosvenor, T. *et al.* (1985) Houston myopia control study: a randomized clinical trial. Part 1. Background and design of the study. *Am. J. Optom. Physiol. Opt.* **62**, 605–613.

Myopia and the near-point stress model

Martin H. Birnbaum

8.1 Introduction

The relative importance of nearwork, hereditary, dietary, metabolic and psychological factors in the aetiology of myopia is still uncertain. However, considerable evidence suggests that the extensive nearwork demands of our society play a significant role. Myopia increases in prevalence and degree throughout the school years (e.g. Donders, 1864; Cohn, 1867; Sorsby, 1932; Morgan, 1967; Goldschmidt, 1968). Additionally, myopes read more, perform more nearwork (Ochapovsky, 1935; Young *et al.*, 1954; Peckham *et al.*, 1977; Angle and Wissmann, 1978; Richler and Bear, 1980), and reach higher academic levels than non-myopes (Ochapovsky, 1935; Baldwin, 1967, 1981; Goldschmidt, 1968; Dunphy *et al.*, 1968; Grosvenor, 1971). It has been argued that individuals do not become myopic because they read more, but rather that they read more because they are myopic (Morgan, 1967; Borish, 1970). However, it appears that in most cases the greater interest in reading and higher academic achievement precede the onset of myopia (Peckham *et al.*, 1977; Birnbaum, 1993).

Several studies have documented the development of myopia in college students and young adults who are engaged in occupations that require extensive nearwork, or who have an imposed visually restricted environment with little opportunity for viewing distant targets. These refractive changes may occur at ages well beyond the point where they can easily be explained by normal ocular growth (Tscherning, 1883; Duke-Elder, 1930; Dunphy *et al.*, 1968; Goldschmidt, 1968;

Zadnik and Mutti, 1987; McBrien and Adams, 1997). Studies of myopia development in association with video display terminals (VDTs) has suggested that the risk of increased myopia onset or progression from VDTs is at least comparable with other forms of nearwork (Canadian Labour Congress, 1983; Bergqvist, 1984; Kajiwara, 1984; Yeow and Taylor, 1991; Cole *et al.*, 1996; Mutti and Zadnik, 1996). A restricted near visual environment has also been reported to induce myopia development in laboratory animals (Young, 1961; Rose *et al.*, 1974; Belkin *et al.*, 1977).

Although nearwork may be a significant contributing factor in the aetiology of myopia for many individuals, neither the conditions that must exist for nearwork to trigger myopia onset, nor the mechanisms by which such ametropia might develop have been established. Two major theories have been proposed: the use–abuse theory and the near-point stress theory, with the latter being attributed principally to Skeffington. These theories, although not mutually exclusive, differ significantly and present somewhat disparate implications for clinical management. Accordingly, an understanding of these differences is important to both the clinician and clinical researcher.

The use–abuse theory holds that myopia results from excessive use of the eyes for nearwork. This theory is often attributed to Cohn (1867), who ascribed myopia to repetitive overuse of accommodation. In more recent times, greater impetus for this theory has been derived from the work of Sato (1957) and Young (1971, 1977). Variations of this theory also emphasize the roles of convergence, gravity and posture as potential aetiological agents (Stilling, 1885; Jackson, 1931; Luedde, 1932; Greene, 1980, 1981).

In the Skeffington near-point stress model (Skeffington, 1928–74; Birnbaum 1985a, 1993), myopia is held to result not from the mechanical overuse of accommodation or convergence, as postulated in the use–abuse theory, but rather to adaptation processes which permit efficient visual function in the presence of a drive for convergence to localize closer than accommodation. Skeffington postulated that the nearwork tasks imposed by our culture generate a physiological stress response, the effect of which is to generate a discrepancy between the convergence and accommodative responses. Sympathetic nervous system activation has been proposed as a mechanism underlying this effector system mismatch (Birnbaum, 1984). In the Skeffington model, myopia is viewed not as an isolated condition, but rather as one of a variety of adaptive pathways which may be undertaken, frequently in concert, by the individual exposed to the near-vision demands of industrialized societies (Skeffington, 1928-74; Birnbaum, 1985b, 1993).

The purpose of this chapter is principally to review the Skeffington near-point stress theory, and to consider myopia from the perspective of this theory. Additional purposes are to overview the evidence for and against the notion of myopia as an adaptation to near-point stress, to discuss how the model relates to the clinical management of myopia and to consider the implications for further myopia research.

8.2   The Skeffington near-point stress model: an overview

A. M. Skeffington served as Director of Education for the Optometric Extension Program Foundation (OEPF), an organization dedicated to postgraduate education in functional and behavioural optometry. The near-point stress model promulgated by Skeffington, and the system of case analysis based upon this model, are closely associated with OEPF. In contrast with traditional models that attribute refractive and oculomotor deviations to hereditary factors, growth and random biological variation, Skeffington proposed that the near-point task demands of our society lead to a broad variety of refractive, binocular and behavioural problems.

Reading introduces a combination of demands which are not normally present in nature, namely to maintain vigilant attention, to sustain relative immobility, and to process information derived from symbols in an artificial, non-stereoscopic, two-dimensional plane. Skeffington postulated that demands for sustained concentration, immobilization and mental effort intrinsic to such nearwork provoke a stress response characterized by a drive for convergence to localize closer than accommodation. The resulting effector system mismatch causes visual inefficiency which may lead to discomfort, avoidance of nearwork, or adaptation within the visual system.

Efficient reading requires that vergence and accommodation localize at the plane of regard. Without some means of compensation, the model predicts that the drive for convergence to localize closer than accommodation leads to blurred vision or diplopia. In order to maintain clear, single binocular vision, individuals make appropriate changes in the pattern of relationships between vergence and accommodation. The model implies that effort directed towards resolution of the mismatch between vergence and accommodation impairs comprehension and decreases efficiency of task performance, with the concurrent risk of asthenopia and an inability to perform near tasks for sustained periods. Consequently, affected individuals may avoid close work, and demonstrate patterns of disinterest and withdrawal. Others adapt within the visual system, developing myopia and/or vergence and accommodative anomalies as means of resolving the discrepancy between the oculomotor responses.

In the Skeffington model, acquired myopia is viewed as adaptive in nature, regardless of whether it is early-onset and stabilizes in the teen years, early-onset with progression into adulthood, or adult-onset. The differences in age of onset are not held to reflect alternative aetiologies, but rather to result from differences in nearwork demand at varying ages.

The prescription of low powered plus near addition lenses is a key element of the Skeffington model. It is proposed that this strategy resolves the drive towards overconvergence, improves visual efficiency, minimizes interference with cognitive function, and eliminates the need for adaptation.

8.3   Physiology of overconvergence

Birnbaum (1984) suggested that the uncoupling of convergence and accommodation proposed by Skeffington is consistent with general stress physiology, arising from the activation of neuroendocrine mechanisms that accompany stress (Cannon,

1929; Selye, 1956). He considers that the requirement for attention and mental effort intrinsic to nearwork are not passive processes, but are mediated through enhanced sympathetic activation similar in nature to the emergency fight-or-flight stress response described by Cannon (1929), although lesser in degree. Heightened sympathetic arousal has been demonstrated during visual attention (Kahneman, 1973; Libby *et al.*, 1973; Pribram and McGuinness, 1975) and during enhanced cognitive processing (Hess and Polt, 1964; Beatty and Wagoner, 1978).

Randle *et al.* (1980) and Malmstrom *et al.* (1980) reported that heightened attention and mental effort produced a reduction in the magnitude of the accommodative response, and considered that this shift may be mediated via enhanced sympathetic innervation to the ciliary muscle. Birnbaum (1984) suggested that to maintain conjugate focus, a parasympathetically induced increase in the innervation to accommodation must occur to override the sympathetically driven negative shift that accompanies increased mental effort. Increased parasympathetic innervation to achieve conjugate focus generates increased accommodative convergence, and hence convergence tends to localize closer than accommodation. Birnbaum (1984) suggested that this effect may be exacerbated by sympathetic activation resulting from the high level of psychological stress that pervades contemporary society.

The essence of the near-point stress model is that the effect of technology on the modern visual environment may have created a task demand that is inconsistent with our physiology. Cognition and mental effort generate sympathetic reflexes which act to mobilize attention and preparation for action (Cannon, 1929; Malmo *et al.*, 1950; Kahneman, 1973; Mountcastle, 1974; Pribram and McGuiness, 1975). Pupillary dilatation (Hess and Polt, 1964; Nunnally *et al.*, 1967; Kahneman, 1973; Libby *et al.*, 1973) and a negative accommodative shift (Malmstrom *et al.*, 1980; Randle *et al.*, 1980; Gilmartin 1986) are the visual components of these autonomic reflexes, and they may be enhanced by sympathetic activation in response to psychological stress, as well as by the attentional intensity of a susceptible individual (Forrest, 1988).

8.4   Clinical evidence for overconvergence

The uncoupling of accommodation and convergence may not become manifest as esophoria at near, since some individuals adapt by creating an exophoric 'buffer'. Although Skeffington did not discuss how such an adaptation might take place, vergence adaptation would seem to be a likely mechanism. Forrest (1960, 1988) reported a shift towards increased esophoria when the near heterophoria is measured before and immediately after a brief period of reading. Ehrlich (1987) reports a similar esophoric shift following prolonged nearwork. Similar trends towards increased esophoria with sustained attention have been also noted by Stenhouse-Stewart (1945), Vaegan (1979) and Birnbaum (1985a).

Birnbaum (1985b) attributed this esophoric shift to increased sympathetic activation, with consequent increase in the accommodative effort required to maintain conjugate focus at the plane of regard. In contrast, Schor and Narayan (1982) suggested that the eso shift in associated phoria at near resulted from the interaction between accommodative convergence (AC) and convergent accommodation (CA). It is possible that each of these factors may contribute to overconvergence during daily nearwork, with the overconvergence tendency triggered by sympathetic activation being exacerbated by AC/CA interactions, so that overconvergence under associated conditions is greater than that reflected by the dissociated near heterophoria (Schor and Narayan, 1982). For example, the associated phoria frequently measures less exophoria or more esophoria than the dissociated heterophoria, whereas many patients who show exophoria at near under dissociated conditions demonstrate eso fixation disparity (Ogle *et al.*, 1967). Such findings are consistent with the existence of a drive towards overconvergence under associated binocular conditions that would be predicted by Skeffington's model.

8.5   Vergence and accommodative disorders

Skeffington (1928–74) indicated that individuals may utilize adaptive processes to alter the innervational pattern to accommodation and/or convergence, thereby avoiding blurred vision and diplopia. Depending upon the specific adaptive pattern, the clinical oculomotor findings may become altered in a variety of syndromes that are known as case types. In the Skeffington model, these changes are not viewed as the primary functional vision problem, but rather as products of adaptation secondary to near-point stress. The shifts in vergence and accommodation reflect the best oculomotor equilibrium that the individual is capable of achieving. A more optimal equilibrium may either be restored through the application of the appropriate near-point plus lenses, which resolve the effector system mismatch, or alternatively in the absence of any intervention, through the development of myopia (Skeffington, 1950–51).

In the presence of a drive for convergence to localize closer than accommodation, variations in the magnitude of the clinical vergence range measurements (Borish, 1970) will be observed. For example, during convergence testing, an increased blur point is frequently found, whereas during divergence testing, a reduced blur point is often recorded. According to Skeffington (1947, 1950–51), the characteristic response to the drive for convergence to localize closer is an attempt to prevent diplopia by blocking or inhibiting this drive. When this inhibition is conditioned and habituated, the convergence break and recovery become reduced. Thus, the usual response to near-point stress is for the convergence blur value to be increased while the break and recovery points are reduced. For divergence testing, decreased blur and increased break and recovery findings are typical. This syndrome is referred to as the B1 case (Skeffington, 1947, 1950–51).

In contrast, Skeffington (1947, 1950–51) indicated that some individuals demonstrate a reversed pattern in which the divergence break and recovery are reduced in comparison with the convergence findings. This pattern is referred to as the B2 case, and is viewed as a distortion of the B1 case that results from the intensified impact of near-point visual activity.

Birnbaum (1985a) viewed accommodative and convergence insufficiency as varieties of adaptation to near-point stress. Accommodative insufficiency, characterized by low positive relative accommodation (PRA) and/or low amplitude of accommodation, is traditionally considered to reflect a weakness of accommodation (Daum, 1983). Convergence insufficiency, characterized by high exophoria at near, low positive fusional convergence, and/or a receded near-point of convergence, is traditionally attributed to a weakness of convergence (Cooper and Duckman, 1978; Daum, 1984). In contrast to these explanations, Birnbaum suggested that these conditions constitute adaptive patterns in which accommodation and convergence are inhibited to reduce overconvergence during near-point visual activity. Thus these syndromes

are a product, rather than a determinant of near-point stress.

Birnbaum (1985a) suggested that accommodative insufficiency occurs as a result of inhibition of accommodative function, thereby creating a lag of accommodation to reduce associated overconvergence. The lag of accommodation reflects the reduced accommodative effort, and reduces overconvergence without inducing blur. A larger lag of accommodation that exceeds the magnitude of the depth-of-focus of the eye will produce blur, but may still be preferable to diplopia. The individual who inhibits accommodation responds poorly to clinical testing that requires localization of accommodation closer than convergence. Consequently, low PRA findings may be observed. When this inhibition becomes sufficiently conditioned, the response to blur induced following the introduction of minus lenses will be poor even during monocular testing, and hence the minus lens amplitude of accommodation (Rosenfield, 1997) will also be reduced (Birnbaum, 1993).

In the Skeffington model, near exophoria of between 4 and 6Δ is viewed as desirable and necessary to buffer overconvergence. Higher exophoria is not considered to represent increased demand upon fusional convergence, as in traditional models, but rather as an alteration in innervational pattern, i.e., an adaptive recalibration to permit alignment under associated conditions, despite the tendency to overconvergence induced by intense near-point activity. Although high exophoria may develop adaptively to buffer overconvergence, it is usually an inefficient adaptation. And often, high exophores either demonstrate asthenopia or tend to avoid reading (Skeffington, 1947, 1950–51; Forrest, 1960; Birnbaum, 1993).

8.6 Clinical vergence and accommodative findings in acquired myopia

In patients who develop myopia as an adaptation to near-point stress, esophoria at near is typically observed, especially in incipient myopia or in myopia that is progressing (Goss, 1990, 1991). Some patients adapt by developing high exophoria to buffer the overconvergence that exists under associated conditions. These individuals frequently inhibit fusional convergence so that the convergence ranges at near become low (Skeffington, 1928–74). In the Optometric Extension Program

(OEP) system of case analysis, this is typical of the B1 case. In traditional terms, such individuals are diagnosed as having convergence insufficiency. Under conditions that require increased concentration or attention, such as repeated heterophoria measures or cheiroscopic tracing, these individuals frequently demonstrate a significant shift towards esophoria.

Birnbaum (1985a, 1993) suggested that the inhibition of accommodation is another adaptive strategy to deal with a tendency towards overconvergence. Individuals who inhibit accommodation to reduce overconvergence adopt a strategy of accommodating as little as possible during near visual tasks. Such individuals will demonstrate a reduced amplitude of accommodation, as they inhibit their response to blur stimuli, an increased lag of accommodation and lower PRA. Additionally, these subjects will typically exhibit signs of overconvergence at near, i.e., either esophoria at near, or exophoria at near which becomes esophoria during conditions of high attentional demand.

Skeffington (1952) indicated that as adaptation proceeds, the relationships between the binocular findings change in consistent characteristic patterns referred to as stages of deterioration. Further, when stress is prolonged, the individual seeks to increase visual efficiency and rebuild visual skills to levels that permit satisfactory function. The individual frequently succeeds in reorganizing so that the clinical findings rebound from the lower measurements found immediately following the near-point stress, but still remain below the expected levels. This process, termed embedding, is characterized by an increase in vergence ranges, PRA reaching near-normal levels, and stabilization of myopia. Accordingly, reduced myopic progression is often accompanied by normal (or nearnormal) clinical oculomotor measurements (especially PRA).

8.7 Anisomyopia, astigmatism and asthenopia

Myopia may be viewed as an adaptation in which an individual sacrifices distance visual acuity in order to achieve heightened visual efficiency at near. Although the degree of refractive error is usually similar in the two eyes, anisomyopia may develop when the maintenance of distance acuity is more important to the individual than the retention of binocularity. In anisomyopia, the emmetropic or less myopic eye is used for distance vision, while the more myopic eye is used for near, thereby reducing the accommodative demand and associated overconvergence (Birnbaum, 1985a).

The onset of myopia is frequently preceded by the development of low degrees of against-the-rule astigmatism (Hirsch, 1964a). Birnbaum (1978) speculated that such astigmatism may serve as an early component of the adaptation process. In the presence of a lag of accommodation during nearwork, accommodation is localized beyond the plane of regard. Against-the-rule astigmatism produces vertically oriented blur circles, which permit resolution of the vertically oriented characters that predominate in the Roman alphabet, with reduced accommodation, and hence with reduced overconvergence. Against-the-rule astigmatism therefore reduces the accommodative demand, while still maintaining adequate resolution at near. However, when near-point stress persists or visual efficiency is unsatisfactory, myopia will still follow. Several studies have reported that the magnitude of against-the-rule astigmatism either reduced or disappeared following near-point plus lens prescription or vision therapy to treat accommodative dysfunction (Weisz, 1978; Garzia and Nicholson, 1988).

Individuals who demonstrate near-point stressinduced shifts in oculomotor findings frequently report significant near-point asthenopia. When nearwork causes discomfort and frustration, many individuals avoid it whenever possible. While they present with abnormal vergence and accommodative findings, these patients may remain asymptomatic, principally because they undertake little nearwork. Asymptomatic individuals may have adequate binocular function, avoid reading, or become myopic. When asthenopia is absent, many practitioners assume that existing functional visual problems do not require treatment. Recognition that such patients may be asymptomatic because they avoid nearwork or exhibit adaptation leads the clinician to consider treatment in such cases to eliminate the need for continued avoidance or further development of adaptive vision disorders (Birnbaum, 1993).

8.8 Early-onset versus adult-onset myopia

It is widely recognized that myopia progression frequently continues into the twenties and beyond, especially in college students and individuals whose occupations require intensive nearwork (Hayden, 1941; Hynes, 1956; Dunphy *et al.*, 1968; O'Neal and Connon, 1987; Zadnik and Mutti, 1987; McBrien and Adams, 1997). Early-onset and late-onset myopes demonstrate differences in tonic accommodation (Ebenholtz, 1985; Bullimore and Gilmartin, 1987a, 1987b; Gilmartin and Bullimore, 1987; McBrien and Millodot, 1987), amplitude of accommodation (McBrien and Millodot, 1986a), accommodative response (McBrien and Millodot, 1986b), and response AC/A ratio (Rosenfield and Gilmartin, 1987). These differences in accommodative function have led several authors to suggest that these conditions differ in aetiology, attributing early-onset myopia principally to genetic factors, and late-onset myopia to nearwork (Goldschmidt, 1968; McBrien and Millodot, 1987).

The Skeffington model holds that those individuals who are most intense in their nearwork application, and those with the greatest drive towards achievement in their nearwork, will develop myopia, unless a near-point plus lens is provided at the appropriate time, since this is the adaptation that best resolves the mismatch and permits optimal efficiency at near. If the demands for nearwork and the drive for achievement persist, and a near-point lens prescription is not provided, then the cycle of increased minus lens prescription and progressing myopia may continue well into adulthood (Skeffington, 1928–74; Birnbaum, 1979, 1985a, 1993).

Some of the previously reported differences in accommodative function between early- and late-onset myopes (Goldschmidt, 1968; Stevenson, 1984; McBrien and Millodot, 1987) may have reflected differences in stages of myopia progression rather than aetiological differences. For example, the early-onset myopes may have had stable myopia, whereas the late-onset myopes may still have been progressing. Therefore, reported differences in accommodative function may reflect differences between progressing and stable myopia, regardless of age of onset. Further studies are required to determine whether the pattern of accommodative function in late-onset myopia truly differs from that found in developing early-onset myopia.

8.9 Psychological factors, near-point stress and myopia

The relationship between myopia, psychological status and personality has long been a subject of controversy. Several studies have reported an association between myopia and personality. These correlations are generally weak, and findings are frequently inconsistent between investigations. Several authors have hypothesized that myopia is caused by psychological factors such as personality, introversion, anxiety, emotional attitude, desire to reduce contact with the external world and stress. This literature has been reviewed by Lanyon and Giddings (1974), Baldwin (1981), Curtin (1985) and Birnbaum (1993), although a detailed summary is beyond the scope of this chapter.

In modern society, psychological stress is pervasive and extreme, and the body becomes habituated to high levels of stress activation (Pelletier, 1977). Near-point activity thus takes place in a milieu of conditioned sympathetic activation arising from psychological stress. Furthermore, individuals frequently engage in nearwork under stressful conditions. Adults study or read under time pressure, and view material that either generates emotional stress or is related to business pressures and decision making. Additionally, they may also read for relaxation when emotionally stressed. Children also experience pressure to achieve, and may experience stress during reading instruction, especially when required to read aloud, during prolonged reading or when they are criticized or feel embarrassed as a result of reading errors. Each of these factors serves to heighten sympathetic activation when reading, and hence to exacerbate the near-point stress response (Birnbaum, 1993).

The frequently cited work of Bates (1920) postulated that myopia and other refractive errors are caused by anxiety, stress, emotional attitudes, effort and strain. He believed that this effort produced abnormal contraction of the extraocular muscles, thereby leading to distortion of the globe. Bates advocated treatment procedures such as blinking, breathing, relaxation and visualization exercises to aid in learning to see effortlessly, without strain or tension. Gottlieb (1982) suggested that axial elongation and myopia result from chronic isometric contraction of the extraocular muscles, occurring as part of a more generalized muscular activity associated with attention, mental processing and problem solving.

Van Alphen (1961,1990) proposed that stress, emotion, or extreme autonomic activity may interfere with the emmetropization mechanism. He indicated that sustained near-visual tasks related to studying and learning create different psychological effects when compared with near-point tasks of a less demanding nature. Birnbaum (1985a, 1993) suggested that myopia be viewed as a stress-induced illness. He indicated that myopia and other adaptations to near-point stress arise from the activation of autonomic reflexes that are linked with physiological arousal, but are incompatible with the extensive demands for sustained concentration intrinsic to our culture. These provoke a drive for convergence to localize closer than accommodation, which will interfere with efficient task performance.

8.10   Clinical procedures and the near-point stress model

8.10.1   Near-point plus lens prescription

The Skeffington model holds that appropriate plus near-vision addition lenses serve to resolve the near-point stress-induced effector system mismatch, and thereby eliminate the need for adaptation. The OEP system of case analysis is designed to determine the magnitude of near-addition required. However, near addition lenses will be only be effective in the early stages of the near-point visual problem, before deterioration and embedding occur. In those cases where additional plus power is no longer accepted, vision therapy is indicated to restore acceptance of the near addition (Skeffington, 1928–74; Manas, 1965; Birnbaum, 1993).

In the OEP approach, the plus lens addition to be prescribed is determined by case analysis of the clinical binocular findings. The goal is to prescribe a lens which will allow vergence and accommodation to localize in the same plane. For patients with B1 and B2 case typings, the maximum near-point addition prescribed is the fused dynamic cross-cylinder finding (Rosenfield, 1997), which will equalize the accommodative stimulus and response. However, the amount of prescribed plus power is reduced if it produces excessive exophoria, or reverses the habitual pattern of either the positive and negative relative vergence blur findings at near, or the NRA and PRA findings. Often the plus lens addition is that which balances the NRA and PRA findings, and in most cases the addition ranges from +0.50 to +1.25 D. This is in contrast with models that link myopia progression with an excessive accommodative response, and hence seek to prescribe high-add bifocals, typically

+1.50 to +3.00 D (Kelly *et al.*, 1975; Oakley and Young, 1975).

8.10.2   Visual hygiene and stress reduction

Birnbaum (1990, 1993) recommends the practitioner to counsel myopic patients regarding nearwork habits to minimize tension and reduce stress activation. Prolonged concentration may generate tension, physiological activation and near-point stress. Accordingly, patients are advised to read in a relaxed manner, adopt good posture with proper lighting, relax muscular tension, maintain general awareness of their surround, take short breaks and frequently look up at distant targets. Birnbaum (1990) suggested the use of deep breathing and progressive relaxation to reduce body tension. Additionally, individuals who work or read intensely should develop the habit of looking up frequently, at the end of each page, to shift focus to distance (Birnbaum, 1990). These suggestions are designed not only to reduce the accommodative demand, as in other nearwork theories of myopia development, but also to reduce the intensity of application, and hence to lower the near-point stress response that is held to underlie the development of myopia.

8.11   Implications for further research

Consistent with the Skeffington postulate of a drive towards overconvergence, incipient and progressing myopes usually demonstrate esophoria (or exophoria lower than the expected 4–6Δ) at near, and reduced PRA (Goss, 1990, 1991). Goss (1991) has demonstrated that these findings typically exist prior to the onset of myopia. Research comparing near phorias and PRA findings in incipient and progressing myopes with those of emmetropes and stable myopes will provide additional data as to the existence of a drive towards overconvergence in the various stages of myopia progression. The near-point stress model would predict that near esophoria will be greater and PRA lower in incipient and progressing myopes, when compared with emmetropes and stable myopes.

It has been suggested that early-onset and late-onset myopia arise from different causes, with genetic factors being of greatest import in early-onset and nearwork in late-onset myopia (Goldschmidt, 1968; McBrien and Millodot, 1987). In contrast, Birnbaum has suggested that early-onset and late-onset myopia each arise as adaptations to near-point stress, but that late-onset myopes are frequently individuals who avoid nearwork as much as possible in the early years, but eventually encounter a level of nearwork demand (e.g. VDT, graduate school, secretarial work) which is unavoidable, and hence adapt by becoming myopic. Research to compare near heterophoria and PRA in early- and late-onset myopes at comparable stages of myopia development (e.g. incipient, progressing, stable) would help to determine whether early- and late-onset myopia occur in response to the same processes, or are indeed discrete conditions having different origins.

Consistent with the Skeffington model, several studies (Roberts and Banford, 1967; Goss, 1986; Goss and Grosvenor, 1990) have indicated that bifocals are most effective in slowing myopia progression in myopes who demonstrate esophoria at near and low PRA. Typically these studies have used low plus addition bifocals consistent with an analysis of their clinical findings. Conversely, other studies which used higher near-addition bifocals prescribed independently of the clinical findings produced even more impressive findings (Kelly *et al.*, 1975; Oakley and Young, 1975). Further research is indicated to determine the optimal procedure to prescribe near addition lenses for myopia control. Such research must consider possible differences in near heterophoria as well as the various stages of myopia development.

Myopia is often preceded by the following: transient distance vision blur after nearwork, reduced near working distance, low PRA, esophoria or reduced exophoria at near, increased lag of accommodation and low against-the-rule astigmatism (Hirsch, 1964b; Birnbaum, 1978; Goss, 1991; Birnbaum, 1993). These patients have lost any low hyperopia that may have existed previously, and sometimes present as emmetropes. Many clinicians, including the author, believe that myopia development can be prevented when near addition lenses are prescribed and used before myopia becomes clinically manifest. Relatively little research has yet been performed to document the ability to prevent myopia development and controlled studies are strongly indicated.

References

Angle, J. and Wissmann, D. A. (1978) Age, reading, and myopia. *Am. J. Optom. Physiol. Opt.* **55**, 302–308.

Baldwin, W. (1967) Clinical research and procedures in refraction. In: *Synopsis of the Refractive State of the Eye: A Symposium* (M. J. Hirsch, ed.). Burgess, pp. 39–59.

Baldwin, W. R. (1981) A review of statistical studies of relations between myopia and ethnic, behavioral and psychological characteristics. *Am. J. Optom. Physiol. Opt.* **58**, 516–527.

Bates, W. (1920) *The Cure of Imperfect Sight by Treatment Without Glasses.* Central Fixation Publishers.

Beatty, J. and Wagoner, B. L. (1978) Pupillometric signs of brain activation vary with level of cognitive processing. *Science* **199**, 1216–1218.

Belkin, M., Yinin, N., Rose L. *et al.* (1977) Effect of visual environment on refractive error of cats. *Doc. Ophthalmol.* **42**, 433–437.

Bergqvist, U. O. (1984) Video display terminals and health: a technical and medical appraisal of the state of the art. *Scand. J. Work Environ. Hlth* **10**, 1–87.

Birnbaum, M. H. (1978) Functional relationship between myopia, accommodative stress, and against-the-rule astigmia: a hypothesis. *J. Am. Optom. Assoc.* **49**, 911–914.

Birnbaum, M. H. (1979) Management of the low myopia pediatric patient. *J. Am. Optom. Assoc.* **50**, 1281–1289.

Birnbaum, M. H. (1984) Nearpoint visual stress: a physiological model. *J. Am. Optom. Assoc.* **55**, 825–835.

Birnbaum, M. H. (1985a) Nearpoint visual stress: clinical implications. *J. Am. Optom. Assoc.* **56**, 480–490.

Birnbaum, M. H. (1985b) An esophoric shift associated with sustained fixation. *Am. J. Optom. Physiol. Opt.* **62**, 732–735.

Birnbaum, M. H. (1990) The use of stress reduction concepts and techniques in vision therapy. *J. Behav. Optom.* **1**, 3–7.

Birnbaum, M. H. (1993) *Optometric Management of Nearpoint Vision Disorders.* Butterworth-Heinemann.

Borish, I. M. (1970) *Clinical Refraction*, 3rd edn. Professional Press.

Bullimore, M. A. and Gilmartin, B. (1987a) Tonic accommodation, cognitive demand, and ciliary muscle innervation. *Am. J. Optom. Physiol. Opt.* **64**, 45–50.

Bullimore, M. A. and Gilmartin, B. (1987b) Aspects of tonic accommodation in late-onset myopia. *Am. J. Optom. Physiol. Opt.* **64**, 499–503.

Canadian Labour Congress, Labour Education and Studies Centre (1983) *Toward a More Humanized Technology; Exploring the Impact of Video Display Terminals on the Health and Working Conditions of the Canadian Work-place: Problems and Prospects.* Institute for Research on Public Policy (Montreal).

Cannon, W. B. (1929) *Bodily Changes in Pain, Hunger, Fear and Rage: An Account of Recent Researches into the Function of Emotional Excitement.* Appleton.

Cohn, H. L. (1867) *Untesuchen der augen von 10060 schulkendern nebst vorschlagen zur verbesserung der den nachtheiligen schuleinrichtungen. Eine atiologische studies.* F. Fleischer.

Cole, B., Maddocks, J. D. and Sharpe, K. (1996) Effect of VDUs on the eyes: report of a 6-year epidemiological study. *Optom. Vis. Sci.* **73**, 512–528.

Cooper, J. and Duckman, R. (1978) Convergence insufficiency: incidence, diagnosis and treatment. *J. Am. Optom. Assoc.* **49**, 673–680.

Curtin, B. J. (1985) *The Myopias. Basic Science and Clinical Management.* Harper & Row.

Daum, K. M. (1983) Accommodative insufficiency. *Am. J. Optom. Physiol. Opt.* **60**, 352–359.

Daum, K. M. (1984) Convergence insufficiency. *Am. J. Optom. Physiol. Opt.* **61**, 16–22.

Donders, F. C. (1864) *On the Anomalies of Accommodation and Refraction of the Eye: With a Preliminary Essay on Physiological Dioptrics.* New Syndenham Society. (Reprinted 1952, Hatton Press.)

Duke-Elder, W. S. (1930) An investigation of the effect upon the eyes of occupations involving close work. *Br. J. Ophthalmol.* **14**, 609–620.

Dunphy, E. B., Stoll, M. R. and King, S. H. (1968) Myopia among American male graduate students. *Am. J. Ophthalmol.* **65**, 518–521.

Ebenholtz, S. M. (1985) Accommodative hysteresis: relation to resting focus. *Am. J. Optom. Physiol. Opt.* **62**, 755–762.

Ehrlich, D. L. (1987) Near vision stress: vergence adaptation and accommodative fatigue. *Ophthal. Physiol. Opt.* **7**, 353–357.

Forrest, E. B. (1960) A modern philosophy of vision. IV. The story of stress. *Optom. Weekly* **51**, 332–334; 635–636.

Forrest, E. B. (1988) *Stress and Vision.* Optometric Extension Program Foundation.

Garzia, R. P. and Nicholson, S. B. (1988) Clinical aspects of accommodative influences on astigmatism. *J. Am. Optom. Assoc.* **59**, 942–945.

Gilmartin, B. (1986) A review of the role of sympathetic innervation of the ciliary muscle in ocular accommodation. *Ophthal. Physiol. Opt.* **6**, 23–37.

Gilmartin, B. and Bullimore, M. A. (1987) Sustained near-vision augments inhibitory sympathetic innervation of the ciliary muscle. *Clin. Vis. Sci.* **1**, 197–208.

Goldschmidt, E. (1968) On the aetiology of myopia. *Acta Ophthalmol.* Suppl. 98, 1–171.

Goss, D. A. (1990) Variables related to the rate of childhood myopia progression. *Optom. Vis. Sci.* **67**, 631–636.

Goss, D. A. (1991) Clinical accommodation and heterophoria findings preceding juvenile onset of myopia. *Optom. Vis. Sci.* **68**, 110–116.

Goss, D. A. (1986) Effect of bifocal lenses on the rate of childhood myopia progression. *Am. J. Optom. Physiol. Opt.* **63**, 637–640.

Goss, D. A. and Grosvenor, T. (1990) Rates of childhood myopia progression with bifocals as a function of

nearpoint heterophoria: consistency of three studies. *Optom. Vis. Sci.* **67**, 637–640.

Gottlieb, R. L. (1982) Neuropsychology of myopia. *J. Optom. Vis. Dev.* **13**, 3–27.

Greene, P. R. (1980) Mechanical considerations in myopia: relative effects of accommodation, convergence, intraocular pressure and the extraocular muscles. *Am. J. Optom. Physiol. Opt.* **57**, 902–914.

Greene, P. R. (1981) Myopia and the extraocular muscles. *Doc. Ophthalmol. Proc. Ser.* **28**, 163–169.

Grosvenor, T. (1971) The neglected hyperope. *Am. J. Optom.* **48**, 376–382.

Hayden, R. (1941) Development and prevention of myopia at the United States Naval Academy. *Arch. Ophthalmol.* **25**, 539–547.

Hess, E. H. and Polt, J. M. (1964) Pupil size in relation to mental activity during simple problem-solving. *Science* **143**, 1190–1192.

Hirsch, M. J. (1964a) Predictability of refraction at age 14 on the basis of testing at age 6. Interim report from the Ojai longitudinal study of refraction. *Am. J. Optom. Arch. Am. Acad. Optom.* **41**, 567–573.

Hirsch, M. (1964b) The longitudinal study in refraction. *Am. J. Optom.* **41**, 137–141.

Hynes, E. A. (1956) Refractive changes in normal young men. *Arch. Ophthalmol.* **56**, 761–767.

Jackson, E. (1931) Norms of refraction. *Trans. Sec. Ophthalmol. Am. Med. Assoc.* pp. 174–190.

Kahneman, D. (1973) *Attention and Effort.* Prentice-Hall, pp. 1–49.

Kajiwara, S. (1984) *Work and Health in VDT Workplaces.* In-service Training Institute for Safety and Health of Labour (Osaka), pp. 5–82.

Karlsson, J. L. (1973) Genetic relationship between giftedness and myopia. *Hereditas* **73**, 85–88.

Kelly, T. S. B., Chatfield, C. and Tustin, G. (1975) Clinical assessment of the arrest of myopia. *Br. J. Ophthalmol.* **59**, 529–538.

Lanyon, R. I. and Giddings, J. W. (1974) Psychological approaches to myopia: a review. *Am. J. Optom. Physiol. Opt.* **51**, 271–281.

Libby, W. L., Lacey, B. C. and Lacey, J. I. (1973) Pupillary and cardiac activity during visual attention. *Psychophysiology* **10**, 270–294.

Luedde, W. H. (1932) Monocular cycloplegia for the control of myopia. *Am. J. Ophthalmol.* **15**, 603–609.

Malmo, R. B., Shagass, C. and Davis, H. (1950) Symptoms specificity and bodily reactions during psychiatric interview. *Psychosom. Med.* **12**, 362–376.

Malmstrom, F. W., Randle, R. J., Bendix, J. S. *et al.* (1980) The visual accommodation response during concurrent mental activity. *Percept. Psychophysiol.* **28**, 440–448.

Manas, L. (1965) *Visual Analysis.* Professional Press.

McBrien, N. A. and Adams, D. W. (1997) A longitudinal investigation of adult-onset and adult-progression of myopia in an occupational group. *Invest. Ophthalmol. Vis. Sci.* **38**, 321–333.

McBrien, N. A. and Millodot, M. (1986a) Amplitude of accommodation and refractive error. *Invest. Ophthalmol. Vis. Sci.* **27**, 1187–1190.

McBrien, N. A. and Millodot, M. (1986b) The effect of refractive error on the accommodative response gradient. *Ophthal. Physiol. Opt.* **6**, 145–149.

McBrien, N.A. and Millodot, M. (1987) The relationship between tonic accommodation and refractive error. *Invest. Ophthalmol. Vis. Sci.* **28**, 997–1004.

Morgan, M. W. (1967) A review of the major theories of the genesis of refractive state. In: *Synopsis of the Refractive State of the Eye: A Symposium* (M. J. Hirsch, ed.). Burgess, pp. 8–12.

Mountcastle, V. B. (1974) *Medical Physiology.* Vol. 1, 13th edn. Mosby, pp. 788–792.

Mutti, D. O. and Zadnik, K. (1996) Is computer use a risk factor for myopia? *J. Am. Optom. Assoc.* **67**, 521–530.

Nunnally, J. C., Knott, P. D., Duchowski, A. *et al.* (1967) Pupillary response as a general measure of activation. *Percept. Psychophysiol.* **2**, 149–155.

Oakley, K. H. and Young, F. A. (1975) Bifocal control of myopia. *Am. J. Optom. Physiol. Opt.* **52**, 758–764.

Ochapovsky, S. (1935) Genesis of the refraction of the human eye. *Arch. Ophthalmol.* **14**, 412–420.

Ogle, K. N., Martens, T. G. and Dyer, J. A. (1967) *Oculomotor Imbalance in Binocular Vision and Fixation Disparity.* Lea & Febiger, pp. 108–113, 175–184, 195–230.

O'Neal, M. R. and Connon, T. R. (1987) Refractive error changes at the United States Air Force Academy Class of 1985. *Am. J. Optom. Physiol. Opt.* **64**, 344–354.

Parssinen, T. O. (1987) Relation between refraction, education, occupation and age among 26- and 46-year-old Finns. *Am. J. Optom. Physiol. Opt.* **64**, 136–143.

Peckham, C. S., Gardiner, P. A. and Goldstein, H. (1977) Acquired myopia in eleven year old children. *Br. Med. J.* **1**, 542–544.

Pelletier, K. R. (1977) *Mind as Healer, Mind as Slayer: A Holistic Approach to Preventing Stress Disorder.* Delacort.

Pribram, K. and McGuinness, D. (1975) Arousal, activation and effort in the control of attention. *Psychol. Rev.* **82**, 116–149.

Randle, R., Roscoe, S. N. and Petitt, J. C. (1980) Effects of magnification and visual accommodation on aim-point estimation in simulated landings with real and virtual image displays. NASA Technical Paper 1635. National Aeronautics and Space Administration, Ames Research Center.

Richler, A. and Bear, J. C. (1980) Refraction, nearwork and education: a population study in Newfoundland. *Acta Ophthalmol.* **58**, 468–477.

Roberts, W. and Banford, R. (1967) Evaluation of bifocal correction techniques in juvenile myopia. *Optom. Weekly* **58**, 25–31, 21 Sept.; **58**, 21–30, 28 Sept; **58**, 23–28, 5 Oct.; **58**, 27–34, 12 Oct.; **58**, 19–26, 26 Oct.

Rose, L., Yinon, U. and Bulkin, M. (1974) Myopia induced in cats deprived of distance vision during development. *Vision Res.* **14**, 1029–1032.

Rosenfield, M. (1997) Accommodation. In: *The Ocular Examination. Measurement and Findings* (K. Zadnik, ed.). Saunders, pp. 87–121.

Rosenfield, M. and Gilmartin, B. (1987) Effect of a near-vision task on the response AC/A of a myopic population. *Ophthal. Physiol. Opt.* **7**, 225–233.

Sato, T. (1957) *The Causes and Prevention of Acquired Myopia.* Kanehata Shuppan.

Schor, C. M. and Narayan, V. (1982) Graphical analysis of prism adaptation, convergence accommodation and accommodative convergence. *Am. J. Optom. Physiol. Opt.* **59**, 774–784.

Selye, H. (1956) *The Stress of Life.* McGraw-Hill.

Skeffington, A. M. (1928–74) Optometric Extension Program Continuing Education Courses. Optometric Extension Program Foundation.

Skeffington, A. M. (1947) *Near Point Optometry.* Optometric Extension Program Continuing Education Courses. Optometric Extension Program Foundation, vol. 2, no. 4–12, Jan.–Sept.

Skeffington, A. M. (1950–51) *Near Point Optometry.* Optometric Extension Program Continuing Education Courses. Optometric Extension Program Foundation, Oct. 1950–Sept. 1951.

Skeffington, A. M. (1952) Myopia. In: *Practical Applied Optometry.* Optometric Extension Program Continuing Education Courses. Optometric Extension Program Foundation, vol. 24, no. 12, Dec., pp. 109–120.

Slataper, F. (1950) Age norms of refraction and vision. *Arch. Ophthalmol.* **43**, 466–481.

Sorsby, A. (1932) School myopia. *Br. J. Ophthalmol.* **16**, 217–224.

Stenhouse-Stewart, D. D. (1945) Some observations on a tendency to nearpoint esophoria, and possible contributory factors. *Br. J. Ophthalmol.* **29**, 37–42.

Stevenson, R. W. W. (1984) The development of myopia and its relationship with intra-ocular pressure. In: *Transactions of the First International Congress, 'The Frontiers of Optometry'* vol. 2. (W. N. Charman, ed.). British College of Ophthalmic Opticians, pp. 43–50.

Stilling, J. (1885) Eine studie zur kurzsichtigkeit frage. *Arch. Augenheilkd* **15**, 133.

Tscherning, M. (1883) Studien uber die aetiology der myopie. *Graefe's Arch. Ophthalmol.* **29**, 201–272.

Vaegan, J. L. (1979) Convergence and divergence show large and sustained improvement after short isometric exercise. *Am. J. Optom. Physiol. Opt.* **56**, 23–33.

Van Alphen, G. W. H. M. (1961) On emmetropia and ametropia. *Ophthalmologica* (Suppl), pp. 1–92.

Van Alphen, G. W. H. M. (1990) Emmetropization in the primate eye. In: *Myopia and the Control of Eye*

Growth. Ciba Foundation Symposium No. 155. Wiley, pp. 115–125.

Weisz, C. L. (1978) Induced against-the-rule astigmatism in accommodative disorders. *J. Am. Optom. Assoc.* **49**, 335–336.

Yeow, P. T. and Taylor, S. P. (1991) Effects of long-term visual display terminal usage on visual function. *Optom. Vis. Sci.* **68**, 930–941.

Young, F. A. (1961) The development and retention of myopia by monkeys. *Am. J. Optom. Arch. Am. Acad. Optom.* **38**, 545–555.

Young, F. A. (1971) The development of myopia. *Contacto* **15**, 36–42.

Young, F. A. (1977) The nature and control of myopia. *J. Am. Optom. Assoc.* **48**, 451–457.

Young, F. A., Beattie, R., Newby, F. J. *et al.* (1954) The Pullman study: a visual survey of Pullman school children. *Am. J. Optom.* **31**, 111–121; **31**, 192–203.

Zadnik, K. and Mutti, D. O. (1987) Refractive error changes in law students. *Am. J. Optom. Physiol. Opt.* **64**, 558–561.

9

Myopia control procedures

Theodore Grosvenor

The methods of myopia control presented in this chapter are those designed to control refractive development by functional means such as reducing the demands upon either accommodation or convergence, or by controlling intraocular pressure. Other methods of myopia control including the wearing of conventionally fitted rigid contact lenses, orthokeratology and keratorefractive surgery, which control myopia by reshaping the cornea, will not be discussed here. Although contact lenses also alter the stimuli to accommodation and convergence when compared with spectacles, due to their closer vertex distance and the absence of induced prismatic effects, these differences are relatively small and are not usually considered to be important in myopia control.

Functional methods of myopia control which will be considered here are:

1 vision therapy;
2 biofeedback training;
3 distance undercorrection;
4 distance overcorrection;
5 bifocals;
6 base-in prisms;
7 various pharmaceutical agents.

9.1 Vision therapy

Vision therapy attempts to reduce the pre-existing amount of myopia by training the patient to improve the accuracy of his or her accommodative response. Unfortunately, in most published reports where these techniques have been studied, the quantified test variable was not refractive error but unaided visual acuity. The literature, beginning in the 1940s, contains many limited reports which cite only one or two cases. Two studies which used larger population samples will also be discussed, namely the Baltimore Myopia Project (Ewalt, 1946) and that of Lin and Ko (1988).

9.1.1 Case reports

During the Second World War, many myopes requested vision training in order to meet the entry criteria for one of the armed services. Typical of the case reports during this period were those of Bannon (1946) and Walton (1946). Bannon (1946) cited a case in which uncorrected visual acuity improved from 6/12 to 6/6 following vision training, although no decrease in myopia was noted. Walton (1946) reported that the uncorrected visual acuity of two naval officers improved following stereoscopic card exercises and rotations with a Myoculator (an instrument which randomly projected images in varying positions of gaze to 'exercise' the extraocular muscles). Observed improvements in unaided visual acuity were two lines of letters for each eye of the first patient (right eye from 6/12 to 6/6, and left eye from 6/9 to 6/4.5); and for the second patient, no change in acuity for the right eye and a change from 6/60 to 6/12 for the left eye.

9.1.2 The Baltimore Myopia Control Project

This large-scale prospective study recruited 111 subjects. The vision training procedures were conducted by optometrists and technicians, while the results were evaluated by ophthalmologists. Subjects were between 9 and 32 years of age, with refractive corrections ranging from −0.50 to −9.00 D. A mean of 25 training sessions were undertaken over a 13-week period. Both before and after the therapy, visual acuity and cycloplegic refraction were assessed. While the training techniques were not described in the literature, it was understood by those familiar with the project that the procedures used were those recommended by the Optometric Extension Program, which were designed to train patients to relax their accommodation. These procedures included accommodative facility training, known at that time as 'accommodative rock', and exercises with 'distance motivators' such as Plateau's Spiral. This test consisted of a black spiral on a white background. When the subject views the spiral as it is rotated, it appears to move inward toward the subject, but after the rotation is stopped the subject is instructed to view a distant object, which rapidly moves outward, thereby relaxing accommodation. These procedures were described mainly in literature published by the Optometric Extension Program which, unfortunately, is not widely available.

In the official optometric report, Ewalt (1946) commented that the subjects, being unselected, were completely unmotivated. He pointed out that many of the subjects were not desirable candidates for vision training on the basis of standards established in most private practices. For example, some of the subjects were in poor health, and it is not likely that a practitioner would have accepted for training a patient over the age of 30 years or one who had as much as 9 D of myopia. Ewalt published scatterplots showing the initial and final unaided monocular and binocular visual acuities. Visual inspection of the graphs indicates an average improvement of about two lines of letters. For example, a subject with an initial uncorrected acuity of 6/120 had a final acuity of 6/30, while a subject with initial uncorrected acuity of 6/12 had a final acuity of 6/7.5. Ewalt concluded that there was a significant change in visual acuity in many subjects. However, he provided no data showing changes in the degree of myopia. When the sole criterion adopted is an improvement in uncorrected visual acuity, it is possible that the subject has simply learned to interpret a blurred retinal image (Bannon, 1946).

In the official ophthalmological report, Woods (1945) evaluated the results of the project in terms of changes in percentage acuity (decimal acuity expressed as a percentage). For 103 subjects on whom data were available, he divided these individuals into four categories:

1 a group of 30 subjects showing a consistent improvement in acuity, with an increase (average of both eyes) of 27 percentage points;
2 a group of 31 subjects showing an average increase of 14.7 percentage points;
3 a group of 32 subjects showing practically no change in acuity;
4 a group of 10 subjects showing an average decrease in acuity of 10.8 percentage points.

Woods concluded that these changes in acuity lay within the limits of measurement error of visual acuity testing, although he failed to define these 'limits of error'. Therefore, one might conclude that for those subjects exhibiting the greatest improvement in visual acuity, these findings could be explained by enhanced blur interpretation.

In addition, Woods (1945) published a table of pre- and post-training cycloplegic retinoscopy findings for 67 subjects. If these results are analysed on the basis that clinical refraction can be considered to be accurate within a range of ±0.25 to ±0.50 D (Bannon, 1977; Perrigin *et al.*, 1982), then one may conclude that there was no significant change in the refractive error for 57 subjects, an increase in myopia for 6 subjects and a decrease in myopia for 5 subjects. Unfortunately, Woods (1945) did not provide any information concerning the time interval between the pre- and post-training examinations. If the elapsed period of time was approximately 6 months or greater, then one might expect a measurable increase in myopia to occur even if no training or other intervention had taken place.

Betts (1947) published a critique of the Baltimore study, noting that:

1 subject selection was performed by ophthalmologists who were not experienced in vision training;
2 subjects were accepted for training regardless of their prognosis;
3 no objective data were available concerning the reliability of the refractive determinations;
4 the number of training sessions varied from a minimum of only five sessions for two subjects to a maximum of 37 sessions for one subject;
5 there was no control group.

Additionally, Hackman (1947) presented further statistical analysis of the Baltimore data and concluded that there were no appreciable changes in refractive error as determined by retinoscopy, although there was a statistically significant difference ($P<0.01$) between pre- and post-training visual acuity for the whole group.

Shepard (1946) summarized the reports of Ewalt (1946) and Woods (1945) and analysed the changes in visual acuity for 71 subjects from the Baltimore study who were examined before the training, at the conclusion of the training and about 5 months later. He converted the visual acuity findings to decimal equivalents, and reported mean (± 1 standard deviation) decimal acuity before and after 5 months of training of 0.16 (± 0.15) and 0.37 (± 0.36), respectively. This change is equivalent to an improvement from 6/37 to 6/16. Shepard suggested that any subject showing a gain in decimal acuity of 0.10 or greater after 5 months had achieved a significant improvement in visual acuity. He concluded that 90% of the myopes may experience significantly improved acuity after training, but because there was no actual reduction in myopia, 'it has been shown that optometry cannot control myopia'. However, he also noted that improvement was shown in school grades and there was greater ease in doing school work, greater achievement and enjoyment of sports, and improvements in general demeanour and maturation after the vision training regime.

9.1.3   Reports after the Baltimore Myopia Control Project

During the half century that has elapsed since the Baltimore Myopia Control Project, relatively few reports of conventional vision therapy for myopia control have appeared. Betts and Dorris (1948) noted that they had trained 16 navy and marine corps officer candidates, most of whom improved by approximately one line in visual acuity. However, no study actually claimed that the pre-existing amount of myopia had been reduced. Kennedy (1951) described the results of a 3-month training programme in which the patient's myopia actually increased during the therapy. Before training, an 8-year-old patient had approximately 1.00 D of myopia in each eye, with uncorrected visual acuities of 6/18. At the conclusion of vision training, retinoscopy indicated an additional −0.25 D sphere while 1 year later the subjective refraction was −1.50 D for each eye, with uncorrected visual acuity of 6/60.

In what appears to be the only large-scale study of vision therapy to retard myopic progression which included a control group, Lin and Ko (1988) described an 18-month study of 604 Taiwanese primary school children in the same grade (ages not reported), who were randomly assigned to two groups. The experimental group, consisting of 390 children, practised 'far gazing and eyeball exercises' three times a day, while the control group of 214 children did not perform any therapy. In this investigation, mean changes in cycloplegic refraction during the 18-month period were assessed. For all subjects (i.e., hyperopes, emmetropes and myopes totalling 1208 eyes), the mean increase in myopia was 0.55 D for the experimental group and 0.57 D for the control group. When considering only the 565 myopic eyes, the mean myopic shifts were 0.96 D for the experimental group and 0.91 D for the control group. Clearly these differences were not significant. Accordingly, one must conclude that while vision training procedures can improve unaided visual acuity, there is no published evidence to support the conclusion that vision training can reduce myopia.

9.2   Biofeedback training

Biofeedback training seeks to reduce myopia by improving accommodative accuracy. The patient is provided with non-visual feedback (typically an auditory tone) to indicate the magnitude of the accommodative response. Trachtman (1978) described an instrument consisting of an optometer which monitored accommodation, and provided feedback to the subject via a change in the pitch of an auditory stimulus, occurring 134 msec following the initiation of an accommodative response. He reported the results of biofeedback training using this instrument on a 30-year-old subject who had been diagnosed with functional myopia. Therapy consisted of seven sessions totalling 34 minutes of biofeedback training (from 4 to 6 minutes per session). The subject's pre- and post-biofeedback visual acuity (for each eye) was 6/15 and 6/9, respectively. Static retinoscopy findings are shown in Table 9.1. Trachtman concluded that the results obtained with this subject and with three prior subjects show that biofeedback of accommodation is a useful tool to reduce functional myopia and teach voluntary control of accommodation. However, this conclusion is supported only by analysis of the subjective findings, and is not consistent

Table 9.1 Refractive correction for a single patient in terms of sphere (D), cylinder (D) and axis (°) as reported by Trachtman (1978) before and after biofeedback training for myopia control

	Right eye	Left eye
Pre-biofeedback retinoscopy	$-0.75 - 0.75 \times 100$	$-1.25 - 0.75 \times 90$
Post-biofeedback retinoscopy	-1.00 sph	-1.25 sph
Pre-biofeedback subjective	$-0.75 - 0.50 \times 90$	-0.75 sph
Post-biofeedback subjective	plano	-0.25 sph

with the pre- and post-training retinoscopy results.

Balliet *et al.* (1982) reported a biofeedback myopia control study which included 17 myopic subjects between 20 and 46 years of age. The accommodative response was monitored while subjects viewed a 20 cycle per degree grating. Training sessions, each of which lasted 45 minutes, were held 3–5 days per week for an average of 35 sessions. Only the right eye of each subject was trained, although binocular visual acuities were recorded. The mean change in visual acuity was from 6/64 to 6/13. No changes in refractive error were found.

Subsequently, Berman *et al.* (1985) used the instrument devised by Trachtman in a study of myopia control. This device was now available commercially as the Accommotrac Vision Trainer. Berman *et al.* reported the results from 16 myopic subjects between 9 and 37 years of age, all of whom received seven 30 minute biofeedback training sessions during a period averaging 7 weeks. Following training, all subjects experienced gains in visual acuity. Mean values for the initial and final uncorrected visual acuity were 6/27 and 6/10.5, respectively. Unfortunately, no refractive error data were reported. Nevertheless, the authors concluded that their findings replicated Trachtman's work, thereby offering additional support for the notion that myopia can be successfully treated using biofeedback training.

In a further study using the Accommotrac Vision Trainer, Gallaway *et al.* (1987) included 11 myopic subjects between 23 to 42 years of age, all of whom had no more than 4.0 D of myopia. After biofeedback training, unaided visual acuity had improved for most of the experimental subjects, but there were no significant changes in refractive error. For the nine experimental subjects who completed at least 12 training sessions, one subject showed an improvement in acuity from 6/21 to 6/6, five subjects exhibited between two and four lines

of improvement (for example, from 6/21 to 6/9) while three subjects did not demonstrate any improvement in acuity. However, of the two control subjects who did not receive biofeedback training (although their visual acuity was measured at the same intervals as the experimental subjects), one improved from 6/36 to 6/18 while the other showed no change in acuity. Gallaway *et al.* (1987) concluded that the increases in visual acuity may have been due to learning effects as shown by the changes in one of the control subjects. Furthermore, when visual acuity was measured several times before the training began, in order to establish a baseline, acuity improved for a number of subjects with repeated testing. For example, two individuals exhibited changes in acuity from 6/60 to 6/36, and 6/24 to 6/12, respectively, while the baseline measures were being established.

Perhaps the best controlled study to examine the efficacy of biofeedback training for myopia control was that of Koslowe *et al.* (1991), who employed a double-masked study using the Accommotrac instrument. Fifteen experimental subjects and 15 control subjects received identical treatment with the exception that control subjects were provided with a false feedback signal from a pre-recorded tape generated by a different subject, which therefore provided erroneous feedback data. Subjects' ages ranged from 20 to 40 years, and subjects were randomized to the experimental and control groups. The training procedures used were precisely those specified by the inventor (Dr Trachtman), and the equipment and technical staff for the project were provided by Trachtman's authorized agents. Treatment consisted of ten sessions, each lasting approximately one hour, together with home exercises. The authors observed no significant differences between the experimental and control groups in terms of unaided visual acuity, cycloplegic and non-cycloplegic retinoscopy, subjective refraction and amplitude or flexibility of accommodation.

Trachtman (1992) criticized the Koslowe *et al.* (1991) study, stating that with further statistical analysis a post-training improvement in accommodative flexibility was found. However, Koslowe *et al.* (1992) replied that no amount of statistical manipulation could conceal the fact that Accommotrac vision training had no appreciable effect on either the amount of myopia as measured by subjective refraction or on aided or unaided visual acuity, and is therefore of questionable value for the control of myopia.

More recently, Angi *et al.* (1996) employed biofeedback procedures on myopic secondary school students over a 10-week training period. For the 21 experimental subjects who were examined 1 year later, the mean amount of myopia had actually increased by 0.09 D and 0.18 D for the right and left eyes, respectively. Interestingly, despite the increased ametropia, mean unaided acuity had improved from 6/14 to 6/10 and 6/15 to 6/12 for the right and left eyes, respectively. For 17 control subjects who were examined at 1 year, their myopia increased by a mean of 0.17 D for the right eye with no change being recorded for the left eye, while their mean unaided visual acuity was unchanged, being approximately 6/18 for the right eye and 6/12 for the left eye. It must be noted that because the rate of myopia progression tends to level off in girls during the early teenage years (Goss and Winkler, 1983), one might have predicted relatively little myopic development for these secondary school students even in the absence of biofeedback training.

In a critical review of studies making use of biofeedback training for the control of myopia, Gilmartin *et al.* (1991) commented that repeated measurements of visual acuity are particularly vulnerable to individual differences in one's ability to discriminate and interpret blurred retinal images. They concluded that positive results from controlled clinical trials are needed before accommodative biofeedback can be considered an established method for the clinical management of myopia.

The results of studies using vision therapy and biofeedback training for myopia control are summarized in Table 9.2. With one exception, success was based only upon an improvement in visual acuity. As noted previously, this change may be explained by an improved ability to interpret a blurred retinal image. Additionally, if repeated use is made of the same acuity chart, then the subject may have simply memorized the letters.

9.3   Distance undercorrection

Distance undercorrection has been recommended as a procedure to control myopia progression since it will reduce the accommodative stimulus. The appeal of this procedure is undoubtedly its simplicity, particularly when compared with other methods such as vision training or the prescribing of bifocals. Unfortunately, during the past 50 years there have not been any large-scale clinical trials to test the efficacy of this technique. In one of the few studies involving undercorrection, Tokoro and Kabe (1964, 1965) compared myopia progression rates during a 3-year period for 33 children who entered with low myopia. Of these individuals, 13 were given a full correction to be worn at all times, 10 children were given an undercorrection of one dioptre or more, while a further 10 children were given a full correction 'to be worn in case of need'. Noting that some of the Tokoro and Kabe subjects were also receiving pharmaceutical agents as a means of myopia control, Goss (1994) calculated the myopia progression rates for those individuals not receiving any pharmacological treatment. He reported that for 11 subjects who were fully corrected on a full-time basis, the mean annual rate of myopia progression ($\pm$1SD) was 0.83 D ($\pm$0.18 D), while for five subjects who were undercorrected the mean annual rate of progression was 0.47 D ($\pm$0.09). Goss reported that the difference in means was statistically significant ($P<0.001$), but he suggested that a bifocal would be a more practical alternative due to the significant reduction in distance visual acuity associated with undercorrection.

In an analysis of their own private-practice data, Roberts and Banford (1963) found that mean myopia progression for 234 myopic children wearing single-vision lenses with a full correction was 0.45 D per year, whereas for 153 children wearing single-vision lenses with an undercorrection, mean progression was 0.40 D/yr. In most cases the undercorrection was no greater than 0.37 D. Although the number of subjects in each group was quite large, this small difference (0.05 D/yr) is well within the $\pm$0.25 to $\pm$0.50 D range of repeatability reported previously for clinical refraction (Bannon, 1977; Perrigin *et al.*, 1982) and therefore is not likely to be clinically significant.

9.4   Distance overcorrection

The rationale for overcorrecting myopes comes from studies examining the rate of change of

Table 9.2 Summary of the results of studies using vision therapy or biofeedback training for myopia control

Study	Subjects	Results
Vision therapy		
Baltimore project Ewalt (1946)	111 experimental No controls	Mean improvement in visual acuity was approximately 2 lines of letters, e.g. from 6/120 to 6/30 or from 6/12 to 6/7.5
Lin and Ko (1988)	390 experimental 214 controls	After 18 months of training, mean increases in myopia were 0.96 D for experimental group and 0.91 D for controls
Biofeedback training		
Balliet *et al.* (1982)	17 experimental	Mean improvement in acuity was from 6/64 to 6/13
Berman *et al.* (1985)	16 experimental No controls	Mean improvement in acuity was from 6/27 to 6/10.5
Gallaway *et al.* (1987)	9 experimental 2 controls	Acuity improved for 6 of 9 experimental subjects, e.g. from 6/21 to 6/9; and for one control, from 6/36 to 6/18
Koslowe *et al.* (1991)	15 experimental 15 controls	No significant difference between the two groups in improvement of visual acuity, retinoscopy, subjective refraction, amplitude or flexibility of accommodation
Angi *et al.* (1996)	21 experimental 17 controls	After 1 yr the mean increase in myopia was <0.25 D for both experimental and control groups; and a mean increase in acuity from 6/14 to 6/10 for the experimental group

refractive error in young hyperopes. For example, Hirsch (1961) reported that hyperopes typically changed by no more than about 0.25 D between 6 and 12 years of age, although myopic children typically progressed by as much as 2.00 D or more during the same age period. In view of the refractive stability of young hyperopes, one might argue that young myopes should be overcorrected, thereby making them effectively hyperopic. In a prospective clinical trial (Goss, 1984), 36 myopic children between the ages of 7 and 16 years were overcorrected by 0.75 D, while a control group of 36 myopic children (matched for age, sex, and initial amount of myopia) received a full refractive correction. Most members of the experimental group were overcorrected for a period of 1.5–2 years, although a few were overcorrected for less than one year. Mean annual rates of myopic progression assessed by subjective refraction for the experimental and control groups were 0.52 D/yr and 0.47 D/yr, respectively. Accordingly, Goss (1984) concluded that distance overcorrection in young myopes did not produce any significant change in the rate of refractive development, although there did appear to be an increased rate of myopic progression in female subjects who were overcorrected as compared with those who were not overcorrected.

9.5 Correction with bifocal lenses

9.5.1 Rationale

The rationale for the use of bifocal lenses in myopia control is to reduce the accommodative demand. However, to date, the precise mechanism whereby accommodation might lead to the development of myopia is unclear (*see* Chapter 5). One proposal is that myopia results from an increased lag of accommodation during nearwork (Gwiazda *et al.*, 1993), with the presence of retinal blur leading to increased ocular growth. Accordingly, bifocal lenses could be used to reduce the accommodative error, thereby decreasing the diameter of the retinal blur circle. One might suggest that if bifocals are used to reduce the accommodative stimulus, then the resulting accommodative response may also be reduced, thereby leaving the magnitude of accommodative error unchanged. However, Goss and Zhai (1994) indicated that the clinical test most commonly used to measure the lag of accommodation, namely the binocular crossed-cylinder test, has been shown by Fry (1940) and by Goodson and Afanador (1974) to yield the lens powers which equalize the accommodative stimulus and response. Therefore, if the prescribed bifocal add is equal to the binocular crossed-cylinder finding, there will be no lag of accommodation during nearwork.

For many years, the literature concerning the use of bifocal lenses to control myopia progression was in the form of case reports and retrospective studies. However, beginning in the early 1980s, a number of prospective clinical trials have also examined this method of myopia control.

9.5.2 Retrospective studies

Following a review of patient records, Mandell (1959) reported rates of progression in 59 myopes fitted with bifocals and 116 myopes fitted with single-vision spectacle lenses. Initial mean ages for the bifocal and single-vision groups were 14.3 and 17.1 years, respectively. Mandell concluded that bifocals did not reduce the progression of myopia to a greater extent than might have been predicted on a chance basis. However, inspection of his graphs indicated that many of the single-vision wearers were more than 20 years of age when they first entered the study, and therefore were beyond the age at which a significant increase in their myopia might have been expected.

In an editorial footnote to Mandell's paper, Hirsch (1959) stated that he had used the chi-square statistic to analyse Mandell's data, using a 2×2 table with degree of change categorized as either less than, or greater than 1 D of myopia. He concluded that those patients who wore bifocals had a significantly greater increase in myopia. Furthermore, Hirsch suggested that this difference may have been unrelated to the mode of refractive correction, since the determination as to which patients in the study received bifocals was made on the basis of the individual's age and initial refractive error.

Later, Miles (1962) reported retrospective data from a group of patients who originally wore single-vision lenses but were later fitted with bifocal spectacles, and therefore were assumed to serve as their own controls. During a 2-year period, 103 myopes wearing single-vision lenses (between 6 and 14 years of age) progressed at a mean rate of 0.75 D/yr. When 48 of these myopes subsequently wore bifocal lenses (now between 8 and 16 years of age), the annual progression rate over the 2-year period was 0.40 D/yr. The reduction in annual progression rate of 0.35 D/yr while wearing bifocals may have been due to the fact that the children were 2 years older when they wore bifocals. This is particularly significant in light of the report by Goss and Winkler (1983) who observed that the rate of myopic progression tends to level off between 14 and 16 years of age for females, and between 15 and 17 years of age for males.

Roberts and Banford (1963, 1967) reported annual myopic progression rates for 85 myopes wearing bifocals having adds ranging from +0.75 to +2.00 D, and 396 myopes wearing single-vision lenses. All subjects had been examined on at least two occasions before 17 years of age. Whilst subjects in the two groups were not matched for age on entering the study, the authors stated that age was factored out by using the appropriate estimating equations, and the mean computed accordingly (however they provided no information concerning the 'appropriate estimating equations'). The authors concluded that bifocals produced a significantly lower rate of refractive change (0.31 D/yr) when compared with single-vision lenses (0.41 D/yr), even when the age and sex distributions of the two groups were equivalent.

In another retrospective analysis of patient records, Oakley and Young (1975) compared the progression rates for 269 bifocal wearers and 275 single-vision wearers. Ages at the time of the initial refractive correction varied between 6 and 21 years. Of the 544 myopes, 441 were Caucasians and 156 were Native Americans living on a reservation in central Oregon. The two treatment groups were matched on the basis of sex, initial age and initial amount of myopia. The distance prescription for bifocal wearers was undercorrected by about 0.50 D, and additions ranged from +0.75 D to +2.00 D in the form of flat-top bifocals with the segment top splitting the pupil. The amount of the bifocal add was apparently determined individually for each patient. After a period of 3–4 years, the mean rates of progression for the Caucasian bifocal (*n* = 226) and single-vision (*n* = 192) wearers were 0.02 D/yr and 0.53 D/yr, respectively. The mean progression rates for Native American bifocal (*n* = 43) and single-vision (*n* = 104) wearers were 0.10 D/yr and 0.38 D/yr, respectively. For the Caucasian children, the mean difference in progression rate of 0.51 D/yr was statistically significant. Oakley and Young attributed the success of the bifocals in Caucasian children to the high segment position, and suggested that the greater progression for the Native American bifocal wearers may have been due to the fact that they tended not to wear their glasses on a regular basis. However, they also commented that there could have been some experimental bias, because all of the refractions were performed by the first author, i.e., no masking was included in the study design.

Later, Neetens and Evans (1985) presented a report based upon a review of the records of myopic children who had been examined in Antwerp, Belgium over a period of more than 20 years. The subject pool comprised 543 children wearing bifocals and 733 children wearing single-vision lenses. Their refractive errors were followed from 8 or 9 years of age (with myopia of less than 0.50 D) until age 18, at which time the mean amounts of myopia were 3.55 D for the bifocal wearers and 5.07 D for the single-vision wearers. Thus the mean progression rates were approximately 0.30 D/yr for the bifocal wearers and 0.45 D/yr for the single-vision wearers. The authors reported that this difference was highly significant (*P*<0.001). Since all of the children entered the study with the same amount of myopia, a mean difference of 1.50 D in the magnitude of refractive correction required at 18 years of age would seem to be clinically significant. Goss

(1986) reported a review of the records in three optometric practices where bifocals were sometimes prescribed for myopes. The examined records described patients who had received four or more refractions between 6 and 15 years of age, and had either worn bifocals (*n* = 60) or single-vision lenses (*n* = 52) for the entire period. Mean rates of myopic progression for the bifocal and single-vision wearers were 0.37 D/yr and 0.44 D/yr, respectively. This difference was not statistically significant.

The results of these retrospective clinical trials of bifocals for the control of myopia progression are summarized in Table 9.3. The greatest difference in progression rates between single-vision (SV) and bifocal wearers was the 0.51 D/yr change shown by the Caucasian subjects in the Oakley and Young study. However, it should also be noted that in that particular investigation, since the subject's entering ages ranged between 6 and 17 years, it was likely that by the end of the 2–4-year study period many of the myopes had reached the age when their myopia would no longer be expected to progress. The same problem exists for the Miles (1962) cross-over study where a difference in progression rates of 0.35 D/yr was observed between single-vision and bifocal wearers. As noted earlier, these myopes were 2 years older when they wore bifocals than when they wore single-vision lenses. Perhaps the most impressive results are those of Neetens and Evans, showing a difference of approximately 1.50 D in the amount of myopia for bifocal and single-vision lens wearers by the age of 18. The credibility of the Neetens and Evans study is enhanced by the number of subjects (1276), which is larger than the number reported in any other study, and by the period of time (between 10 and 11 years) that each subject was followed.

9.5.3   Prospective clinical trials

Following completion of the Oakley and Young (1975) study, a prospective clinical trial was begun at the University of Houston. To avoid the problem of examiner bias, the study design made use of an evaluation team and a patient care team. The evaluation team examined each subject prior to being enrolled in the study and at the end of each year for 3 years. Each evaluation consisted of keratometry, A-scan ultrasound measurements, phakometry and both retinoscopy and Dioptron Nova autorefraction under 1% cyclopentolate cycloplegia. The patient care team was responsible for all patient care aspects of the study including

Table 9.3 Summary of retrospective studies examining the use of bifocals for myopia control (SV = single vision controls)

Study	Duration (yr)	Initial ages (yr)	Groups	Mean rate of myopic progression
Mandell (1959)	Variable[a]	Mean 17.1	SV	See below[a]
		Mean 14.3	Bifocal	See below[a]
Miles (1962)	2	6–14[b]	SV	0.75 D/yr
		8–16[b]	Bifocal	0.35 D/yr
Roberts and Banford (1967)	See below[c]	See below[c]	SV	0.41 D/yr
Oakley and Young (1975)			Bifocal	0.31 D/yr
Native Americans	3–4	6–17	SV	0.37 D/yr
			Bifocal	0.11 D/yr
Caucasians	3–4	6–17	SV	0.52 D/yr
			Bifocal	0.02 D/yr
Neetens and Evans (1985)	9–10	8–9	SV	0.45 D/yr
			Bifocal	0.30 D/yr
Goss (1986)	See below[d]	See below[d]	SV	0.44 D/yr
	See below[d]		Bifocal	0.37 D/yr

[a] Subjects had two or more refractions before age 30. Mean changes in refraction were not reported, but it was concluded that bifocals did not reduce progression of myopia more than would have occurred on a chance basis.
[b] A cross-over study, in which the same subjects wore single-vision lenses for 2 years and then wore bifocals for 2 years.
[c] Subjects had at least two refractions before age 17.
[d] Subjects had four or more refractions between the ages of 6 and 15 years.

examination, prescribing and follow-up care. The patient care team routine included manifest retinoscopy, subjective refraction and Dioptron Nova refraction but no biometric measurements.

In this 3-year prospective clinical trial (Grosvenor *et al.*, 1985; Young *et al.*, 1985; Grosvenor *et al.*, 1987), 207 myopic children between 6 and 15 years of age were enrolled. The selection criteria were:

1 myopia of at least 0.25 D (spherical equivalent);
2 corrected visual acuity of at least 6/6 in each eye;
3 normal binocular vision, i.e., no strabismus or amblyopia;
4 normal ocular health.

Candidates having more than about 2.00 D of corneal astigmatism were not included because of the difficulty in obtaining biometric data. Each child was randomly assigned to one of three treatment groups, i.e., single-vision, +1.00 D add bifocal, or +2.00 D add bifocal. The three groups were matched on the basis of sex, initial age and the initial amount of myopia.

The bifocal wearers were fitted with Executive bifocals, with the segment top located 2 mm below the centre of the pupil. Subjects in the three treatment groups were instructed to wear their glasses at all times. At follow-up examinations, conducted at 6 monthly intervals during the 3-year period, the spectacles were adjusted to ensure that the correct bifocal height was maintained. Additionally, subjects were asked the following questions: 1 Do you wear your glasses all the time? 2 Do you do all your reading through the bifocal segments (for bifocal wearers)? 3 Are you having any problems with your glasses? 4 Are you having any other problems today? Subjects not wearing their glasses full time or not reading through the bifocals were discontinued from the study. However, compliance was at such a high level that very few subjects were discontinued for these reasons; most subjects who failed to complete the study discontinued voluntarily, either because of moving from the Houston area or because of the inability or unwillingness of their parents to bring them to the clinic for follow-up examinations.

Of the 124 subjects who completed the 3-year study, the mean myopia progression rates (right eye) were 0.34 D/yr for the single-vision lens wearers, 0.36 D/yr for the +1.00 D add bifocal wearers, and 0.34 D/yr for the +2.00 D add bifocal wearers. As expected, biometric data showed axial length increases for virtually all of the children whose myopia progressed. The distributions of changes in refractive error for the three treatment groups, shown in Figure 9.1, differed mainly in their modal progression rates, which were 0.25 D/yr for the single-vision and +1.00 D add bifocal wearers, but 0.50 D/yr for the +2.00 D add bifocal wearers. On the basis of these findings, Grosvenor *et al.* (1987) concluded that regardless of whether single-vision or bifocal lenses were worn, the rate of progression depended primarily upon the age of myopic onset. As shown in Figure 9.2, for both single-vision (*n* = 23) and +2.00 D add bifocal wearers (*n* = 22), those individuals with 1 or 2 D of myopia around 9 years of age tended to progress at rates of between 0.50 and to 1.00 D/yr, whereas subjects whose myopia began around 11 years of age or later progressed by no more than approximately 0.25 D/yr.

In another prospective clinical trial (Hemminki and Parssinen, 1987; Parssinen and Hemminki, 1988; Parsinnen *et al.*, 1989) 240 children (initial ages between 9 and 11 years of age, myopia between 0.25 and 3.00 D, and no more than 2.00 D of anisometropia or astigmatism) were randomly allocated to three groups:

1 a single-vision group wearing their lenses full-time;
2 a second single-vision group wearing their lenses for distance vision only;
3 a bifocal group, wearing +1.75 D add flat-top bifocals with the segment top fitted 2–3 mm below the centre of the pupil.

Cycloplegic subjective refraction was quantified with subjects being followed for periods ranging between 2 and 5 years (95% of subjects were followed for 3 years). The mean rates of progression were 0.49 D/yr for the full-time single-vision group, 0.63 D/yr for the distance-only single-vision group and 0.53 D/yr for the bifocal group.

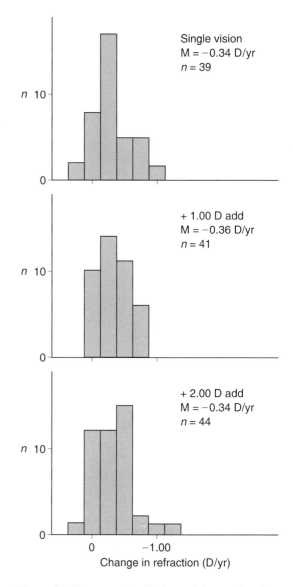

Figure 9.1 Frequency distributions of changes in spherical equivalent refractive correction (right eye), for subjects wearing single-vision lenses, +1.00 D add bifocals and +2.00 D add bifocals. M = mean progression rate. (From Grosvenor *et al.*, 1987)

These differences were not statistically significant. Subjects completed a questionnaire indicating the amount of time spent on nearwork and outdoor activities. A low but significant positive correlation was found between myopia progression and the time spent performing nearwork (*r* = 0.25), whilst a low negative correlation was found between myopia progression and the time spent undertaking outdoor activities (*r* = −0.17).

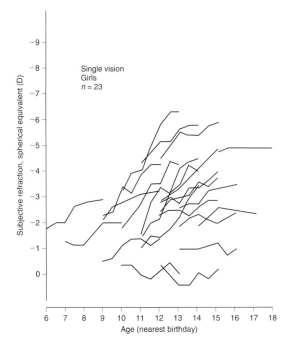

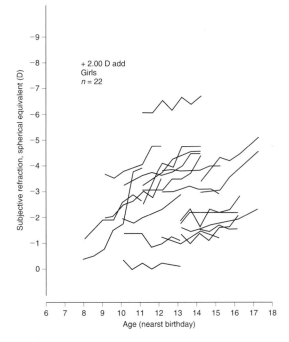

Figure 9.2 Progression of myopia during a 3-year period, (A) for girls wearing single-vision lenses and (B) for girls wearing +2.00 D add bifocals. (From Grosvenor *et al.*, 1987)

Additionally, Jensen (1991) conducted a 2-year prospective clinical trial using both bifocals and the non-selective beta-adrenergic antagonist timolol maleate (0.5%). Subjects were 159 Danish children between 9 and 12 years of age, having between 1.25 and 6.00 D of myopia. Subjects were randomly assigned to one of three treatment groups: a bifocal group, a timolol group and a single-vision (SV) control group. Members of the bifocal group wore 38 mm flat-top bifocals with the segment top located at the lower edge of the pupil when the child looked straight forward. All subjects were instructed to wear their glasses constantly, and to read at a distance not less than 30 cm. At the end of the 2-year period, the mean rates of progression for 145 children who completed the study were 0.48 D/yr for the bifocal group, 0.59 D/yr for the timolol group and 0.57 D/yr for the SV group. The differences in progression rates were not statistically significant. However, it is of interest to note that the bifocals were more successful in those subjects having higher levels of intraocular pressure (i.e., greater than 17 mmHg).

The results of these three randomized prospective clinical trials, summarized in Table 9.4, are not supportive of the proposal that bifocal lenses retard myopic progression, and additionally are not consistent with the slightly more favourable results observed in the retrospective studies (*see* Table 9.3).

9.5.4   Effects of near-point esophoria and high lags of accommodation on myopia control with bifocals

In a review of studies associating myopia with accommodation, Rosenfield (1994) suggested that the myopic population may not be homogenous, and that a single aetiological mechanism cannot be assigned to all myopia. He further suggested that while a particular treatment regime may work successfully in a subgroup of myopes, if it is applied indiscriminately to a larger population, then the mean findings for the group may not demonstrate any significant effect. Two subgroups of myopes which have received attention in recent years are those having near-point esophoria or a poor accommodative response, with the latter being demonstrated clinically as a relatively high lag of accommodation.

The rationale for the use of bifocal lenses in myopes having a high near-point esophoria was presented in Chapter 7, where Goss suggested that

Table 9.4 Summary of prospective studies examining the use of bifocals for myopia control

Study	Duration (yr)	Initial ages (yr)	Groups	Mean rate of myopic progression
Grosvenor *et al.* (1985, 1987)	3	6–15	SV	0.34 D/yr
			+1.00 D add	0.36 D/yr
			+2.00 D add	0.34 D/yr
Parsinnen *et al.* (1988, 1989)	3[a]	Mean 10.9	SV full time	0.49 D/yr
			SV dist. only	0.63 D/yr
			+1.75 D add	0.53 D/yr
Jensen (1991)	2	9–12	SV	0.57 D/yr
			+2.00 add	0.48 D/yr
			Timolol	0.59 D/yr

[a] Subjects were followed for periods of 2–5 years (3 years for 95% of subjects).

children who have near-point esophoria tend to have higher lags of accommodation when compared with subjects having either near-point orthophoria or exophoria. In order to achieve and maintain single binocular vision, a person who is esophoric at near must use fusional divergence (negative fusional vergence). The latter will produce a reduction in convergent accommodation, thereby producing an increased lag of accommodation. This error of accommodation will place the image formed by the eye's optical system behind the retina. The presence of a defocused retinal image may stimulate scleral growth to produce an increase in axial length, thus repositioning the image back onto the retina (*see* Chapter 3).

In a survey of the records from three optometric practices, Goss (1986) analysed the data in terms of initial near-point phoria findings. Phoria findings were considered in terms of three categories, namely, greater than 6 Δ of exophoria, between orthophoria and 6 Δ of exophoria – i.e., Morgan's (1944) 'normal' range for the phoria at 40 cm – and any amount of esophoria. For patients in either of the two exophoria groups, the mean rate of myopia progression did not differ significantly between single-vision and bifocal wearers, with both groups showing mean rates of progression slightly less than 0.50 D/yr. However, for the esophoria group, the mean progression rate for the single-vision and bifocal wearers was 0.54 D/yr and 0.32 D/yr, respectively. This difference was statistically significant.

In the same population, Goss (1986) also analysed the near binocular dynamic crossed-cylinder findings. This test quantifies the lag of accommodation, with typical findings ranging from 0.25

to 0.75 D. For those patients demonstrating lags of accommodation of less than 0.50 D, the mean progression rates were 0.39 D/yr for the single-vision group and 0.41 D/yr for the bifocal group. In contrast, in those patients exhibiting accommodative lags of 0.50 D or greater, the mean progression rate was 0.48 D/yr for single-vision wearers, but only 0.25 D/yr for bifocal wearers. This difference was statistically significant. Goss concluded that bifocals may be successful in controlling myopia in patients with either near-point esophoria or a high lag of accommodation.

Subsequently, Goss and Grosvenor (1990) reanalysed data from the Grosvenor *et al.* (1987), Roberts and Banford (1967) and Goss (1986) retrospective studies in terms of the heterophoria at near. They indicated that for children who were initially esophoric at near through their distance refractive correction, the mean rate of myopia progression was approximately 0.20 D/yr lower for bifocal wearers when compared with single-vision wearers. However, for children with either orthophoria or exophoria at near, there were no significant differences between the rates of progression for bifocal and single-vision wearers. These results are summarized in Table 9.5. Goss and Grosvenor observed that there was a high degree of consistency between the reanalysed findings of the three studies.

In a prospective clinical trial examining the use of bifocals for myopia control in individuals demonstrating esophoria at near, Fulk and Cyert (1996) recruited 32 children who had near-point esophoria as well as at least 0.50 D of myopia in the principal meridia of each eye. Subjects were randomly allocated either to a +1.25 D add bifocal treatment

Table 9.5 Summary of three bifocal studies, showing mean progression of myopia (D/yr) on the basis of initial near-point phoria findings

Study	>6 Δ exophoria		0–6 Δ exophoria		Esophoria	
	SV	Bif	SV	Bif	SV	Bif
Roberts and Banford (1967)	See below[a]		See below[a]		0.48	0.28
Goss (1986)	0.47	0.48	0.43	0.46	0.54	0.32
Grosvenor *et al.* (1987)	0.50	0.43	0.43	0.42	0.51	0.31

[a] For exophoria and orthophoria combined, mean progression rates were 0.41 D/yr for single-vision (SV) and 0.38 D/yr for bifocals (Bif).
From Goss and Grosvenor (1990)

group or a single-vision control group. The +1.25 D add was chosen on the basis that it would cause most subjects to become slightly exophoric at near. Objective cycloplegic autorefraction was measured at 6 monthly intervals during an 18-month period.

The mean progression rates (± 1SEM) were 0.57 (±0.11) D/yr for the single-vision group ($n = 14$) and 0.39 (±0.12) D/yr for the bifocal group ($n = 14$). This difference was not statistically significant ($P = 0.26$). However, the increase in axial length for each subject was closely correlated with increase in myopia ($r = 0.84$). Progression rates were calculated for each 6-month interval within the test period, and it was noted that during the first 12 months of the study bifocals produced no significant change in myopic development. During the 12–18-month period of the investigation, the mean rates of progression were 0.37 D/yr for the bifocal group and 0.80 D/yr for the single-vision group. Fulk and Cyert concluded that bifocals did appear to slow myopic progression in children with near-point esophoria, although a longer term study with more subjects was needed to confirm this finding.

9.6 The use of base-in prisms

The rationale for the use of base-in prisms for myopia control is the reduction or elimination of the demand upon convergence. The base-in prisms may be combined with a bifocal add to reduce or eliminate both the vergence and accommodative stimulus simultaneously. However, the ophthalmic literature contains no reports of large-scale prospective (or retrospective) clinical studies examining this procedure.

Rehm (1975) designed an instrument called the Myopter Viewer, which provided sufficient plus power and base-in prism so that no accommodation or convergence were required for nearwork. To avoid the large amounts of distortion which would come from using high prism values, this device incorporated a system of mirrors and lenses with a beam-splitter to allow the subject to read without any need for accommodation or convergence. Rehm (1981) published only a few case reports in which the degree of myopia decreased by approximately 0.25 to 0.50 D.

The use of base-in prism combined with a bifocal add is an appealing procedure, but the problems with the procedure are numerous. For example, as Rehm (1975) observed, high powered prisms can cause significant distortion, often referred to as prism blur. Additionally, even if sufficient base-in prism and plus lens power are used to reduce the stimuli for both disparity vergence and blur-induced accommodation to zero, the fact that the reading material is close will stimulate both proximal vergence and accommodation, possibly leading to diplopia or blur. Thirdly, children whose myopia progresses at the fastest rates tend to be esophoric at near (Goss, 1994). Use of base-in prism will obviously increase the amount of near-point esophoria, although the use of plus lens power will also decrease the esophoria by an amount that varies with the AC/A ratio. Finally, although Rehm's Myopter Viewer solves the problem of prism blur, the other difficulties will still remain, together with the discomfort and inconvenience of having to read through this instrument.

9.7 Instillation of pharmaceutical agents

The rationale for the use of pharmaceutical agents is that myopia progression can be controlled either by the relaxation of accommodation (cycloplegic agents) or the reduction of intraocular pressure (adrenergic blocking agents).

9.7.1 Cycloplegic agents

Since myopia is considered by many practitioners to be produced by accommodation during nearwork, the literature contains a number of studies making use of cycloplegic agents for myopia control. Problems which might arise during the long-term use of cycloplegic agents include:

1 The necessity for patients to remove their distance glasses for reading, or to wear a near-vision addition.
2 The inconvenience of instilling drops on a daily basis for a period of several years.
3 Pupillary mydriasis producing photophobia, possible ultra-violet or infra-red radiation damage and raised intraocular pressure.
4 The possibility of an adverse reaction to the cycloplegic agent or interaction with systemic medication.
5 The ethical dilemma of prescribing long-term medication for a child or a young adult who is in good health.

Tropicamide
Abraham (1966) examined the rate of myopic progression for 68 myopic children between 7 and 18 years of age who instilled 1% tropicamide drops at night, and a control group of 82 myopic children. The two groups were matched for age, sex and family history of myopia. Bifocals were not used, and the children were apparently encouraged to read without their glasses if necessary. Abraham commented that the children's pupils were seldom still dilated upon arising in the morning, and if nearwork was required early in the morning 'the uncorrected nearsightedness took care of the problem'. His rationale was that the use of the eyes for nearwork during the daytime resulted in a 'spastic ciliary muscle' during the night; and the advantages of instilling tropicamide drops at bedtime were that the children were not likely to be bothered by pupillary dilation or poor accommodation during the daytime. Over an 18-month observation period, the mean progression rates for the experimental and control groups were 0.27 D/yr and 0.57 D/yr, respectively. Jensen and Goldschmidt (1991) suggested that it is difficult to draw any

conclusions from this study because all children who were not treated, regardless of reason, were placed in the control group.

Schwartz (1976, 1981) described an 8.5-year study involving the use of both tropicamide and bifocals. Subjects for the study were 25 pairs of myopic monozygotic twins between 7 and 13 years of age. One twin in each pair wore bifocals with a +1.25 D add and was given two drops of 1% tropicamide in each eye at night, while the other twin wore single-vision lenses and did not receive tropicamide. Schwartz reported that the mean rate of progression for all subjects was 0.26 D/yr; and that the mean progression rate was 0.03 D/yr less for the treatment group than for the control group. This small difference is obviously not clinically significant. In view of the extended duration of this study combined with the use of identical twins, this investigation provides convincing evidence that the use of tropicamide in conjunction with a +1.25 D add bifocal was not effective in controlling the progression of myopia.

Atropine
Amongst the many studies to examine the use of atropine for myopia control was that of Gimbel (1973), who compared myopic progression rates in 279 experimental subjects and 572 controls. The mean ages of the control and experimental subject groups were 11.0 and 9.7 years, respectively. The typical dosage was one drop of 1% atropine in each eye at night, but this was sometimes reduced if reading difficulties were reported. Additionally, the dosage either reduced or increased depending upon whether the myopia had stabilized or was progressing. Gimbel's (1973) report is confusing and contradictory with the result that it is difficult to interpret. He stated that 53% of the patients had stopped treatment, usually because of 'annoying side effects', but he also stated that only 22 of the original 279 treated subjects were followed for 3 years. Furthermore, Gimbel reported results for only those treated subjects who initially presented with no more than 2.00 D of myopia, and those for control subjects whose initial refraction was not greater than 1.50 D of myopia. For the 22 treated subjects, the mean change in ametropia was 0.07 D less myopia, whereas for the control subjects (number not reported) there was a mean increase in myopia of 1.22 D. Interpretation is further complicated by the fact that refractive error was measured under atropine for the treated subjects but with tropicamide cycloplegia for the control subjects.

Later, Bedrossian (1979) used a cross-over study, in which subjects instilled atropine (1%) into one eye for a 1-year period, and in the fellow eye during the following year. Again, refraction was measured under atropine cycloplegia for the treated eye and tropicamide cycloplegia for the control eye. For 90 subjects who remained in the study for 2 years, the mean change in refractive error was 0.20 D less myopia for the treated eyes and 0.94 D more myopia for the control eyes. For the two eyes of each subject, this indicates a mean rate of myopic progression of 0.5×(−0.20 +0.94) or 0.37 D/yr. For the 28 subjects who remained in the study for an additional 2 years, the mean changes in refractive correction were 0.30 D less myopia and 0.90 D more myopia for the treated eye and control eyes, respectively, indicating a mean myopic progression rate of 0.5×(−0.30 +0.90) or 0.30 D/yr. For the 57 subjects who were examined between 1 and 6 years following completion of the study, the mean progression rate was 0.06 D/year.

The value of atropine treatment in the Bedrossian (1979) study is questionable, since the mean myopic progression rates of 0.37 D/yr for the first two years and 0.30 D/yr for the third and fourth years of the study differed little from the expected progression rate for children of comparable ages who did not receive any treatment. For example, in the Grosvenor *et al.* (1987) bifocal study, members of the single-vision lens-wearing control group progressed at a mean rate of 0.34 D/yr. Moreover, Bedrossian's mean post-treatment progression rate of 0.06 D/yr, which occurred for subjects between 12 and 22 years of age is consistent with the finding that myopic progression generally comes to a halt during the late teen years (Goss and Winkler, 1983).

Gruber (1979) reported results from a treatment group of 100 myopic children who received one drop of 1% atropine daily, and a control group of 100 myopic children who did not receive any treatment. The drop-out rate was reported to be 12%. The treatment group progressed at a mean rate of 0.11 D/yr during the treatment period of 1–2 years, and at a mean rate of 0.46 D/yr after treatment. The control group progressed at a mean rate of 0.28 D/yr. Thus for the treated subjects, the mean progression rate during the 2-year period was 0.5×(0.11 +0.46), or 0.29 D/yr. This is similar to the expected progression rates in the absence of treatment, indicating that the retarded rate of myopic progression during atropine treatment was fully compensated by the accelerated rate of progression once treatment had ceased.

The effect of combining both atropine and bifocals for myopia control was examined by Brodstein *et al.* (1984). Here, the treatment group consisted of 435 myopic children who were fitted with +2.25 D add bifocals and given one drop of 1% atropine into each eye every morning. The control group consisted of 146 myopic children, who wore single-vision lenses and did not receive atropine. The follow-up period averaged 33 months for the treated subjects and 49 months for the control subjects. The treatment group progressed at a mean rate of 0.16 D/yr during the treatment period and 0.39 D/yr after treatment, for a mean progression rate of 0.23 D/yr. The control group progressed at a mean rate of 0.25 D/yr. Again, this study fails to demonstrate that atropine reduces the rate of myopic progression.

In view of the difficulties resulting from the regular instillation of cycloplegic drugs already described, i.e., inconvenience, reading problems, discomfort and possible danger from pupillary mydriasis, the possibility of an adverse reaction to the drug, and the ethical problems associated with the instillation of a potentially harmful pharmaceutical agent into a healthy eye, as well as the lack of clearcut evidence that these agents are effective in reducing the rate of myopic progression, there appears to be little reason to persist with this form of therapy.

9.7.2 Adrenergic blocking agents

The rationale for the use of adrenergic antagonists in myopia control is to reduce the intraocular pressure. Whilst these agents might also alter the accommodative response (*see* Chapter 6), this has not generally been stated as a primary reason for their use.

Adrenergic blocking agents that have been used for manipulation of intraocular pressure include labetalol, a beta-adrenoceptor antagonist that also exhibits weak alpha-adrenoceptor antagonist action, and the non-specific beta-adrenoceptor antagonist timolol maleate. Hosaka (1988) reported that 0.5% and 0.25% labetalol was given twice daily to 50 myopic children between 6 and 14 years of age. After 2–4 months of treatment the mean refractive correction decreased from −0.64 D to −0.24 D, with a decrease of at least −0.25 D in 68% of the patients. In the same paper, Hosaka (1988) reported that 0.25% timolol drops were given twice daily to 20 myopic children between 7 and 14 years of age. After 2–6 months of treatment, there was no significant effect upon myopia

Table 9.6 Summary of studies using pharmaceutical agents for myopia control

Study	Subjects	Duration (yr)	Rate of myopia progression (D/yr)
Tropicamide			
Abraham (1966)	68 treatment	1.5	0.27
	82 controls	1.5	0.57
Schwartz (1976, 1981)	25 treatment	8.5	0.24
	25 controls[a]	8.5	0.27
Atropine			
Gimbel (1973)	22 treatment	3	0
	? controls[b]	3	0.41
Gruber (1979)	100 treatment	1–2	0.11
	100 controls	(Variable)	0.28
Bedrossian (1979)	90 treatment[c]	1	−0.20[d]
	90 controls	1	0.94
Brodstein *et al.* (1984)	435 treatment	Mean 2.75	0.16
	146 controls	Mean 4.08	0.25
Labetolol			
Hosaka (1988)	50 treatment	0.17–0.33	−0.24 to −0.62[d]
	No controls		
Timolol			
Hosaka (1988)	20 treatment	0.17–0.50	No effect
	No controls		
Jensen (1991)	45 treatment	2	0.59
	48 controls		0.57

[a] Subjects were monozygotic twins; one twin in each pair was in the treatment group and the other was in the control group.
[b] The number of control subjects who completed the study was not given. Data were reported only for experimental subjects who initially had less than 2.00 D of myopia and for control subjects who initially had less than 1.50 D of myopia.
[c] Cross-over study in which each subject was given atropine in one eye during the first year and in the other eye during the second year.
[d] A minus rate of progression indicates a hyperopic shift in refractive error.

progression, with only 28% of patients having a reduction in myopia of at least 0.25 D. In neither of these studies were post-treatment data reported, nor was there any mention of a control group.

In the study by Jensen (1991) cited earlier, children between 9 and 12 years of age were randomly assigned to either a bifocal group, a timolol group, or a single-vision control group. At the end of the 2-year period, the difference in the mean myopic progression rates for the timolol group (0.59 D/yr) and the single-vision control group (0.57 D/yr)

were not statistically significant, although a decrease in mean intraocular pressure was found in the timolol group. Although timolol instillation was discontinued after 2 years, both the timolol and control groups were examined after an additional year, during which both groups were found to progress at a mean rate of 0.42 D/yr.

The results of studies making use of cycloplegic agents and adrenergic blocking agents for myopia control are summarized in Table 9.6. It is clear from these results that neither of these pharmacological agents has been demonstrated to control myopic progression successfully.

9.8 What do these attempts to control myopia tell us about the relationship between myopia and nearwork?

The most promising method of myopia control appears to be that offered by the use of bifocal lenses for young myopes who are either esophoric at near (Roberts and Banford, 1967; Goss, 1986; Goss and Grosvenor, 1990) or who have large lags of accommodation (Goss, 1986). The success of this form of myopia control is all the more impressive when it is understood that for myopes wearing single-vision lenses, those individuals having near-point esophoria typically exhibit significantly higher rates of myopic progression when compared with subjects who are either orthophoric or exophoric at near (Goss, 1986). The results suggest that the relationship between myopia and nearwork involves not only the accommodative system but also, and of either equal or greater importance, the vergence system (*see* Chapter 7).

Evidence for the relationship between myopia and vergence was reported by Flom and Takahashi (1962). They observed that previously uncorrected or undercorrected myopes tended to be esophoric at near through their full refractive correction. However, they found that if the full correction was worn for a week, then the mean near heterophoria changed by 2Δ in the exophoric direction, while the mean calculated AC/A ratio decreased by 1Δ/D. Flom and Takahashi concluded that when myopia is uncorrected, there is a reduction in the accommodative stimulus–and thus in the accommodative response–by the amount of the undercorrection, with an associated decrease in accommodative convergence. To maintain bifixation at the reading distance, accommodative convergence is supplemented by positive relative convergence (positive fusional or disparity convergence) which becomes conditioned and is therefore still in play when the new, and stronger, lenses are worn. As described by Rosenfield (1997), the sustained output of slow fusional vergence shifts the phoria in the eso direction when the full correction is first worn. However, with continued wearing of the full correction, the output of slow fusional vergence will decline, thereby shifting the phoria in the exo direction.

We may now ask the question, how does the induced near-point esophoria demonstrate a link between myopia and vergence? More specifically, does the myopia cause the near-point esophoria, or does the near-point esophoria cause the myopia? The explanation given by Flom and Takahashi (1962) can be interpreted as showing that *the uncorrected myopia is the cause of the near-point esophoria*, which would not have been present had the patient remained emmetropic. On the other hand, Goss (Chapter 7) has provided evidence that *the near-point esophoria may be the cause of the myopia*. As shown by Goss and Jackson (1996), children who later became myopic were found to have near-point esophoria while they were still emmetropic. Furthermore, many researchers (e.g. Maddock *et al.*, 1981; Bullimore and Gilmartin, 1987; Gwiazda *et al.*, 1993) have shown that myopes tend to have a poorer accommodative response than emmetropes or hyperopes. Additionally, Goss noted that myopic children who have near-point esophoria tend to have higher lags of accommodation than those having near-point orthophoria or exophoria. The reduced accommodative response places the image of a near object behind the retina, causing retinal defocus, which may stimulate scleral growth to produce axial elongation, thereby placing the image back on the retina (Goss and Zhai, 1994). If both of these conditions prevail, i.e., if near-point esophoria is both a *cause* and a *result* of myopia, then this might explain the inexorable progression that is typical of myopia.

Even though many of the methods advocated for myopia control described in this chapter have proved to be ineffective, this does not constitute sufficient evidence for us to conclude that there is no relationship between myopia and nearwork. That both heredity and environmental factors play important roles in the causation of myopia seems beyond doubt. While it may be virtually impossible to separate the relative roles of heredity and environment, some insight may be gained by considering the differences in the prevalence of myopia in societies where little or no nearwork is done, as compared with the much higher prevalence found in 'advanced' societies such as those in North America, Europe, and Asia.

Researchers from the University of Auckland, New Zealand, conducted two visual surveys in the South Pacific island nation of Vanuatu. Formerly known as New Hebrides, Vanuatu consists of some 70 islands located approximately 3000 km north of

New Zealand. Agriculture, conducted at a subsistence level, employs about 70% of the economically active population. Garner *et al.* (1985) examined 977 Melanesian schoolchildren in Vanuatu between 6 and 17 years of age, most of whom lived in the smaller rural islands. Only 13 (1.3%) of the children were found to have myopia of 0.50 D or greater. This is remarkably low considering that the prevalence of myopia in the United States has been shown to be about 2% at 6 years of age, increasing to about 15% by aged 15 years (Blum *et al.*, 1959).

Additionally, Garner *et al.* (1988) and Grosvenor (1988) reported a survey conducted in Port Vila, the capital of Vanuatu (and the only city of any size). Of 788 Melanesian children between 6 and 18 years of age, only 23 (2.9%) had myopia of 0.50 D or more. When the 479 primary schoolchildren (between 6 and 13 years of age) were considered separately, the prevalence of myopia was only 0.6%. Even though these children attended school regularly, reading was not an important part of their lives. Furthermore, many houses had no electricity, and little if any reading was done outside of school. There was no television broadcasting, and the children spent much of their after-school time working in the family gardens, tending the chickens and pigs, and fishing in nearby streams. There was an obvious lack of stress in their lives. In contrast, the prevalence of myopia for the 309 secondary schoolchildren was 7.8%. These children attended Malapola College, a preparatory school for tertiary education which had the highest entry standards of any secondary school on the islands.

These extremely low prevalences of myopia contrast strikingly with the high values reported by Lin *et al.* (1988) for Taiwanese children. In a survey of more than 4000 Taiwanese schoolchildren, Lin *et al.* reported a prevalence of myopia (at least 0.50 D) of 8% for 7-year-old children living in metropolitan areas, which increased to 70% by 15 years of age. For children who lived in more rural Taiwanese villages, the prevalence at 7 and 15 years of age was 3% and approximately 42%, respectively. While discussing these results, Lin *et al.* stated that most schoolchildren in Taiwan are under a great amount of stress due to the highly competitive college entrance examination, spending more than 10 hours reading and studying every day. They concluded that when all members of a society are exposed to a high-risk environment, genetic susceptibility becomes less important when

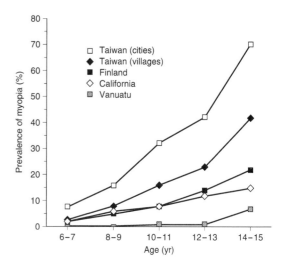

Figure 9.3 Prevalence of myopia on the basis of age for schoolchildren in Taiwan (Lin *et al.*, 1988), Finland (Laatikainen and Erkkila, 1980), California (Blum *et al.*, 1959) and Vanuatu (Garner *et al.*, 1988)

compared with environmental factors. The prevalences of myopia reported for children in Taiwan, Finland, California and Vanuatu are shown graphically in Figure 9.3.

In conclusion, the fact that various methods of myopia control have achieved very limited success should not necessarily be interpreted as proving the absence of any relationship between myopia and nearwork. It is possible that once axial elongation (which is not compensated by a reduction in either corneal or lens power) has begun, continued near-visual activity will produce additional axial elongation irrespective of any form of external intervention.

References

Abraham, S. V. (1966) Control of myopia with tropicamide. A progress report. *Ophthalmol.* **3**, 10–22.

Angi, M. R., Caucci, S., Pilotto, E., Racano, E., Rupolo, G. and Sabbadin, E. (1996) Changes in myopia, visual acuity, and psychological distress after biofeedback visual training. *Optom. Vis. Sci.* **73**, 35–42.

Balliet, R., Clay, A. and Blood, K. (1982) The training of visual acuity in myopia. *J. Am. Optom. Assoc.* **53**, 719–724.

Bannon, R. E. (1946) Comments on orthoptics. *Am. J. Optom. Arch. Am. Acad. Optom.* **23**, 483–497.

Bannon, R. E. (1977) A new automated subjective optometer. *Am. J. Optom. Physiol. Opt.* **54**, 443–458.

Bedrossian, R. H. (1979) The effect of atropine on myopia. *Ophthalmol.* **86**, 713–717.

Berman, P. E., Levinger, S. I., Massoth, N. A. *et al.* (1985) Effectiveness of biofeedback training as a viable method of treatment and reduction of myopia. *J. Optom. Vis. Devel.* **16**, 17–21.

Betts, E. A. (1947) An evaluation of the Baltimore Myopia Control Project. Part A. Experimental procedures. *J. Am. Optom. Assoc.* **17**, 481–485.

Betts, E. A. and Dorris, V. (1948) Maintaining visual acuity in the navy. *Optom. Weekly* **39**, 691–692.

Blum, H. L., Peters, H. B. and Bettman, J. W. (1959) *Vision Screening for Elementary Schools: The Orinda Study.* University of California Press.

Brodstein, R. S., Brodstein, D. E., Olson, R. J. *et al.* (1984) The treatment of myopia with atropine and bifocals. *Ophthalmol.* **91**, 1373–1379.

Bullimore, M. A. and Gilmartin, B. (1987) Aspects of tonic accommodation in emmetropia and late onset myopia. *Am. J. Optom. Physiol. Opt.* **64**, 499–503.

Ewalt, W. H. Jr (1946) The Baltimore Myopia Project. *J. Am. Optom. Assoc.* **17**, 167–185.

Flom, M. C. and Takahashi, E. (1962) The AC/A ratio and undercorrected myopia. *Am. J. Optom. Arch. Am. Acad. Optom.* **39**, 305–312.

Fry, G. A. (1940) Significance of the fused cross-cylinder test. *Optom. Weekly* **31**, 16–19.

Fulk, G. W. and Cyert, L. A. (1996) Can bifocals slow myopia progression? *J. Am. Optom. Assoc.* **67**, 749–754.

Gallaway, M., Pearl, S. M., Winkelstein, A. M. and Scheiman, M. (1987) Biofeedback training of visual acuity and myopia: a pilot study. *Am. J. Optom. Physiol. Opt.* **64**, 62–71.

Garner, L. F., Kinnear, R. F., Klinger, J. D. and McKellar, M. J. (1985) Prevalence of myopia in school children in Vanuatu. *Acta Ophthalmol.* **63**, 323–326.

Garner, L. F., Kinnear, R. F., McKellar, M. J., Klinger, J. D., Hovander, M. and Grosvenor, T. (1988) Refraction and its components in Melanesian school children in Vanuatu. *Am. J. Optom. Physiol. Opt.* **65**, 182–189.

Gilmartin, B., Gray, L. S. and Winn, B. (1991) The amelioration of myopia using biofeedback of accommodation: a review. *Ophthal. Physiol. Opt.* **11**, 304–313.

Gimbel, H. V. (1973) The control of myopia with atropine. *Can. J. Ophthalmol.* **8**, 527–532.

Goodson, R. A. and Afanador, A. J. (1974) The accommodative response to the near point crossed cylinder test. *Optom. Weekly* **65**, 1138–1140.

Goss, D. A. (1984) Overcorrection as a means of slowing myopia progression. *Am. J. Optom. Physiol. Opt.* **61**, 85–93.

Goss, D. A. (1986) Effect of bifocal lenses on rate of childhood myopia progression. *Am. J. Optom. Physiol. Opt.* **63**, 135–141.

Goss, D. A. (1991) Clinical accommodation and heterophoria findings preceding juvenile onset of myopia. *Optom. Vis. Sci.* **68**, 110–116.

Goss, D. A. (1994) Effect of spectacle correction on the progression of myopia in children–a literature review. *J. Am. Optom. Assoc.* **65**, 117–128.

Goss, D. A. and Grosvenor, T. (1990) Rates of childhood myopia progression with bifocals as a function of nearpoint phoria: consistency of 3 studies. *Optom. Vis. Sci.* **67**, 637–640.

Goss, D. A. and Jackson, T. (1996) Clinical findings before the onset of myopia in youth: 3. Heterophoria. *Optom. Vis. Sci.* **73**, 269–278.

Goss, D. A. and Winkler, R. L. (1983) Progression of myopia in youth: age of cessation. *Am. J. Optom. Physiol. Opt.* **60**, 651–658.

Goss, D. A. and Zhai, H. (1994) Clinical and laboratory investigations of the relationship of accommodation and convergence function with refractive error. *Doc. Ophthalmol.* **86**, 349–380.

Grosvenor, T. (1988) Myopia in Melanesian school children in Vanuatu. In: *Myopia Workshop* (H. C. Fledelius and E. Goldschmidt, eds). *Acta Ophthalmol.* Suppl. 185, **66**, 24–28.

Grosvenor, T., Maslovitz, B., Perrigin D. M. and Perrigin, J. (1985) The Houston Myopia Control Study: a preliminary report by the patient care team. *J. Am. Optom. Assoc.* **56**, 636–643.

Grosvenor, T., Perrigin, D. M., Perrigin, J. and Maslovitz, B. (1987) Houston Myopia Control Study: a randomized clinical trial. Part 2. Final report of the patient care team. *Am. J. Optom. Physiol. Opt.* **64**, 482–498.

Gruber, E. (1979) The treatment of myopia with atropine: a clinical study. In: *Ophthalmology: Proceedings of the International Congress, Kyoto 1978* (E. T. Shimizu and J. A. Oosterhuis, eds). Excerpta Medica, pp. 1212–1216.

Gwiazda, J., Thorn, F., Bauer, J. and Held, R. (1993) Myopic children show insufficient response to blur. *Invest. Ophthalmol. Vis. Sci.* **34**, 690–694.

Hackman, R. B. (1947) An evaluation of the Baltimore Myopia Project. Part B. Statistical procedure. *J. Am. Optom. Assoc.* **17**, 416–426.

Hemminki, E. and Parssinen, O. (1987) Prevention of myopia progress by glasses. Study design and first year results of a randomized trial among schoolchildren. *Am. J. Optom. Physiol. Opt.* **64**, 611–616.

Hirsch, M. J. (1959) Editorial footnote to Mandell paper. *Am. J. Optom. Arch. Am. Acad. Optom.* **36**, 657–658.

Hirsch, M. J. (1961) A longitudinal study of refractive state of children during the first six years of school: a preliminary report of the Ojai study. *Am. J. Optom. Arch. Am. Acad. Optom.* **38**, 564–571.

Hosaka, A. (1988) The role of pharmaceutical agents. In: *Myopia Workshop* (H. C. Fledelius and E. Goldschmidt, eds). *Acta Ophthalmol.* Suppl. 185, **66**, 130–131.

Jensen, H. (1991) Myopia progression in young school children. A prospective study of myopia progression and the effect of a trial with bifocal lenses and beta blocker eye drops. *Acta Ophthalmol.* Suppl. 200 (Monograph).

Jensen, H. and Goldschmidt, E. (1991) Management of myopia: pharmaceutical agents. In: *Refractive Anomalies. Research and Clinical Applications* (T. Grosvenor and M. Flom, eds). Butterworth-Heinemann, ch. 21.

Kennedy, J. R. (1951) A case of an uncorrected child myope showing progression in the presence of visual training. *Am. J. Optom. Arch. Am. Acad. Optom.* **28**, 642–644.

Koslowe, K. C., Spierer, S., Rosner, M. and Belkins, M. (1991) Evaluation of Accommotrac feedback training of visual acuity in myopia: a pilot study. *Optom. Vis. Sci.* **68**, 338–343.

Koslowe, K. C., Spierer, S., Rosner, M. and Belkins, M. (1992) Reply to letter to the editor. *Optom. Vis. Sci.* **69**, 254.

Laatikainen, L. and Erkkila, H. (1980) Refractive errors and other findings in school children. *Acta Ophthalmol.* **58**, 129–136.

Lin, L. L.-K. and Ko, L.-S. (1988) The effect of distance gazing and eyeball exercise on the prevention of myopia progression. In: *Myopia Workshop* (H. C. Fledelius and E. Goldschmidt, eds). *Acta Ophthalmol.* Suppl 185, **66**, 139–140.

Lin, L. L.-K., Chen, C.-J., Hung, P.-T. and Ko, L.-S. (1988) Nation-wide survey of myopia among schoolchildren in Taiwan, 1986. In: *Myopia Workshop* (H. C. Fledelius and E. Goldschmidt, eds). *Acta Ophthalmol.* Suppl. 185, **66**, 29–33.

Maddock, R. J., Millodot, M., Leat, S. and Johnson, C. A. (1981) Accommodation responses and refractive error. *Invest. Ophthal. Vis. Sci.* **20**, 387–391.

Mandell, R. B. (1959) Myopia control with bifocal correction. *Am. J. Optom. Arch. Am. Acad. Optom.* **36**, 652–658.

Miles, P. W. (1962) A study of heterophoria and myopia in children, some of whom wore bifocal lenses. *Am. J. Ophthalmol.* **54**, 111–114.

Morgan, M. W. (1944) Analysis of clinical data. *Am. J. Optom. Arch. Am. Acad. Optom.* **21**, 477–491.

Neetens, A. and Evans, P. (1985) The use of bifocals as an alternative in the management of low grade myopia. *Bull. Soc. Belge Ophthalmol.* **214**, 79–85.

Oakley, K. A. and Young, F. A. (1975) Bifocal control of myopia. *Am. J. Optom. Physiol. Opt.* **52**, 758–764.

Parsinnen, O. and Hemminki, E. (1988) Spectacle use, bifocals, and prevention of myopic progression–two years' results of a randomized trial among schoolchildren. In: *Myopia Workshop* (H. C. Fledelius and E. Goldschmidt, eds). *Acta Ophthalmol.* Suppl. 185, **66**, 156–161.

Parsinnen, O., Hemminki, E. and Klemetti, A. (1989) Effect of spectacle use and accommodation on myopic progression: final results of a three-year randomized

clinical trial among schoolchildren. *Br. J. Ophthalmol.* **73**, 747–751.

Perrigin, J., Perrigin, D. M. and Grosvenor, T. (1982) A comparison of clinical refractive data obtained by three examiners. *Am. J. Optom. Physiol. Opt.* **59**, 515–519.

Rehm, D. (1975) The Myopter Viewer: an instrument for treating and preventing myopia. *Am. J. Optom. Physiol. Opt.* **52**, 347–350.

Rehm, D. S. (1981) *The Myopia Myth.* Braden Press.

Roberts, W. L. and Banford, R. D. (1963) Evaluation of bifocal correction technique in juvenile myopia. O.D. dissertation, Massachusetts College of Optometry.

Roberts, W. L. and Banford, R. D. (1967) Evaluation of bifocal correction technique in juvenile myopia. *Optom. Weekly* **58**(38), 25–31; (39), 21–30; (40), 23–28; (41), 27–34; (43), 19–26.

Rosenfield, M. (1994) Accommodation and myopia, are they related? *J. Behavioral Optom.* **5**, 3–11, 25.

Rosenfield, M. (1997) Tonic vergence and vergence adaptation. *Optom. Vis. Sci.* **74**, 303–328.

Schwartz, J. T. (1976) A monozygotic cotwin control study of a treatment for myopia. *Acta Genet. Med. Gemellol.* **25**, 133–136.

Schwartz, J. T. (1981) Results of a monozygotic cotwin control study on a treatment for myopia. In: *Twin Research 3: Epidemiological and Clinical Studies.* Liss, pp. 249–258.

Shepard, C. F. (1946) The Baltimore project. *Optom. Weekly* **37**, 133–135.

Tokoro, T. and Kabe, S. (1964) Treatment of the myopia and the changes in optical components. Report 1. Topical application of neosynephrine and tropicamide. *Acta Soc. Ophthalmol. Jpn* **68**, 1958–1961.

Tokoro, T. and Kabe, S. (1965) Treatment of the myopia and the changes in optical components. Report II. Full- or under-correction of myopia by glasses. *Acta Soc. Ophthalmol. Jpn* **69**, 140–144.

Trachtman, J. N. (1978) Biofeedback of accommodation to reduce functional myopia: a case report. *Am. J. Optom. Physiol. Opt.* **55**, 400–406.

Trachtman, J. N. (1992) Biofeedback training for myopia control (Letter to the editor). *Optom. Vis. Sci.* **69**, 252–254.

Walton, W. G. (1946) Two case histories of orthoptic training to improve visual acuity. *Am. J. Optom. Arch. Am. Acad. Optom.* **23**, 526–529.

Woods, A. C. (1945) Report from the Wilmer Institute on the results obtained in treatment of myopia by visual training. *Trans. Am. Acad. Ophthalmol. Otolaryngol.* **49**, 37–65.

Young, F. A., Leary, G. A., Grosvenor, T. *et al.* (1985) Houston myopia control study: a randomized clinical trial. Part 1. Background and design of the study. *Am. J. Optom. Physiol. Opt.* **62**, 605–613.

10

Myopia and nearwork: causation or merely association?

Mark Rosenfield and Bernard Gilmartin

This book has sought to consider the proposal that the performance of sustained nearwork leads to the development of myopia; a condition which affects billions of people worldwide, and has substantial socio-economic and public health implications. There are few topics in ocular physiology which evoke more controversy than the suggestion that nearwork is a precursor to the development or progression of myopia (Curtin, 1985). Indeed, trying to extricate genetic from environmental factors in the aetiology of this refractive error is an onerous task. There is compelling evidence for the influence of heredity, as demonstrated by the similar prevalence levels observed amongst monozygotic twins when compared with dizygotic twins (Waardenberg, 1950; Sorsby *et al.*, 1963; Goldschmidt, 1968; Borish, 1970; Karlsson, 1974). Additionally, Zadnik *et al.* (1994) noted that children with two myopic parents had longer axial lengths and less hyperopia than children with one or no myopic parents, even before the onset of myopia. While there seems little doubt that myopia has a strong hereditary component, this book has examined the evidence as to whether environmental influences in general, and nearwork in particular, also act as a catalyst for myopic development. As suggested by Raviola and Wiesel (1985), while the refractive state of the eye may be programmed on a genetic basis, visual experiences may disrupt the process of ocular growth and influence the refractive error, that is, a genetic propensity to myopia can be modulated by the visual environment. A particular problem is that it may not be possible to separate genetic from environmental factors completely, since family members share not only common genetic backgrounds but also similar environmental experiences (Framingham Offspring Eye Study Group, 1996). Accordingly, this concluding chapter weighs up the current evidence for the proposal that myopia results from prolonged periods of nearwork, speculates on possible mechanisms whereby the two might be related and considers what conclusions are appropriate in the light of our present knowledge base.

10.1 Myopia and nearwork are associated

10.1.1 Occupational evidence

The association between the development of myopia and the performance of sustained near-vision tasks dates back at least to Kepler, who noted in 1604 that people who used their eyes a great deal for reading and writing tended to become myopic (Duke-Elder and Abrams, 1970). Many subsequent studies have demonstrated that higher prevalences of myopia are associated with tasks involving significant amounts of nearwork. However, as Zadnik and Mutti indicated in Chapter 2, care must be taken to differentiate between association and causation. Simply because nearwork appears to be associated with myopia does not prove that one causes the other. For example, Zadnik and Mutti noted the potential confounding effect of intelligence, whereby subjects with higher intelligence levels might spend more time reading. If intelligence is indeed an inherited characteristic, then the inheritance of both myopia and intelligence may be associated, with the result that those individuals who exhibit inherited myopia may also read more than average. This might also at least partially explain why some individuals whose visual requirements demand substantial periods of near-work do not become myopic: they may lack the genetic predisposition to undergo axial elongation. It should also be noted that studies examining a possible association between intelligence and myo-pia have reported mixed results (for review, *see* Curtin, 1985), although both Rosner and Belkin (1987) and Teasdale *et al.* (1988) observed that the prevalence of myopia increased with intelligence test score. However, increasing intelligence did not correlate with the degree of refractive error for myopia greater than 2.0 D (Teasdale *et al.*, 1988).

Furthermore, any hypothesis must also account for the lower prevalence of myopia in occupations such as fine-work craftsmen when compared with university students (*see* Table 2.3; Tscherning, 1882; Goldschmidt, 1968). The tasks performed by the craftsmen will require substantial amounts of nearwork, necessitating accurate accommodation, although some are performed monocularly, thereby eliminating the need for accurate convergence. One explanation may be that the visual require-ments (e.g. the magnitude and duration of accom-modative and vergence demands) found in these occupations are more varied, when compared with, for example, a video display terminal (VDT) oper-ator, whose visual working distance may remain relatively fixed for several hours. Another possibil-ity is that the mental effort, intellectual demand and psychological stress associated with craft workers and artists is significantly different from that required of the university student, lawyer or accountant. For example, Shulkin and Bari (1986) reported that the prevalence of myopia amongst medical and art students was 70% and 36.5%, respectively. These differences would suggest that myopia may not simply result from a cumulation of 'dioptre-hours' over time.

The dramatic increase in computer utilization in recent years, both in the workplace and domestic environment, has led many practitioners to suggest that VDT use may be associated with the develop-ment or progression of myopia. However, a review of the literature by Mutti and Zadnik (1996) noted a high prevalence of asthenopia amongst computer users but no clear evidence of any association with myopia progression. Furthermore, two reports by Yeow and Taylor (1989, 1991) examined changes

in refractive error and visual acuity in groups of VDT and non-VDT workers over both short- (2–4 hours) and long-term (2-year monitoring period) intervals, and observed no significant difference in these parameters between the two occupational groups. More recently, Cole *et al.* (1996) reported that a population of computer users were signifi-cantly more myopic than the control group (mean difference = 0.35 D, standard deviation not pro-vided), but the authors did not feel that this differ-ence was clinically significant. Rather, they considered that the difference in refractive error may have resulted from the sample population, i.e., that myopes either tend to select, or alternatively are selected for occupations involving VDTs (Cole *et al.*, 1996).

10.1.2 Educational evidence

The higher prevalence of myopia associated with increased educational demands also suggests that nearwork produces myopia. For example, a retro-spective study by O'Neal and Connon (1987) assessed refractive error development in 497 cadets (ages on entry ranged from 17 to 21 years of age) at the United States Air Force Academy. This programme was considered to be academically challenging, with a graduation rate of approxi-mately 67%. After 2.5 years of attendance at the Academy, a myopic shift of at least 0.50 D was observed in 21%, 25% and 55% of eyes classified initially as being hyperopic, emmetropic and myopic, respectively.

Later, Zylbermann *et al.* (1993) examined the prevalence of myopia amongst male and female Jewish students (between 14 and 18 years of age) who attended either general or Orthodox religious schools. Whilst the prevalence of myopia was sim-ilar for students of both genders who attended the general schools and for females attending the Orthodox schools (prevalence rates for these three groups varied between 27 and 36%), the preva-lence of myopia in males attending the Orthodox schools was 81.3%. The authors suggested that this higher level was due to the fact that the Orthodox males studied religious texts for up to 16 hours a day, with some type being as small as 1 mm in height. Additionally, many of these students have a habit of swaying back and forth during studying (*shokling*), thereby necessitating constant changes in both the accommodation and vergence responses which would be substantial at close working distances. Since the male and female Orthodox students are likely to have similar diet, intelligence and genetic characteristics and had equivalent mean ages, then the most likely explanation for the high prevalence of myopia amongst the male Orthodox population would appear to be related to their prolonged studying. However, it remains unclear whether the myopia was produced by the extended periods of nearwork, or by the constant changes in oculomotor stimuli.

Other investigations which have reported myopia to be associated with increased educational demands may also have been confounded by non-visual factors. For example, Young *et al.* (1969) examined the prevalence of myopia amongst Eskimo families. They investigated 41 family units in Barrow, Alaska comprising 197 subjects. It was noted that the Eskimo families consisted of parents who were illiterate, while their children had learned to read and were required to attend schools comparable to those in the contiguous USA. Young *et al.* observed that out of 130 parents, only two were clearly myopic. The remaining parents had refractive errors between emmetropia and 3.00 D of hyperopia, with the majority having hyperopia greater than 1.50 D. However, around 60% of the schoolchildren examined were myopic. Whilst the increased near-visual demands are the obvious explanation for the change in refractive status, other factors besides schoolwork may have been related to the increased myopia in the Eskimo children, such as the introduction of a Western type diet. Young *et al.* suggested that as the refractive changes occurred in the offspring but not in the parents, then it is unlikely that a change in diet played a major role in myopic development. However, the degree of susceptibility to refractive error development varies with age, since ametropia tends to become more stable during the adult years (Curtin, 1985). It does seem improbable that these generational differences can be accounted for by variations in intelligence or other inherited characteristics. Other factors such as an increase in lifestyle stress and anxiety, or a switch from a mobile outdoor lifestyle to more sedentary indoor activities may also be associated with the reported change in refractive error.

Furthermore, as stated by Zadnik and Mutti in Chapter 2, attempting to estimate accurately the amount of nearwork performed by an individual is extremely difficult. Indeed, Schaeffel and Howland (1995) stated that unless the degree of exposure to nearwork can be quantified (in terms of both magnitude and duration), one cannot reliably conclude that nearwork produces myopia. Quantifying years of education is inadequate, since it will be confounded by intelligence and socio-economic status. The latter is also associated with variations in diet and physical wellbeing. An additional factor to consider is that rather than myopes performing more nearwork, it may be that emmetropes and particularly hyperopes perform less, possibly due to their higher accommodative demands. A common clinical impression is that many myopic individuals remove their refractive correction during sustained nearwork, thereby reducing further the blur-driven accommodative stimulus. Thus myopes may be able to perform near tasks for longer periods of time than other refractive groups, resulting in greater educational success. Tiffin (1943) demonstrated that the production of hosiery loopers increased with declining distance visual acuity, with the most experienced workers being approximately 3.0 D myopic. This might imply that the presence of uncorrected myopia improves occupational visual efficiency.

A further investigation linking the development of myopia with occupational demands necessitating substantial amounts of nearwork was that of McBrien and Adams (1997), who measured refractive error development on a longitudinal basis over a 2-year period in clinical microscopists. The sample population was aged between 21 and 63 years, i.e., significantly older than the previously reported age of cessation of ocular growth (Goldschmidt, 1968). Of the 95 eyes that were emmetropic at the start of the study, 37 eyes (39%) underwent an increase in myopia of at least 0.37 D, with 23 eyes (24%) becoming clinically myopic (i.e., having a refractive error of at least 0.37 D of myopia). The remaining 14 eyes initially had small amounts of hyperopia (up to 0.625 D), hence their myopic shift did not render them clinically myopic. The structural correlate associated with the myopic shift was an increase in vitreous chamber depth, with no significant change in corneal curvature or crystalline lens power being observed. It is also of interest to note that the median age of myopia onset for previously emmetropic subjects who developed clinical myopia was 26.3 years with a range of 22–42 years. This finding confirms that myopia may become manifest at any time during young adulthood.

10.1.3 Increased prevalance of myopia in younger generations

Additional indirect evidence for the association between myopia and nearwork may be drawn from those studies which have reported that the prevalence of myopia observed amongst population cohorts between 20 and 40 years of age is significantly higher than for older population groups (Johnson *et al.*, 1979; Fledelius, 1983; Aine, 1984; Dib, 1990; Goh and Lam, 1994; Lam *et al.*, 1994; Framingham Offspring Eye Study Group, 1996). For example, the Framingham Offspring Eye Study Group (1996) indicated that, for both sexes, the prevalence of myopia decreased from about 60% for subjects between 23 and 34 years of age to 20% for subjects over 65 years of age. This decline could result from either a hyperopic shift with increasing age, or increased prevalence of myopia in the younger subjects. The Framingham study noted that myopia does not usually improve over time, and indeed Hirsch (1958) reported that the prevalence of myopia increased from 6.7% at 45 years of age to 15.3% at 75 years of age or older. Hirsch attributed this increase in myopia to changes in the crystalline lens. Additionally, a longitudinal investigation of refractive changes between 20 and 40 years of age (Grosvenor, 1977a, 1977b) indicated that only 11 out of the 111 subjects examined (10%) exhibited a decrease in myopia (or more hyperopia) of at least 0.50 D over the 20-year period, whereas 16 subjects (14%) showed an increase in myopia (or less hyperopia) and 84 individuals (76%) demonstrated no change in refractive status greater than ±0.50 D.

Accordingly, one must conclude that there is no evidence for a marked hyperopic shift after 40 years of age, and that the prevalence of myopia has indeed increased in recent generations. This would strongly suggest an environmental cause. The question therefore becomes what external factor has changed most over the past 50 years? The investigation of Young *et al.* (1969) noted that the prevalence of myopia increased following the introduction of formal schooling, a proposal which has been supported elsewhere (Peckham *et al.*, 1977; Richler and Bear, 1980a, 1980b; Au Eong *et al.*, 1993a, 1993b; Pärssinen and Lyyra, 1993). Increased nearwork would certainly appear to be the most compelling explanation for the increased prevalence of myopia in younger subgroups.

Thus the epidemiological finding of a higher prevalence of myopia amongst those occupations requiring substantial amounts of nearwork (e.g. university students, military cadets and microscopists), combined with the observation of increasing numbers of myopes amongst younger generations, provide support for the proposal that nearwork produces myopia.

10.2 Mechanisms linking nearwork and myopia

Whilst a number of aetiological models based upon various components of the near-vision response have been proposed, the evidence for many of them is indirect and circumstantial. Variations in accommodation (*see* Chapter 5), intraocular pressure (Chapters 3, 5 and 6), autonomic balance (Chapter 6) and vergence (Chapter 7) have been cited as possible mechanisms, yet, in common with all putative models of myopia development, it is still uncertain whether, or how, any of them could produce vitreous chamber elongation, which has been demonstrated to be the structural change producing almost all myopia (Chapter 3).

10.2.1 Evidence from animal studies

The animal studies reviewed by Smith in Chapter 4 confirm that myopia can be induced by changes in the visual environment. Three procedures have been used principally to induce experimental myopia, namely: restriction to a close viewing distance (Young, 1961; Miles and Wallman, 1990), form deprivation (Raviola and Wiesel, 1985; Wallman, 1991) and the introduction of negative spectacle lenses (Schaeffel *et al.*, 1988; Irving *et al.*, 1992). These animal studies have provided results which were unlikely to have been observed in human investigations where laboratory controlled manipulations of visual experience could not have been undertaken (Schaeffel and Howland, 1995). A key question for this chapter to address is how these animal studies might be related to nearwork-induced myopia in humans.

Wallman *et al.* (1987) speculated that since printed text largely consists of achromatic text containing only high spatial frequencies at a relatively small range of luminance levels, then the non-foveal retina would receive reduced stimulation during reading which might result in form deprivation. However, a more likely explanation might be that axial elongation results from extended periods of hyperopic retinal defocus, i.e., when the image of the object of regard lies posterior to the retina. This concept will be explored further in Section 10.2.2. However, caution must be exercised when associating experimentally induced myopia in animals with refractive error development in humans. In a comprehensive review of this topic, Zadnik and Mutti (1995) listed three specific factors suggesting difficulties in applying the animal findings to human juvenile and young-adult-onset myopia.

Firstly, the degree of visual deprivation provided in the animal studies with either translucent occluders or lid suture provides a much greater degree of contrast reduction when compared with anything typically found in the naturalistic human visual experience.

Secondly, the sensitive period for producing myopia in animal models does not correspond with the typical age for the development of nearwork-induced myopia in humans. For example, Zadnik and Mutti noted that the sensitive period in primates corresponds to between birth and 7 years of age in humans (Young, 1961).

Studies investigating changes in refractive error in humans between these ages have reported somewhat inconsistent findings. For example, Gwiazda *et al.* (1993a) in a longitudinal observation of 72 children reported a mean increase in hyperopia between birth and 1 year of age, but subsequently the mean ametropia remained relatively stable until around 7 or 8 years of age. Mean refractive stability has also been reported using cross-sectional data between 5 and 7 years of age (Zadnik *et al.*, 1993) and between 3 and 5 years of age (Sorsby *et al.*, 1961). In contrast, Brown (1938) observed an increase in hyperopia each year between birth and 7 years of age. Most investigators of myopia which appears to be related to nearwork have assumed that this would become manifest at an age where nearwork demands (e.g. schooling) become substantial, typically after 14 years of age. One might question whether this is reasonable, since children under 5 years of age undoubtedly spend much of their time performing near-visual activities requiring significant amounts of accommodation and convergence, although possibly of lower cognitive demand. Nevertheless, many studies where myopia has been induced, particularly in chicks, have been performed on neonatal animals. However, a recent report has documented the development of form-deprivation myopia in 1-year-old chicks (approximately equivalent to a 30-year-old human, Wildsoet, personal communication), although the growth response was attenuated (Papastergiou *et al.*, 1997).

Thirdly, the ocular response in chicks to the imposed retinal defocus produced by ophthalmic lenses appears to be mediated, at least in the initial stages, by changes in choroidal thickness (Wallman *et al.*, 1992; Wildsoet and Wallman, 1995), although subsequent growth of the sclera makes the refractive changes more permanent and allows the choroid to return to its original thickness (Wildsoet, 1997). Zadnik and Mutti (1995) suggested that changes in choroidal thickness are not significant factors in human refractive error development, although this has not been tested directly. An investigation of human myopic eyes using magnetic resonance imaging (MRI) revealed a mean difference in choroidal thickness between groups of hyperopes and myopes of only 0.4 mm (equivalent to approximately 1.3 D), whereas the mean difference in refractive error was 10.25 D (Cheng *et al.*, 1992).

Interestingly, Reiner *et al.* (1995) demonstrated that myopia induced in chicks by ocular occlusion was accompanied by a reduction in choroidal blood flow resulting from a decline in the volume of the choroidal vascular bed. Choroidal blood flow was still reduced in chicks whose occluders had been removed for 2 days before measurements were taken. Additionally, when choroidal blood flow was reduced in chicks by transecting the choroidal nerves, no significant change in axial length was observed. Thus decreases in choroidal blood flow do not promote ocular growth, but rather, the axial elongation associated with visual deprivation leads to reduced choroidal blood flow.

Reiner *et al.* also reported the effect of instilling either intravitreal or subconjunctival nicotine in the chick eye to stimulate prolonged accommodation. Chick ciliary muscle is striated, and hence an increase in accommodation will result from the agonist action of nicotine on nicotinic receptors. The administered dose was found to produce an accommodative response of between 1 and 2 D that lasted approximately 4–6 hours. Daily subconjunctival nicotine produced a small increase in myopia (mean = 0.75 D) in the treated eye, whereas intravitreal nicotine did not produce any significant change in refractive error. The authors indicated that these findings may provide preliminary support for the notion that excessive periods of accommodation may lead to myopic development. In considering why intravitreal nicotine failed to stimulate refractive changes, Reiner *et al.* suggested that the direct effect of nicotine on the retina may have interfered with vitreal elongation.

It should also be noted that the degree of form-deprivation myopia (and associated morphological degenerative changes) induced in chicks very rapidly reaches orders of magnitude that would be considered pathological in humans. For example, Wallman and Adams (1987) observed up to 20.0 D of myopia after just 2 weeks of form deprivation.

Furthermore, the ability to recover from induced refractive errors declines with both increasing age and species, being slower in primates for example, when compared with chicks, although the degree of ametropia induced in primates by visual deprivation is also lower in magnitude (*see* Chapter 4).

In noting the absence of a clearly defined physiological process linking nearwork with myopic development in humans (*see* section 10.1), it must be pointed out that the precise mechanism whereby visual degradation in animals leads to axial elongation is also uncertain (Reiner *et al.*, 1995). Further, the mechanisms responsible for deprivation myopia appear to be different from those associated with axial elongation following retinal defocus (Schaeffel *et al.*, 1994; Schaeffel and Howland, 1995; Zadnik and Mutti, 1995). Additionally, the visual demands of neonatal chicks and primates are clearly very different from the varying oculomotor, cognitive and intellectual stimuli encountered by, for example, the student or medical microscopist. It will be clear that there are many discrepancies when attempting to make inferences from these animal models to human nearwork-induced myopia, although some mechanisms may be common to both.

Nevertheless, these investigations of environmentally induced myopia in animals have demonstrated the presence of a so-called emmetropizing process, whereby the axial length of the eye is adjusted to focus emergent rays from the object of regard onto the retina (Wildsoet, 1997). As noted by Wildsoet in Chapter 3, the term emmetropization may be inappropriate, since the distance which is desired to be conjugate with the retina in the absence of accommodation may not lie at optical infinity. The data illustrated in Figure 4.1 clearly demonstrate that a variety of different ground-foraging species have developed varying degrees of lower-field myopia which correspond closely with the height of the eye above the ground. The results of lens-induced myopia in animals suggest that the sign of the retinal defocus can be determined, with axial elongation occurring when the image of the object of regard is posterior to the retina. However, as noted in section 5.9.1, inconsistent results have been found, with both inter- and intra-species variations being reported. Notwithstanding these differences, the animal myopia studies may provide great insight into the biochemical and histological changes taking place during axial elongation, which might parallel those occurring in human myopia, and may ultimately lead to a pharmacological treatment designed to control or prevent myopic development.

10.2.2 Evidence from human studies

Several recent reports (e.g. Goss, 1988; Goss and Wickham, 1995; Ong and Ciuffreda, 1997) have suggested that the presence of retinal defocus during periods of nearwork may be the most likely environmental factor to stimulate myopic development (*see* Section 5.9.1). This notion is consistent with those animal studies which demonstrated that when the conjugate point to an object of regard lies posterior to the retina (i.e., hyperopic defocus), relative axial elongation occurs to image these rays onto the retina (Schaeffel *et al.*, 1988; Irving *et al.*, 1991, 1992).

Similarly, when the conjugate point to the fixation target lies anterior to the retina (myopic defocus), axial growth is attenuated to restore the quality of the retinal image (*see* Chapters 3 and 4). Could a similar mechanism be operating in young-adult humans? One possibility that has been proposed is that an increased lag of accommodation during the course of a sustained near task would create hyperopic defocus (McBrien and Millodot, 1986; Rosenfield and Gilmartin, 1988a; Gwiazda *et al.*, 1993b, 1995). Interestingly, examinations of clinical records by Goss (1991) and Portello *et al.* (1997) both reported an increased lag of accommodation in patients before they developed clinical myopia. However, it must also be noted that most young individuals are constantly varying their accommodative response, so that the position of the point conjugate with the retina may never remain in a single location for an extended period of time.

If the presence of retinal defocus does indeed stimulate refractive development, then this would have significant implications with regard to the correction of ametropia. The hyperopic individual may benefit from being at least partially uncorrected, with the image of an object of regard focused posterior to the retina, since subsequent axial elongation may attenuate the refractive error. Indeed, both Dobson *et al.* (1986) and Ingram *et al.* (1991) reported that infants wearing a full-time hyperopic correction tended to remain hyperopic, in contrast with those individuals whose hyperopia remained uncorrected. Thus the correction of hyperopia in young infants may interfere with the emmetropization process (Medina, 1987; Hung *et al.*, 1995). However, this proposal must be interpreted with extreme caution, since uncorrected hyperopia in children may lead to reduced visual acuity at both distance and near, as well as the development of strabismus, amblyopia, decreased visual perceptual skills and learning disabilities (Grisham and Simons, 1986; Rosner and Rosner, 1986).

In contrast, the defocus hypothesis would suggest that hyperopic retinal defocus must be avoided in the emmetropic or myopic patient. This may be particularly critical at near, where bifocals may be prescribed to reduce, but not necessarily eliminate the lag of accommodation. In order to ensure accurate focusing on a near object of regard, subjects should be cyclopleged and provided with a near addition lens. Additionally, the dilated pupil will minimize the depth-of-focus for the period of cycloplegia. Thus, subjects would typically require a +2.50 or +3.00 D near addition for close work. A similar protocol was reported by Brodstein *et al.* (1984), whereby 435 myopic children were fitted with +2.25 D add bifocals and given one drop of 1% atropine into each eye every morning. The control group consisted of 146 myopic children, who wore single-vision lenses and did not receive atropine. The treatment group progressed at a mean rate of 0.16 D per year during the treatment period (average duration = 33 months) and 0.39 D/yr after treatment, for a mean progression rate of 0.23 D/yr. The control group progressed at a mean rate of 0.25 D/yr (average duration = 49 months). Thus, these results do not provide convincing support for this procedure to control myopic progression.

It must also be noted that a lag of accommodation having magnitude within the depth-of-field of the eye (typically around ±0.3 D; Campbell, 1957; Charman and Whitefoot, 1977) is the expected finding when viewing a near target (Morgan, 1944; Heath, 1956). Thus hyperopic retinal defocus is found in most individuals during nearwork. One might therefore ask why nearwork-induced myopia is not a universal finding? Additionally, the overcorrection of myopia would also induce hyperopic defocus, and therefore might also be expected to stimulate myopic development. However, in a prospective clinical trial (Goss, 1984), 36 myopic children between 7 and 16 years of age were overcorrected by 0.75 D, while a control group of 36 myopic children (matched for age, sex and initial amount of myopia) received a full refractive correction. Most members of the experimental group were overcorrected for a period of 1.5–2 years, although a few were overcorrected for less

than 1 year. Mean annual rates of myopic progression assessed by subjective refraction for the experimental and control groups were 0.52 D/yr and 0.47 D/yr, respectively. This difference was not statistically significant. Interestingly, the overcorrected female subjects exhibited a significantly higher rate of myopic progression when compared with the female controls (0.64 D/yr versus 0.35 D/yr) while the overcorrected males demonstrated a lower, but not significantly different, rate to the male controls (mean rates of 0.40 and 0.58 D/yr for the male experimental and control groups, respectively). However, the amount of nearwork performed by the two groups may not have been equivalent.

The range of results cited above fails to provide convincing evidence that the presence of a relatively large lag of accommodation to a sustained near target is the primary cause of myopic development. However, an extended hypothesis (*see* Section 10.4) is that reduced accommodative adaptation during a sustained near-vision task might represent the primary phase of refractive error development, which would also produce the secondary effect of an increased lag of accommodation to a sustained near stimulus.

10.2.3 Late-onset myopia

Although myopia often stabilizes around the age of 15 years, a significant number of individuals exhibit myopia for the first time later in life. Late- or young-adult onset myopia typically appears in the late teens or early and middle twenties and has no clear hereditary basis (Goss and Winkler, 1983; Grosvenor, 1987; O'Neal and Connon, 1987; National Research Council, 1989; Baldwin *et al.*, 1991). Young-adult onset myopia constitutes around 8% of all myopia, although a prevalence of approximately 25% has been proposed (Fledelius, 1995). It develops over a relatively short period of time, and frequently stabilizes at low dioptric levels of around 1.5 D. Nevertheless, magnitudes of up to 4 D or more are not uncommon (Adams, 1987; Fledelius, 1995) and have allowed ocular biometric studies to demonstrate that the principal structural correlate for both early- and late-onset myopia is increased vitreous chamber depth (McBrien and Millodot, 1987; Bullimore *et al.*, 1992; Grosvenor and Scott, 1991, 1993; Fledelius, 1995; McBrien and Adams, 1997).

Attention has been drawn to late-onset myopia in many studies that have investigated the association between near vision and accommodation, as its incidence often appears to be directly linked with an occupational requirement for significant amounts of nearwork, or alternatively to a change in visual demands within the workplace. A consequence of this association is that the condition has been attributed principally to the influence of the visual environment (Goldschmidt, 1968; McBrien and Adams, 1997), although predisposing genetic factors should not be discounted.

A full account of the accommodative characteristics of late-onset myopia is given in Chapter 5 and indicates that there is no consensus as to whether the group can genuinely be distinguished in this regard from emmetropia or other categories of myopia. Nevertheless, it is likely that late-onset myopia will continue to figure in future research studies on myopia and nearwork. In experimental terms, the category has special advantages in comparison with early-onset myopes. It is readily accessible to researchers (often being drawn from the student population), can participate effectively in relatively complex experimental procedures, and can comply more readily with the strictures of ethical requirements for studies that require informed consent for special investigative procedures.

10.2.4 Anisomyopia

When evaluating the likelihood of a potential association between the performance of nearwork and the development of myopia, a further condition that must also be accounted for is that of anisomyopia, i.e., where one eye is either emmetropic or hyperopic and the other myopic, or where the eyes have differing amounts of myopia. Anisomyopes, like bilateral myopes, demonstrate a structural correlate whereby the interocular difference in refractive error corresponds with a difference in axial length between the two eyes (Sorsby *et al.*, 1962; Fledelius, 1981; Logan *et al.*, 1995). The prevalence in the general population of anisomyopia greater than 2 D is approximately 1.0–1.5%, and this condition is around two to three times more common than anisohyperopia (Jampolsky *et al.*, 1955; Schapero, 1971). In an investigation of anisometropia in strabismic Taiwanese children, Chang and Lin (1992) observed that out of 521 exotropic patients, the prevalance of anisomyopia increased with the degree of ametropia. Thus, 21.3% of the low myopes (between 0.25 and 3.00 D) and 45% of the moderate and high myopes (more than 3.00 D) had anisometropia greater than 2.00 D.

In infants, anisomyopia may arise from differences in the rate of ocular growth (which may correspond with differences in the rate of emmetropization). Additionally, anisomyopes exhibit marked interocular differences in fundus morphology, for example, scleral crescents and generalized tessellation of the fundus are often more marked in the more myopic eye.

It is unclear how anisomyopia could result from differences in accommodation since the accommodative response is generally regarded as being consensual. One possibility is that anisomyopes have previously adopted asymmetrical convergence during nearwork, so that the forces exerted on the globe by the extraocular muscles differ between the two eyes. However, with our current knowledge it is difficult to explain anisomyopia on the basis of nearwork activity.

10.3 Effect of distance fixation during or after nearwork

Refractive changes which might result from sustained near visual activities may also be modified by intervals of distance fixation either during or immediately following nearwork. For example, does distance viewing with minimal accommodation and vergence ameliorate the effects of nearwork? If this is the case, then how much distance viewing is required to counteract each dioptre-hour of nearwork? Napper *et al.* (1995) observed that 130 minutes of normal visual exposure per day was sufficient to reduce occlusion-induced myopia in chicks by 95%. This finding would suggest that if nearwork does indeed stimulate axial elongation, then relatively short periods of distance viewing might be sufficient to prevent myopic development.

Patients are commonly advised to take frequent breaks during sustained near vision, and to view a far target during these rest periods (Birnbaum, 1993). While it is difficult to argue against this advice, which seems likely, as a minimum, to reduce the degree of asthenopia, it would be of interest to determine whether the duration of nearwork activity does indeed have a cumulative effect over time. Again, the difficulty in quantifying nearwork accurately is apparent. Ong and Ciuffreda (1997) have suggested that the myopic retinal defocus (resulting from sustained accommodative adaptation) occurring when individuals view a distant target following sustained near fixation may also be a precursor to axial elongation. While the sign of the defocus would appear to be inappropriate to stimulate axial elongation, Ong and Ciuffreda suggested that its magnitude may be insufficient to provide directional information. Accordingly, all small amounts of retinal defocus might stimulate axial elongation. Thus, myopia could develop from a combination of the hyperopic retinal defocus occurring during the near task, and the myopic defocus exhibited during distance fixation immediately following nearwork (Ong and Ciuffreda, 1995, 1997).

10.4 Could reduced accommodative adaptation lead to myopic development?

The primary cause of nearwork-induced myopia might be associated with the absence of an efficient slow blur-driven accommodative response (SBAR), thereby resulting in reduced accommodative adaptation. Accommodative adaptation reflects the maintained output of SBAR and is most commonly assessed immediately following the removal of a sustained accommodative stimulus. The aggregate blur-driven accommodative response can be subdivided into two temporal components: a fast component which acts rapidly (typically within 1 s) to reduce retinal defocus, and a slow component which acts to maintain the overall blur-driven accommodative response over an extended period of time (Rosenfield and Gilmartin, 1989). According to the model of accommodation–vergence interaction proposed by Schor (1980), the stimulus for SBAR is the sustained output of the fast blur-driven accommodative response (FBAR). When a blur stimulus is introduced, the initial response is mediated via FBAR. However, if this stimulus is maintained for a period of time greater than approximately 30 s (Törnqvist, 1967; Rosenfield and Gilmartin, 1989; Fisher *et al.*, 1990), then the sustained FBAR will initiate SBAR. This onset of SBAR is accompanied by a simultaneous reduction in FBAR in order to maintain the aggregate accommodative response relatively constant.

It has also been demonstrated that the output of SBAR normally serves to reduce the magnitude of the lag of accommodation (Schor *et al.*, 1986; Rosenfield and Gilmartin, 1998), thereby increasing the accuracy of the accommodative response with respect to the stimulus demand (*see* Section 5.6.2). Accordingly, subjects lacking an efficient

SBAR (resulting in reduced accommodative adaptation) would exhibit a larger lag of accommodation, and hence increased retinal defocus during the course of a sustained near task, since their response would result exclusively from FBAR. This is consistent with the finding that myopic individuals demonstrate a reduced accommodative response to a near target both before (Goss, 1991; Portello *et al.*, 1997) and after (McBrien and Millodot, 1986; Rosenfield and Gilmartin, 1988a; Gwiazda *et al.*, 1993b) they develop manifest clinical myopia.

Furthermore, it appears that SBAR receives innervation from both the sympathetic and parasympathetic nervous systems, whereas FBAR is innervated by the parasympathetic system only (Gilmartin and Bullimore, 1987; Rosenfield and Gilmartin, 1989; Gilmartin and Winfield, 1995). Accordingly, subjects lacking adequate SBAR would also exhibit reduced sympathetic innervation to the ciliary muscle (*see* Chapter 6).

One might also predict that subjects having a reduced SBAR would be more likely to develop asthenopic symptoms. This proposal is based upon analogous findings in the vergence system, where symptomatic subjects almost invariably exhibited reduced vergence adaptation (North and Henson, 1981). It is not surprising that subjects with abnormal vergence adaptation should be symptomatic, since the role of the slow disparity vergence mechanism is to maintain the aggregate vergence response over time, thereby relieving the fast controller and making it available to respond to subsequent stimulus changes (Rosenfield and Gilmartin, 1989; Rosenfield, 1997). For those individuals with deficient slow disparity vergence mechanisms, the sustained response may either be maintained solely by the fast fusional controller, or alternatively by the fast controller in conjunction with an inefficient slow fusional controller. Either case may necessitate an increased output of fast fusional vergence, which in turn may lead to the development of symptoms, since the fast system is not designed to provide a sustained output over time. Thus excessive demand upon fast fusional vergence may be responsible for the development of asthenopia in patients lacking an adequate slow fusional vergence response (Rosenfield *et al.*, 1997). Similarly, excessive demand placed upon FBAR may also produce symptoms and ultimately lead to an adaptation designed to reduce the demand upon blur-driven accommodation, namely the development of myopia.

Additionally, Schor and Horner (1989) demonstrated that subjects with convergence excess, i.e., having esophoria at near while being relatively orthophoric at distance, generally exhibited poor accommodative adaptation and a high accommodative convergence to accommodation (AC/A) ratio. Based upon the model of accommodative–vergence interaction proposed by Schor (1983), the oculomotor crosslinks (i.e., accommodative convergence and convergent accommodation) receive input from the fast controllers only. Thus accommodative convergence would be innervated by FBAR, but not by SBAR. An alternative model proposed by both Ebenholtz and Fisher (1982) and Rosenfield and Gilmartin (1988b) suggested that the oculomotor crosslinks were innervated by both FBAR and SBAR. Nevertheless, for those individuals lacking an appropriate SBAR (and therefore having reduced accommodative adaptation), additional demand would be placed upon the FBAR, possibly resulting in an increased AC/A ratio and esophoria at near. Increased AC/A ratios have previously been demonstrated either in both early- and late-onset myopes (Rosenfield and Gilmartin, 1987a) or in early-onset myopes only (Rosenfield and Gilmartin, 1987b), when compared with emmetropic subjects. Interestingly, while attempts to control myopia progression by altering the demands placed upon accommodation have generally been disappointing (*see* Chapter 9), one exception appears to be those subjects who are esophoric at near (approximately 25% of the population between 10 and 20 years of age; Hirsch *et al.*, 1948). Bifocals appear to be more successful in controlling myopic progression in these individuals (*see* section 7.4), suggesting that their myopia may indeed be accommodative in origin and might be related to the absence of an appropriate SBAR. Indeed, a model of emmetropization proposed by Flitcroft and Eustace (1997) predicted that esophoria and reduced blur-driven accommodation should increase the tendency for late-onset myopia to develop.

Thus subjects having reduced SBAR are likely to exhibit a complex synthesis of (i) an increased lag of accommodation to a sustained near stimulus, (ii) reduced sympathetic input to accommodation, (iii) asthenopia, (iv) esophoria at near and (v) an increased AC/A ratio. Each of these five factors has previously been associated with the development of myopia in young adults (Curtin, 1985; Gilmartin and Bullimore, 1987; Rosenfield and Gilmartin, 1987a; Goss and Grosvenor, 1990; Gwiazda *et al.*, 1993b). The precise order whereby these changes take place over time is unclear, and some individuals may not exhibit all of the elements simultaneously. What also remains unclear, however, is how reduced SBAR could lead to axial elongation. As noted in section 5.9.1, it has been speculated that changes in retinal growth factors may result from the abnormal accommodative response. However, no direct linkage has been demonstrated to date in either human or animal studies.

10.5   Concluding comments

Despite the fact that myopia was identified by Aristotle (384–322 BC) more than 2300 years ago, practitioners are still unable to treat this form of refractive error adequately. In fact, 'Aristotle is generally thought to have been the first to provide data on myopia, in that he remarked that short-sighted people blinked and wrote a small hand' (Goldschmidt, 1968, p. 12).

Concave lenses may be used to restore visual acuity, but they fail to alter the progression of this condition. The key to appropriate treatment lies in a greater understanding of the physiological mechanisms which lead to the development of myopia. This book has sought to consider whether the performance of sustained nearwork produces myopia. However, we believe that our current state of knowledge does not allow us to reach a definitive answer to this question. Clearly myopia and nearwork are associated, but as noted earlier, attempts to prove causation may be confounded by a variety of other environmental factors. Furthermore, attempting to distinguish between genetic and environmental influences on refractive development is extremely difficult.

A future answer may come from the rapid progress being made in mapping the human genetic profile (Marshall, 1996). The genes producing such conditions as Huntington's disease (Claes *et al.*, 1995), Parkinson's disease (Polymeropoulos *et al.*, 1996), ovarian and breast cancer (Rubin *et al.*, 1996) have all been identified, and in time a myopia gene–or genes, if myopia exhibits a polymeric inheritance pattern (Goldschmidt, 1968)–may be identified. Should this transpire, then it will be possible to determine whether myopia occurs in those individuals not carrying the relevant genetic information, which would confirm an environmental aetiology. One must also consider which environmental factors other than nearwork could be associated with myopia development. For example, might variations in nutrition, intelligence, general fitness, psychological stress, physical immobility or systemic disease be associated with the onset of myopia? Additionally, ocular factors independent of nearwork such as ocular hypertension or disease in the posterior segment might also stimulate axial elongation. These topics have all been addressed but no consensus currently exists as to their specific role. An alternative hypothesis is that myopia may develop from multiple aetiological factors, one of which might be nearwork. Thus the performance of sustained near-visual activities, in conjunction with one or more additional stimuli, might provide the catalyst for the development of myopia.

In addition to the social and economic costs associated with the correction of myopia (which are now increasing even more rapidly due to the growing use of surgical intervention as a treatment modality), myopia is a leading cause of visual loss throughout the world. In view of the rapidly increasing prevalence of myopia associated with nearwork, it is crucial that we obtain a better understanding of the processes involved in its onset and development in order to evolve and apply effective procedures for its amelioration.

References

Adams, A. J. (1987) Axial length elongation, not corneal curvature, as a basis of adult onset myopia. *Am. J. Optom. Physiol. Opt.* **64**, 150–151.

Aine, E. (1984) Refractive errors in a Finnish rural population. *Acta Ophthalmol.* **62**, 944–954.

Au Eong, K. G., Tay, T. H. and Lim, M. K. (1993a) Race, culture and myopia in 110,236 young Singaporean males. *Singapore Med. J.* **34**, 29–32.

Au Eong, K. G., Tay, T. H. and Lim, M. K. (1993b) Education and myopia in 110,236 young Singaporean males. *Singapore Med. J.* **34**, 489–492.

Baldwin, W. R., Adams, A. J. and Flattau, P. (1991) Young adult myopia. In: *Refractive Anomalies: Research and Clinical Applications* (T. Grosvenor and M. C. Flom, eds). Butterworth-Heinemann, pp. 104–120.

Birnbaum, M. H. (1993) *Optometric Management of Nearpoint Vision Disorders*. Butterworth-Heinemann, pp. 307–309.

Borish, I. M. (1970) *Clinical Refraction*, 3rd edn. Professional Press, pp. 83–114.

Brodstein, R. S., Brodstein, D. E., Olson, R. J. *et al.* (1984) The treatment of myopia with atropine and bifocals. A long-term prospective study. *Ophthalmology* **91**, 1373–1379.

Brown, E. V. L. (1938) Net average yearly change in refraction of atropinized eyes from birth to beyond middle life. *Acta Ophthalmol.* **19**, 719–734.

Bullimore, M. A., Gilmartin, B. and Royston, J. M. (1992) Steady-state accommodation and ocular biometry in late-onset myopia. *Doc. Ophthalmol.* **80**, 143–155.

Campbell, F. W. (1957) The depth of field of the human eye. *Optica Acta* **4**, 157–164.

Chang, S.-W. and Lin, L. L.-K. (1992) Study of refractive status on strabismic patients in Taiwan. *Trans. Ophthalmol. Soc. Repub. China* **31**, 263–272.

Charman, W. N. and Whitefoot, H. (1977) Pupil diameter and the depth-of-field of the human eye as measured by laser speckle. *Optica Acta* **24**, 1211–1216.

Cheng, H. M., Singh, O. S., Kwong, K. K. *et al.* (1992) Shape of the myopic eye as seen with high-resolution magnetic resonance imaging. *Optom. Vis. Sci.* **69**, 698–701.

Claes, S., Van Zand, K., Legius, E. *et al.* (1995) Correlations between triplet repeat expansion and clinical features in Huntington's disease. *Arch. Neurol.* **113**, 749–753.

Cole, B. L., Maddocks, J. D. and Sharpe, K. (1996) Effect of VDUs on the eyes: report of a 6-year epidemiological study. *Optom. Vis. Sci.* **73**, 512–528.

Curtin, B. J. (1985) *The Myopias. Basic Science and Clinical Management*. Harper & Row.

Dib, A. (1990) Distribution of refractive errors in patients from Dominica, West Indies. *J. Am. Optom. Assoc.* **61**, 40–43.

Dobson, V., Sebris, S. L. and Carlson, M. R. (1986) Do glasses prevent emmetropization in strabismic infants? *Invest. Ophthalmol. Vis. Sci.* (Suppl.) **27**, 2.

Duke-Elder, S. and Abrams, D. (1970) *System of Ophthalmology*, Vol. V: *Ophthalmic Optics and Refraction*. C. V. Mosby.

Ebenholtz, S. M. and Fisher, S. K. (1982) Distance adaptation depends upon plasticity in the oculomotor control system. *Percept. Psychophys.* **31**, 551–560.

Fisher, S. K., Ciuffreda, K. J. and Bird, J. E. (1990) The effect of stimulus duration on tonic accommodation and tonic vergence. *Optom. Vis. Sci.* **67**, 441–449.

Fledelius, H. C. (1981) Refractive components in aniso- and isometropia. *Doc. Ophthal. Proc. Series* No. 28 (H. C. Fledelius, P. H. Alsbirk and E. Goldschmidt, eds). Dr W. Junk, pp. 89–95.

Fledelius, H. C. (1983) Is myopia getting more frequent? A cross-sectional study of 1416 Danes aged 16 years +. *Acta Ophthalmol.* **61**, 545–559.

Fledelius, H. C. (1995) Adult-onset myopia–oculometric features. *Acta Ophthalmol.* **73**, 397–401.

Flitcroft, D. I. and Eustace, P. (1997) Emmetropization and late-onset myopia: the role of retinal image quality and the accommodation system. *Invest. Ophthalmol. Vis. Sci.* **38**, S461.

Framingham Offspring Eye Study Group (1996) Familial aggregation and prevalence of myopia in the Framingham offspring eye study. *Arch. Ophthalmol.* **114**, 326–332.

Gilmartin, B. and Bullimore, M. A. (1987) Sustained near-vision augments inhibitory sympathetic innervation of the ciliary muscle. *Clin. Vis. Sci.* **1**, 197–208.

Gilmartin, B. and Winfield, N. R. (1995) The effect of topical β-adrenoceptor antagonists on accommodation in emmetropia and myopia. *Vis. Res.* **35**, 1305–1312.

Goh, W. S. H. and Lam, C. S. Y. (1994) Changes in refractive trends and optical components of Hong Kong Chinese aged 19–39 years. *Ophthal. Physiol. Opt.* **14**, 378–382.

Goldschmidt, E. (1968) On the etiology of myopia. An epidemiological study. *Acta Ophthalmol.* **98** (Suppl.), 1–172.

Goss, D. A. (1984) Overcorrection as a means of slowing myopic progression. *Am. J. Optom. Physiol. Opt.* **61**, 85–93.

Goss, D. A. (1988) Retinal image-mediated ocular growth as a possible etiological factor in juvenile-onset myopia. Vision Science Syposium, A Tribute to Gordon G. Heath. Indiana University, pp. 165–183.

Goss, D. A. (1991) Clinical accommodation and heterophoria findings preceding juvenile onset of myopia. *Optom. Vis. Sci.* **68**, 110–116.

Goss, D. A. and Grosvenor, T. (1990) Rates of childhood myopia progression with bifocals as a function of nearpoint phoria: consistency of three studies. *Optom. Vis. Sci.* **67**, 637–640.

Goss, D. A. and Wickham, M. G. (1995) Retinal-image mediated ocular growth as a mechanism for juvenile onset myopia and for emmetropization. *Doc. Ophthalmol.* **90**, 341–375.

Goss, D. A. and Winkler, R. L. (1983) Progression of myopia in youth: age of cessation. *Am. J. Optom. Physiol. Opt.* **60**, 651–658.

Grisham, J. D. and Simons, H. D. (1986) Refractive error and the reading process: a literature analysis. *J. Am. Optom. Assoc.* **57**, 44–55.

Grosvenor, T. (1977a) A longitudinal study of refractive changes between ages 20 and 40. Part 2: Changes in individual subjects. *Optom. Weekly* **68**, 415–419.

Grosvenor, T. (1977b) A longitudinal study of refractive changes between ages 20 and 40. Part 3: Statistical analysis of data. *Optom. Weekly* **68**, 455–457.

Grosvenor, T. (1987) Review and a suggested classification system for myopia on the basis of age-related prevalence and age of onset. *Am. J. Optom. Physiol. Opt.* **64**, 545–554.

Grosvenor, T. and Scott, R. (1991) A comparison of refractive components in youth-onset and early adult-onset myopia. *Optom. Vis. Sci.* **68**, 204–209.

Grosvenor, T. and Scott, R. (1993) Three-year changes in refraction and its components in youth-onset and early adult-onset myopia. *Optom. Vis. Sci.* **70**, 677–683.

Gwiazda, J., Thorn, F., Bauer, J. and Held, R. (1993a) Emmetropization and the progression of manifest refraction in children followed from infancy to puberty. *Clin. Vis. Sci.* **8**, 337–344.

Gwiazda, J., Thorn, F., Bauer, J. and Held, R. (1993b) Myopic children show insufficient accommodative response to blur. *Invest. Ophthalmol. Vis. Sci.* **34**, 690–694.

Gwiazda, J., Bauer, J., Thorn, F. and Held, R. (1995) A dynamic relationship between myopia and blur-driven accommodation in school-aged children. *Vis. Res.* **35**, 1299–1304.

Heath, G. G. (1956) Components of accommodation. *Am. J. Optom. Arch. Am. Acad. Optom.* **33**, 569–579.

Hirsch, M. J. (1958) Changes in refractive state after the age of forty-five. *Am. J. Optom. Arch. Am. Acad. Optom.* **35**, 229–237.

Hirsch, M. J., Alpern, M. and Schultz, H. L. (1948) The variation of phoria with age. *Am. J. Optom. Arch. Am. Acad. Optom.* **25**, 535–541.

Hung, L. F., Crawford, M. L. J. and Smith, E. L. (1995) Spectacle lenses alter eye growth and the refractive status of young monkeys. *Nature Med.* **1**, 761–765.

Ingram, R. M., Arnold, P. E., Dally, S. and Lucas, J. (1991) Emmetropization, squint, and reduced visual acuity after treatment. *Br. J. Ophthalmol.* **75**, 414–416.

Irving, E. L., Callender, M. G. and Sivak, J. G. (1991) Inducing myopia, hyperopia, and astigmatism in chicks. *Optom. Vis. Sci.* **68**, 364–368.

Irving, E. L., Sivak, J. G. and Callender, M. G. (1992) Refractive plasticity of the developing chick eye. *Ophthal. Physiol. Opt.* **12**, 448–456.

Jampolsky, A., Flom, B. C., Weymouth, F. W. and Moses, L. E. (1955) Unequal corrected visual acuity as related to anisometropia. *Arch. Ophthalmol.* **54**, 893–904.

Johnson, G. J., Matthews, A. and Perkins, E. S. (1979) Survey of ophthalmic conditions in a Labrador community. I. Refractive errors. *Br. J. Ophthalmol.* **63**, 440–448.

Karlsson, J. L. (1974) Concordance rates for myopia in twins. *Clin. Genet.* **6**, 142–146.

Lam, C. S. Y., Goh, W. S. H., Tang, Y. K. *et al.* (1994) Changes in refractive trends and optical components of Hong Kong Chinese aged over 40 years. *Ophthal. Physiol. Opt.* **14**, 383–388.

Logan, N. S., Gilmartin, B. and Dunne, M. C. M. (1995) Computation of retinal contour in anisomyopia. *Ophthal. Physiol. Opt.* **15**, 363–366.

Marshall, E. (1996) Whose genome is it anyway? *Science* **273**, 1788–1789.

McBrien, N. A. and Adams, D. W. (1997) A longitudinal investigation of adult-onset and adult-progression of myopia in an occupational group. *Invest. Ophthalmol. Vis. Sci.* **38**, 321–333.

McBrien, N. A. and Millodot, M. (1986) The effect of refractive error on the accommodative response gradient. *Ophthal. Physiol. Opt.* **6**, 145–149.

McBrien, N. A. and Millodot, M. (1987) Biometric investigation of late-onset myopic eyes. *Acta Ophthalmol.* **65**, 461–468.

Medina, A. (1987) A model for emmetropization. Predicting the progression of ametropia. *Ophthalmologica* **194**, 133–139.

Miles, F. A. and Wallman, J. (1990) Local ocular compensation for imposed local refractive error. *Vis. Res.* **30**, 339–349.

Morgan, M. W. (1944) Accommodation and its relationship to convergence. *Am. J. Optom. Arch. Am. Acad. Optom.* **21**, 83–95.

Mutti, D. O. and Zadnik, K. (1996) Is computer use a risk factor for myopia? *J. Am. Optom. Assoc.* **67**, 521–530.

Napper, G. A., Brennan, N. A., Barrington, M. *et al.* (1995) The duration of normal visual exposure necessary to prevent form deprivation myopia in chicks. *Vis. Res.* **35**, 1337–1344.

National Research Council (1989) *Myopia: Prevalence and Progression.* National Academy Press.

North, R. and Henson, D. B. (1981) Adaptation to prism-induced heterophoria in subjects with abnormal binocular vision or asthenopia. *Am. J. Optom. Physiol. Opt.* **58**, 746–752.

O'Neal, M. R. and Connon, T. R. (1987) Refractive error change at the United States Air Force Academy Class of 1985. *Am. J. Optom. Physiol. Opt.* **64**, 344–354.

Ong, E. and Ciuffreda, K. J. (1995) Nearwork-induced transient myopia. *Doc. Ophthalmol.* **91**, 57–85.

Ong, E. and Ciuffreda, K. J. (1997) *Accommodation, Nearwork and Myopia.* Optometric Extension Program.

Papastergiou, G. I., Schmid, G. F., Laties, A. M. *et al.* (1997) Induction of axial eye elongation and myopic refractive shift in one year old chickens. *Invest. Ophthalmol. Vis. Sci.* **38**, S543.

Pärssinen, O. and Lyyra, A.-L. (1993) Myopia and myopic progression among schoolchildren: a three-year follow-up study. *Invest. Ophthalmol. Vis. Sci.* **34**, 2794–2802.

Peckham, C. S., Gardiner, P. A. and Goldstein, H. (1977) Acquired myopia in 11-year-old children. *Br. Med. J.* **1**, 542–544.

Polymeropoulos, M. H., Higgins, J. J., Golbe, L. I. *et al.* (1996) Mapping of a gene for Parkinson's disease to chromosome 4q21–q23. *Science* **274**, 1197–1199.

Portello, J. K., Rosenfield, M. and O'Dwyer, M. (1997) Clinical characteristics of pre-myopic individuals. *Optom. Vis. Sci.* **74** (Suppl.), 176.

Raviola, E. and Wiesel, T. N. (1985) An animal model of myopia. *N. Engl. J. Med.* **312**, 1609–1615.

Reiner, A., Shih, Y.-F. and Fitzgerald, M. E. C. (1995) The relationship of choroidal blood flow and accommodation to the control of ocular growth. *Vis. Res.* **35**, 1227–1245.

Richler, A. and Bear, J. C. (1980a) Refraction, nearwork and education. A population study in Newfoundland. *Acta Ophthalmol.* **58**, 468–478.

Richler, A. and Bear, J. C. (1980b) The distribution of refraction in three isolated communities in western Newfoundland. *Am. J. Optom. Physiol. Opt.* **57**, 861–871.

Rosenfield, M. (1997) Tonic vergence and vergence adaptation. *Optom. Vis. Sci.* **74**, 303–328.

Rosenfield, M. and Gilmartin, B. (1987a) Effect of a near-vision task on the response AC/A of a myopic population. *Ophthal. Physiol. Opt.* **7**, 225–233.

Rosenfield, M. and Gilmartin, B. (1987b) Beta-adrenergic receptor antagonism in myopia. *Ophthal. Physiol. Opt.* **7**, 359–364.

Rosenfield, M. and Gilmartin, B. (1988a) Disparity-induced accommodation in late-onset myopia. *Ophthal. Physiol. Opt.* **8**, 353–355.

Rosenfield, M. and Gilmartin, B. (1988b) The effect of vergence adaptation on convergent accommodation. *Ophthal. Physiol. Opt.* **8**, 172–177.

Rosenfield, M. and Gilmartin, B. (1989) Temporal aspects of accommodative adaptation. *Optom. Vis. Sci.* **66**, 229–234.

Rosenfield, M. and Gilmartin, B. (1998) Accommodative adaptation during sustained near-vision reduces accommodative error. *Invest. Ophthalmol. Vis. Sci.* **39**, S639.

Rosenfield, M., Chun, T. W. and Fischer, S. W. (1997) Effect of prolonged occlusion on the subjective assessment of heterophoria. *Ophthal. Physiol. Opt.* **17**, 478–482.

Rosner, M. and Belkin, M. (1987) Intelligence, education, and myopia in males. *Arch. Ophthalmol.* **105**, 1508–1511.

Rosner, J. and Rosner, J. (1986) Some observations of the relationship between the visual perceptual skills development of young hyperopes and age of first lens correction. *Clin. Exp. Optom.* **69**, 166–168.

Rubin, S. C., Benjamin, I., Behbakht, K. *et al.* (1996) Clinical and pathological features of ovarian cancer in women with germ-like mutations of BRCA1. *N. Engl. J. Med.* **335**, 1413–1416.

Schaeffel, F. and Howland, H. C. (1995) Guest editorial. *Vis. Res.* **35**, 1135–1139.

Schaeffel, F., Glasser, A. and Howland, H. C. (1988) Accommodation, refractive error and eye growth in chickens. *Vis. Res.* **28**, 639–657.

Schaeffel, F., Hagel, G., Bartmann, M. *et al.* (1994) 6-Hydroxy dopamine does not affect lens-induced refractive errors but suppresses deprivation myopia. *Vis. Res.* **34**, 143–149.

Schapero, M. (1971) *Amblyopia.* Chilton Books.

Schor, C. M. (1980) Fixation disparity: a steady state error of disparity-induced vergence. *Am. J. Optom. Physiol. Opt.* **57**, 618–631.

Schor, C. M. (1983) Fixation disparity and vergence adaptation. In: *Vergence Eye Movements: Basic and*

Clinical Aspects (C. M. Schor and K. J. Ciuffreda, eds). Butterworths, pp. 465–516.

Schor, C. M. (1986) Adaptive regulation of accommodative vergence and vergence accommodation. *Am. J. Optom. Physiol. Opt.* **63**, 587–609.

Schor, C. M. and Horner, D. (1989) Adaptive disorders of accommodation and vergence in binocular dysfunction. *Ophthal. Physiol. Opt.* **9**, 264–268.

Schor, C. M., Kotulak, J. C. and Tsuetaki, T. (1986) Adaptation of tonic accommodation reduces accommodative lag and is masked in darkness. *Invest. Ophthalmol. Vis. Sci.* **27**, 820–827.

Shulkin, D. J. and Bari, M. M. (1986) Deteriorating vision: an occupational risk for the medical student. *Arch. Ophthalmol.* **104**, 1274.

Sorsby, A., Benjamin, B. and Sheridan, M. (1961) *Refraction and Its Components During the Growth of the Eye from the Age of Three.* Medical Research Council Special Reports Series No. 301. HMSO.

Sorsby, A., Leary, G. A. and Richards, M. J. (1962) The optical components in anisometropia. *Vis. Res.* **2**, 43–51.

Sorsby, A., Sheridan, M. and Leary, G. A. (1963) *Refraction and Its Components in Twins.* Medical Research Council Special Reports Series No. 303. HMSO.

Teasdale, T. W., Fuchs, J. and Goldschmidt, E. (1988) Degree of myopia in relation to intelligence and educational level. *Lancet*, **ii**, 1351–1354.

Tiffin, J. (1943) *Industrial Psychology.* Prentice-Hall, pp. 139–142.

Törnqvist, G. (1967) The relative importance of the parasympathetic and sympathetic nervous systems for accommodation in monkeys. *Invest. Ophthalmol.* **6**, 612–617.

Tscherning, M. (1882) *Studier oven myopiens aetiologi.* C. Myhre

Waardenburg, P. J. (1950) Twin research in ophthalmology. *Doc. Ophthalmol.* **4**, 154–200.

Wallman, J. (1991) Retinal factors in myopia and emmetropization: clues from research on chicks. In: *Refractive Anomalies. Research and Clinical Applications* (T. Grosvenor and M. C. Flom, eds). Butterworth-Heinemann, pp. 268–286.

Wallman, J. and Adams, J. I. (1987) Developmental aspects of experimental myopia in chicks: susceptibility, recovery and relation to emmetropization. *Vis. Res.* **27**, 1139–1163.

Wallman, J., Gottlieb, M. D., Rajaram, V. and Fugate-Wentzek, L. A. (1987) Local retinal regions control local eye growth and myopia. *Science* **237**, 73–77.

Wallman, J., Xu, A., Wildsoet, C. *et al.* (1992) Moving the retina: a third mechanism of focusing the eye. *Invest. Ophthalmol. Vis. Sci.* (Suppl.) **33**, 1053.

Wildsoet, C. F. (1997) Active emmetropization–evidence for its existence and ramifications for clinical practice. *Ophthal. Physiol. Opt.* **17**, 279–290.

Wildsoet, C. and Wallman, J. (1995) Choroidal and scleral mechanisms of compensation for spectacle lenses in chicks. *Vis. Res.* **35**, 1175–1194.

Yeow, P. T. and Taylor, S. P. (1989) Effects of short-term VDT usage on visual functions. *Optom. Vis. Sci.* **66**, 459–466.

Yeow, P. T. and Taylor, S. P. (1991) Effects of long-term visual display terminal usage on visual functions. *Optom. Vis. Sci.* **68**, 930–941.

Young, F. A. (1961) The effect of restricted visual space on the primate eye. *Am. J. Ophthalmol.* **52**, 799–806.

Young, F. A., Leary, G. A., Baldwin, W. R. *et al.* (1969) The transmission of refractive errors within Eskimo families. *Am. J. Optom. Arch. Am. Acad. Optom.* **46**, 676–685.

Zadnik, K. and Mutti, D. O. (1995) How applicable are animal myopia models to human juvenile onset myopia? *Vis. Res.* **35**, 1283–1288.

Zadnik, K., Mutti, D. O., Friedman, N. E. and Adams, A. J. (1993) Initial cross-sectional results from the Orinda longitudinal study of myopia. *Optom. Vis. Sci.* **70**, 750–758.

Zadnik, K., Satariano, W. A., Mutti, D. O. *et al.* (1994) The effect of parental history of myopia on children's eye size. *J. Am. Med. Assoc.* **271**, 1323–1327.

Zylbermann, R., Landau, D. and Berson, D. (1993) The influence of study habits on myopia in Jewish teenagers. *J. Ped. Ophthalmol. Strab.* **30**, 319–322.

A note on the dioptric power matrix

William F. Harris

In the familiar clinical representation one writes astigmatic power as sphere (F_s), cylinder (F_c) and axis (a). It turns out that for performing most types of calculations this clinical representation of power is inconvenient or inappropriate (Harris, 1990, 1992, 1997a; Deal and Toop, 1993; Thibos *et al.*, 1994). Long (1976) has shown that calculating the sum of the powers of obliquely crossed thin astigmatic lenses is greatly simplified if the power is represented by what is known as the *dioptic power matrix*. Since then an extensive literature has developed on the subject (*see* Harris, 1997a and the references cited therein). This note briefly describes some basic properties of matrices, defines the dioptric power matrix, shows how power in the clinical representation is converted to the matrix representation and vice versa, and illustrates the use of the matrix for calculating the mean of a set of astigmatic powers. Finally it shows how the calculation can be made slightly more convenient by using the *coordinate vector* **h**, a matrix related to the dioptric power matrix.

Matrices

A matrix is a mathematical entity consisting of numbers arranged in rows and columns. (There are many good introductory texts on the subject, e.g. Anton and Rorres, 1987; Grossman, 1987; Keating, 1988; Nicholson, 1993). In general there can be any number of rows and columns, but the dioptric power matrix has exactly two rows and two columns and is said to be a 2×2 matrix. Here are two examples of 2×2 matrices:

$$\begin{pmatrix} 3 & 2 \\ -2 & 1 \end{pmatrix}$$

and

$$\begin{pmatrix} 2 & 1 \\ 1 & 0 \end{pmatrix}$$

The numbers within the matrix are the *components* of the matrix. The components lying on the diagonal from top left to bottom right (3 and 1 in the first example) are said to be the *diagonal* components; the others are the *off-diagonal* components. If the off-diagonal components are zero then the matrix itself is called *diagonal*. A 2×2 matrix whose two off-diagonal components are the same is *symmetric*. Of the two examples given above the second matrix is symmetric (both off-diagonal components are 1) while the first is asymmetric (the off-diagonals are different, being 2 and –2).

Rules of addition and multiplication are defined for matrices. Addition is straightforward: corresponding components are added. Thus:

$$\begin{pmatrix} 3 & 2 \\ -2 & 1 \end{pmatrix} + \begin{pmatrix} 2 & 1 \\ 1 & 0 \end{pmatrix} = \begin{pmatrix} 5 & 3 \\ -1 & 1 \end{pmatrix}$$

The top left component is the sum of the top left components of the matrices being added, and so on. Multiplication of a matrix by a number is also straightforward: each component is multiplied.

Thus:

$$3\begin{pmatrix} 2 & 1 \\ 1 & 0 \end{pmatrix} = \begin{pmatrix} 6 & 3 \\ 3 & 0 \end{pmatrix}$$

Two matrices can also be multiplied; however that is a much more complicated issue and will not be discussed here.

We are now in a position to calculate averages of matrices. We add the matrices and then divide by the number of matrices. Dividing by a number is equivalent to multiplying by the inverse of the number.

Example 1: Find the average of the following three matrices:

$$\begin{pmatrix} 1 & 1 \\ 0 & 2 \end{pmatrix}, \begin{pmatrix} -1 & 3 \\ 2 & 1 \end{pmatrix} \text{ and } \begin{pmatrix} 3 & 2 \\ 1 & 0 \end{pmatrix}$$

The answer is

$$\frac{1}{3}\left[\begin{pmatrix} 1 & 1 \\ 0 & 2 \end{pmatrix} + \begin{pmatrix} -1 & 3 \\ 2 & 1 \end{pmatrix} + \begin{pmatrix} 3 & 2 \\ 1 & 0 \end{pmatrix}\right] \text{ or } \frac{1}{3}\begin{pmatrix} 3 & 6 \\ 3 & 3 \end{pmatrix}$$

that is

$$\begin{pmatrix} 1 & 2 \\ 1 & 1 \end{pmatrix}$$

Usually a matrix is represented by a bold-face upper-case letter such as **F**. Each of its components is represented by a light-face lower-case letter with two subscripts which specify the row and column in which the component lies. For example one writes:

$$\mathbf{F} = \begin{pmatrix} f_{11} & f_{12} \\ f_{21} & f_{22} \end{pmatrix} \tag{1}$$

where component f_{11} is in the first row and first column of **F**, component f_{12} is in the first row and second column, and so on. (Note that f_{12} is read 'eff one two' not 'eff twelve'.)

The dioptric power matrix

The dioptric power matrix is a matrix **F** with components that are related to sphere, cylinder and axis as follows (Long, 1976):

$$f_{11} = F_s + F_c \sin^2 a \tag{2}$$

$$f_{21} = f_{12} = -F_c \sin a \cos a \tag{3}$$

$$f_{22} = F_s + F_c \cos^2 a \tag{4}$$

We refer to these as Long's equations. Notice that the dioptric power matrix is always symmetric [1] (i.e. $f_{21} = f_{12}$). This means that, although there are four components to a dioptric power matrix, only three of them are distinct. In calculating the matrix one begins with one set of three numbers, namely sphere, cylinder and axis, and ends up with another three, f_{11}, f_{21} (the same as f_{12}) and f_{22}. While sphere and cylinder are usually measured in dioptres and axis in degrees, all the components of the dioptric power matrix are measured in the same units, namely dioptres.

The components in the first column of **F** represent the horizontal meridian or direction. Component f_{11} represents power associated with curvature (Keating, 1986) and is called the *curvital power* (Harris, 1997a) in the horizontal direction. Component f_{21} is the *torsional power* (Keating, 1986) in the horizontal direction. Thus, associated with the horizontal direction are two types of power, curvital and torsional [2]. The same is true of any direction [3]. The components in the second column of **F** represent the vertical direction: we need consider only f_{22}, the curvital power in the vertical meridian.

It follows from equation (3) above that when the principal meridians are vertical and horizontal ($a = 90°$ or $a = 180°$) the torsional power in the horizontal is zero, and hence the dioptric power matrix is diagonal. Otherwise the dioptric power matrix is not diagonal. For a purely spherical power $F_c = 0$, and hence it follows from equations (2) to (4) that the matrix, in addition to being diagonal, has equal diagonal components ($f_{11} = f_{22}$). In particular, a spherical power of 1 D has a dioptric power matrix $\begin{pmatrix} 1 & 0 \\ 0 & 1 \end{pmatrix}$, a matrix called the *identity matrix*. The dioptric power matrix corresponding to plano power is the *null matrix*, the components of which are all zero.

Converting sphere, cylinder and axis to the dioptric power matrix

Given power in the usual form of sphere, cylinder and axis, calculation of the corresponding dioptric power matrix is straightforward; one merely uses equations (2) to (4) to calculate the three distinct components and substitutes the results into equation (1). For the power +3.00 −1.00 × 20, for example, one obtains the matrix

$$\begin{pmatrix} 2.8830 & 0.3214 \\ 0.3214 & 2.1170 \end{pmatrix}$$

The power +2.00 +1.00 × 110 leads to the same matrix, which might have been expected because one representation is simply the sphero-cylindrical transposition of the other.

Converting the dioptric power matrix to sphere, cylinder and axis

The reverse process of converting a dioptric power matrix into power in the clinical form is slightly more complicated. Suppose we have a dioptric power matrix. We check first whether it is symmetric. If it is not, then there is no corresponding power in the clinical form and we cannot proceed [4]. If the matrix is symmetric then there is a corresponding power of the clinical form. Next we check whether the matrix is diagonal. If it is, then the principal meridians are horizontal and vertical and the powers along them are f_{11} and f_{22} respectively. One can write the power as sphere, cylinder and axis directly. If the matrix is not diagonal we calculate what are called the *trace* (t) and *determinant* (d) of the matrix. They are given by

$$t = f_{11} + f_{22} \tag{5}$$

and

$$d = f_{11} f_{22} - f_{21} f_{12} \tag{6}$$

Notice that the units of t are D and the units of d are D². Then the cylinder is calculated using (Keating, 1980)

$$F_c = \pm\sqrt{t^2 - 4d} \tag{7}$$

The sign ± implies that either the positive or the negative power can be chosen for the cylinder. The sphere is calculated using

$$F_s = (t - F_c)/2 \tag{8}$$

and, finally, the axis is given by

$$\tan a = (F_s - f_{11})/f_{21} \tag{9}$$

Equations (7) to (9) are known as Keating's equations.

As examples, consider the three matrices

$$\begin{pmatrix} -2 & 0 \\ 0 & -2 \end{pmatrix}, \begin{pmatrix} 4 & 0 \\ 0 & 2 \end{pmatrix} \text{ and } \begin{pmatrix} 2 & -1 \\ -1 & 1 \end{pmatrix}.$$

Following the procedure described above, we first check for symmetry. We see that all three are symmetric and that each therefore has a power in the familiar clinical form. The first and second are diagonal, implying that the principal meridians are horizontal and vertical. The principal powers are equal in the first showing that it represents the spherical power −2 D. In the second the principal powers are 4 D and 2 D along the horizontal and vertical meridians respectively, implying the power +4.00 −2.00 × 180 or, equivalently, +2.00 +2.00 × 90. The third is not diagonal. Hence, for this matrix, we calculate t and d using equations (5) and (6): the results are $t = 3$ D and $d = 1$ D². Then from equation (7) the cylinder is $F_c = \pm 2.24$ D approximately. Let us choose the negative form, that is $F_c = -2.24$ D. Then, by equation (8), the sphere is $F_s = +2.62$ D. By equation (9) tan $a = -0.6180$. The calculator gives $a = -31.7°$. Whenever the angle is negative (as in this case) we add 180° to make the angle positive. Thus we have −31.7 + 180 = 148.3°. (Notice that 180° can be added because the tangent of any angle is the same as the tangent of the sum of the angle and 180°.) Hence we find the third dioptric power matrix to be equivalent to +2.62 −2.24 × 148.3. Choosing instead the positive cylinder form we find +0.38 +2.24 × 58.3.

When $t = 0$ D the power is Jacksonian (that is, the power is that of a Jackson crossed cylinder) and when $d = 0$ D² the power is purely cylindrical [5]. These conclusions follow from equations (7) and (8).

Calculating the average power

The following two examples illustrate the use of the dioptric power matrix for the calculation of average dioptric power.

Example 2: Calculate the mean of the following three sphero-cylindrical powers: +3.00 −1.00 × 20, +3.00 −2.00 × 20 and +3.00 −1.00 × 180. We convert each of these powers to the corresponding dioptric power matrix, add the three matrices, multiply by 1/3 (or divide by 3) and, finally, convert the resulting matrix back to power in the familiar form. Thus

$$\frac{1}{3}\left[\begin{pmatrix} 2.8830 & 0.3214 \\ 0.3214 & 2.1170 \end{pmatrix} + \begin{pmatrix} 2.7660 & 0.6428 \\ 0.6428 & 1.2340 \end{pmatrix} \right.$$
$$\left. + \begin{pmatrix} 3.0000 & 0.0000 \\ 0.0000 & 2.0000 \end{pmatrix} \right]$$

$$= \frac{1}{3}\begin{pmatrix} 8.6490 & 0.9642 \\ 0.9642 & 5.3510 \end{pmatrix} = \begin{pmatrix} 2.8830 & 0.3214 \\ 0.3214 & 1.7836 \end{pmatrix}$$

The matrix is symmetric but not diagonal. Hence we calculate $t = 4.6667$ D and $d = 5.0390$ D^2. In negative cylinder form one obtains $F_c = -1.27$ D. Then $F_s = 2.97$ D and $\tan a = 0.2709$. Thus the mean power is $+2.97 - 1.27 \times 15.2$.

Example 3: In this example we determine the average of the following two purely cylindrical powers: $+2.00 \times 15$ and $+2.00 \times 165$. The average matrix is

$$\frac{1}{2}\left[\begin{pmatrix} 0.1340 & -0.5000 \\ -0.5000 & 1.8660 \end{pmatrix} + \begin{pmatrix} 0.1340 & 0.5000 \\ 0.5000 & 1.8660 \end{pmatrix} \right]$$

$$= \frac{1}{2}\begin{pmatrix} 0.2680 & 0.0000 \\ 0.0000 & 3.7320 \end{pmatrix} = \begin{pmatrix} 0.1340 & 0.0000 \\ 0.0000 & 1.8660 \end{pmatrix}$$

The resulting matrix is symmetric and diagonal. Hence the principal powers are $+0.134$ D and $+1.866$ D along the horizontal and vertical directions respectively. Thus the average is $+0.13 + 1.73 \times 180$ approximately in the usual representation. Notice that the average of the two cylindrical powers is a sphero-cylindrical power.

The coordinate vector h

The two identical off-diagonal components imply redundancy in the dioptric power matrix. Furthermore the matrix is clumsy: it takes up a good deal of space on the page. The coordinate vector **h** (devised by Harris, 1991) provides a neater method of calculating the average power.

Coordinate vector **h** is a 3×1 matrix, also called a *column vector*. In terms of its components **h** is (Harris 1991):

$$\mathbf{h} = \begin{pmatrix} h_1 \\ h_2 \\ h_3 \end{pmatrix} = \begin{pmatrix} f_{11} \\ \sqrt{2}f_{21} \\ f_{22} \end{pmatrix} \tag{10}$$

In other words, **h** is simply a list of the distinct components of the dioptric power matrix [6], except that component h_2 is f_{21} multiplied by $\sqrt{2}$. It is convenient to use the (matrix) transpose, represented by the prime ($.'$). This allows one to write the vector as a row:

$$\mathbf{h} = (h_1 \ h_2 \ h_3)' \tag{11}$$

In order to calculate the average power using vector **h**, one proceeds as follows: For each power we calculate a vector **h** using:

$$h_1 = F_s + F_c \sin^2 a \tag{12}$$

$$h_2 = -\sqrt{2}F_c \sin a \cos a \tag{13}$$

$$h_3 = F_s + F_c \cos^2 a \tag{14}$$

These equations are merely equations (2) to (4) suitably modified. The vectors **h** are summed in the usual way and the average vector **h** is obtained by dividing by the number of powers under consideration. We examine the average vector **h**. If it has $h_2 = 0$ D then the principal meridians of the average are horizontal and vertical and the corresponding principal powers along those meridians are h_1 and h_3. If $h_2 \neq 0$ D then one calculates t and d according to

$$t = h_1 + h_3 \tag{15}$$

and

$$d = h_1 h_3 - h_2^2/2 \tag{16}$$

Then the corresponding cylinder and sphere are calculated using equations (7) and (8). Finally the axis is calculated using:

$$\tan a = \sqrt{2} \ (F_s - h_1)/h_2 \tag{17}$$

Using vector **h** Example 2 above can be performed as follows:

$+3.00 -1.00 \times 20$	$\Rightarrow (2.8830 \ \ 0.4545 \ \ 2.1170)'$
$+3.00 -2.00 \times 20$	$\Rightarrow (2.7660 \ \ 0.9091 \ \ 1.2340)'$
$+3.00 -1.00 \times 180$	$\Rightarrow (3.0000 \ \ 0.0000 \ \ 2.0000)'$
	$(8.6490 \ \ 1.3636 \ \ 5.3510)'$
$+2.97 -1.27 \times 15.2$	$\Leftarrow (2.8830 \ \ 0.4545 \ \ 1.7836)'$

Each power is converted to a vector **h** using equations (11) to (14). The vectors **h** are summed and the total divided, in this case, by 3. Finally the result is converted back to the clinical form using equations (15), (16), (7), (8) and (17).

Example 3 is performed as follows:

plano +2.00 × 15   ⇒ (0.1340 −0.7071 1.8660)′

plano +2.00 × 165   ⇒ (0.1340   0.7071 1.8660)′

―――――――――――――――――――――

              (0.2680   0.0000 3.7320)′

+0.13 + 1.73 × 180 ⇐ (0.1340   0.0000 1.8660)′

―――――――――――――――――――――

Concluding remarks

This note has provided a brief introduction to the dioptric power matrix. It has demonstrated only one of its many uses. For a more complete account the reader is referred elsewhere (Harris 1997a, 1997b; Keating, 1997; and other papers in *Optometry and Vision Science*, June 1997).

As shown by Example 1, the calculation of an average matrix is simple and straightforward. The only calculational complications arise during the interconversion between power in the form sphere, cylinder and axis and in the form of the matrix. Thus the complications are not associated with the matrix itself but are rather a result of the representation of power as sphere, cylinder and axis. The calculations are a little tedious if performed by hand; a simple computer program can do the job easily. The method described here of calculating average dioptric power via the dioptric power matrix was first described by Keating (1983). There are other methods (*see* the discussion in Saunders, 1982) which all give the same result.[7] A key paper which stimulated work on the basic statistics of dioptric power was that of Saunders (1980).

Calculating the mean via the dioptric power matrix and via vector **h** are essentially doing the same thing. Coordinate vector **h** merely allows a neater representation of the calculation. There are other coordinate vectors (Deal and Toop, 1993; Thibos *et al.*, 1994; *see also* the discussion in Harris, 1997a) in terms of which the same calculation can be performed. Although ostensibly quite different from vector **h**, the calculations are fundamentally the same as those done here.

For the purpose of calculating average power the $\sqrt{2}$ can be omitted from equation (10), as was done originally (Harris, 1989). It must then also be omitted from equations (13) and (17) and the 2 must be omitted from equation (16). It is retained here because vector **h** (with the $\sqrt{2}$) has other uses as

well (Harris, 1991) and seems likely to become standard.

Acknowledgements

I thank the following for advice and assistance: M. Edwards, Hong Kong Polytechnic University; R. D. van Gool, W. D. H. Gillan, A. Rubin and C. A. Blackie of the Optometric Science Research Group, Rand Afrikaans University, South Africa.

Notes

1   For thick lens systems the matrix is asymmetric in general (Keating, 1981a, 1981b, 1997; Harris, 1993, 1997a).
2   Traditionally in optometry one encounters only one type of power in a meridian. It is associated with curvature and is what is called curvital power here.
3   We assume throughout that the reference direction is the horizontal, in keeping with normal practice. There are circumstances in which it is useful to choose other directions as reference (Harris, 1997b). In those circumstances one measures the angle *a* anticlockwise from the reference.
4   For what can be done in such cases, *see* Harris, 1993, 1997a.
5   In the theory of matrices a matrix whose determinant *d* is zero is called a *singular matrix*.
6   h_1 is the curvital power in the horizontal direction, h_2 is called the *scaled* torsional power (Harris 1997a) in the horizontal direction; and h_3 is the curvital power in the vertical direction.
7   There is, however, a method that does *not* give the same result; it leads to what is called the *naive average*. One simply averages sphere, cylinder and axis separately. This method would result in +3.00 − 1.33 × 73 in the case of Example 2 and plano +2.00 × 90 in Example 3. The naive average is not a valid average. For a discussion of the naive average of power and the absurd results that can be obtained, see Harris, 1990.

References

Anton, H. and Rorres, C. (1987) *Elementary Linear Algebra with Applications*. Wiley.

Deal, F. C. and Toop, J. (1993) Recommended coordinate systems for thin spherocylindrical lenses. *Optom. Vis. Sci.* **70**, 409–413.

Grossman, S. I. (1987) *Elementary Linear Algebra*, 3rd edn. Wadsworth.

Harris, W. F. (1989) Simplified rational representation of the dioptric power matrix. *Ophthal. Physiol. Opt.* **9**, 455.

Harris, W. F. (1990) The mean and variance of samples of dioptric powers: the basic calculations. *Clin. Exp. Optom.* **73**, 89–92.

Harris, W. F. (1991) Representation of dioptric power in Euclidean 3-space. *Ophthal. Physiol. Opt.* **11**, 130–136.

Harris, W. F. (1992) Testing hypotheses on dioptric power. *Optom. Vis. Sci.* **69**, 835–845.

Harris, W. F. (1993) Keating's asymmetric dioptric powers expressed in terms of sphere, cylinder, axis, and asymmetry. *Optom. Vis. Sci.* **70**, 666–667.

Harris, W. F. (1997a) Dioptric power: its nature and representation in three- and four-dimensional space. *Optom. Vis. Sci.* **74**, 349–366.

Harris, W. F. (1997b) Meridional profiles of variance-covariance of symmetric dioptric power: classes of variation that are uniform across the meridians of the eye. *Optom. Vis. Sci.* **74**, 397–413.

Keating, M. P. (1980) An easier method to obtain the sphere, cylinder and axis from an off-axis dioptric power matrix. *Am. J. Optom. Physiol. Opt.* **57**, 734–737.

Keating, M. P. (1981a) A system matrix for astigmatic optical systems: I. Introduction and dioptric power relations. *Am. J. Optom. Physiol. Opt.* **58**, 810–819.

Keating, M. P. (1981b) A system matrix for astigmatic optical systems: II. Corrected systems including an astigmatic eye. *Am. J. Optom. Physiol. Opt.* **58**, 919–929.

Keating, M. P. (1983) On the use of matrices for the mean value of refractive errors. *Ophthal. Physiol. Opt.* **3**, 210–213.

Keating, M. P. (1986) Dioptric power in an off-axis meridian: the torsional component. A system matrix for astigmatic optical systems: I. Introduction and dioptric power relations. *Am. J. Optom. Physiol. Opt.* **63**, 830–838.

Keating, M. P. (1988) *Geometric, Physical, and Visual Optics.* Butterworths, Appendix.

Keating, M. P. (1997) Equivalent power asymmetry relations for thick astigmatic systems. *Optom. Vis. Sci.* **74**, 388–392.

Long, W. F. (1976) A matrix formalism for decentration problems. *Am. J. Optom. Physiol. Opt.* **53**, 27–33.

Nicholson, W. K. (1993) *Elementary Linear Algebra with Applications*, 2nd edn. PWS Publishing.

Saunders, H. (1980) A method for determining the mean value of refractive errors. *Br. J. Physiol. Opt.* **34**, 1–11.

Saunders, H. (1982) The mean value of refractive errors. Author's reply. *Ophthal. Physiol. Opt.* **2**, 88–91.

Thibos, L. N., Wheeler, W. and Horner, D. (1994) A vector method for the analysis of astigmatic refractive errors. In: *Vision Science and Its Applications*, Technical Digest Series Vol. 2. Optical Society of America, pp. 14–17.

Index